Public health:
ethical issues

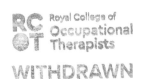
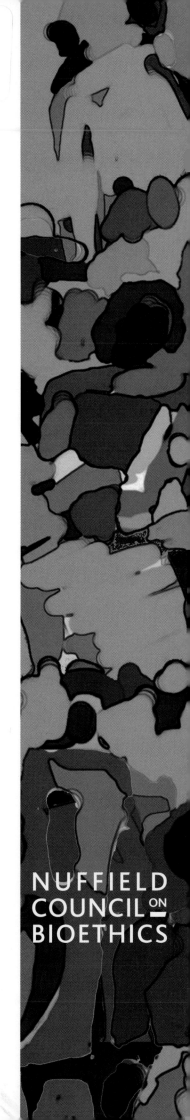

NUFFIELD
COUNCIL ON
BIOETHICS

Nuffield Council on Bioethics

The terms of reference of the Council are:

1 to identify and define ethical questions raised by recent advances in biological and medical research in order to respond to, and to anticipate, public concern;

2 to make arrangements for examining and reporting on such questions with a view to promoting public understanding and discussion; this may lead, where needed, to the formulation of new guidelines by the appropriate regulatory or other body;

3 in the light of the outcome of its work, to publish reports; and to make representations, as the Council may judge appropriate.

**The Nuffield Council on Bioethics is funded jointly by
the Medical Research Council, the Nuffield Foundation and the Wellcome Trust**

Foreword

Whose job is it to ensure that we lead a healthy life? Who should help us not to eat or drink too much, to take exercise, and to protect our children and ourselves against disease? Is it entirely up to us as individuals to choose how to lead our lives, or does the state also have a role to play? Two typical, and contradictory, responses are "We don't want the nanny state interfering with our lives" and "The Government should do more to curb drunkenness amongst young people". This Report presents an ethical framework that aims to help answer the question of when and how the state should act.

The term 'public health' refers to the efforts of society as a whole to improve the health of the population and prevent illness. The emphasis of public health policy on prevention rather than treatment of the sick, on the population as a whole rather than the individual, and the importance of collective effort, poses a particular set of ethical problems. In traditional bioethics, much emphasis is placed on the freedom of the individual, in terms of consent, treatment and information. Whilst these freedoms remain in ethical considerations of public health, they are woven into a complex fabric, in which many different players have roles and responsibilities.

People are much healthier today than they were 150 years ago. Since the turn of the 20th Century, life expectancy has increased by nearly 70%, equivalent to 16 hours per day. Much of this change is a result of what might be seen as quite interventionist public health policies such as provision of clean water, sanitation and mandatory vaccination, as well as protection of workers and children through specific legislation. In all of this the state has played a central role in improving people's health.

People's perception of acceptable risk has changed as we have become healthier. In the 1930s there were about 2,000 deaths per year from bovine tuberculosis, contracted largely through raw milk. Yet parliament decided that the risks did not warrant legislation to prevent these deaths by pasteurising milk. When the Pasteurisation Bill finally came before parliament in 1949, Dr Edith Summerskill said: "Pasteurisation has been prevented by ignorance, prejudice and selfishness." Perhaps something similar will be said in the future about the unsubstantiated MMR-autism scare, which led to the refusal of many parents to vaccinate their children against measles, mumps and rubella. In Chapter 3 we discuss the acceptability of risk and the nature of evidence, as well as the responsibility of the media, all too often not fulfilled, in accurate rather than biased and sensationalist reporting.

It takes only a moment's thought to recognise that many of the 'choices' that individuals make about their lifestyle are heavily constrained as a result of policies established by central and local government, by various industries as well as by various kinds of inequality in society. People's choice about what to eat, whether or not they allow their children to walk to school, or the kinds of products that are marketed to them, are often, in reality, limited. This means that the notion of individual choice determining health is too simplistic. Instead, we develop what we call the 'stewardship model' of the role of the state in relation to public health. This model recognises that the state should not coerce people or restrict their freedoms unnecessarily, but also that the state has a responsibility to provide the conditions under which people can lead healthy lives if they wish. The stewardship state, in addition to protecting its citizens from harm caused by others, sees itself as having a particular responsibility for protecting the health of vulnerable groups such as children, and in closing the gap between the most and least healthy in society (as overall life expectancy has increased, the gap has not closed).

Some may find our ethical framework strays too far away from the freedoms of the individual and toward the value of the community as a whole. But our conclusion is that any state that seriously aims to promote and implement public health policies has to accept a stewardship role. We also note that 'doing nothing' is an active decision by the state that will have an impact on people's ability to lead a healthy life. We describe the different kinds of intervention that the state may use to promote public health, on what we term the 'intervention ladder', from the least to the most coercive or intrusive measures. The further up the ladder the state climbs, the stronger the justification has to be.

We consider four case studies within our stewardship framework: infectious disease, obesity, smoking and alcohol (as a compare and contrast case) and fluoridation of water. Each case highlights different aspects of the stewardship state. Our model does not lead to a set of rules for the stewardship state, but rather a set of guidelines and signposts for the state as well as others involved in public health policy. We have highlighted these in the recommendations and conclusions throughout the report.

I would like to thank all those involved in the preparation of this Report: the members of the Working Party, the Council, the excellent secretariat, in particular Harald Schmidt, Julia Trusler and Caroline Rogers, those who responded to our consultation, and those who came to our fact-finding meetings to brief us and debate their views.

Lord Krebs Kt FRS FMedSci

Chair of the Working Party

Acknowledgements

The Council would like to thank the members of the Working Party for their expertise and contributions to this Report. Also greatly appreciated were the peer review comments from the experts who reviewed an earlier version of this Report (see Appendix 1), and comments from those who have attended fact-finding meetings (see Appendix 1) and responded to our consultation (see Appendix 2). Members are also very grateful to those who provided advice on specific parts of the Report, including Professor Alex Capron, Dr Andreas Reis, Dr Angus Nicoll, Dr Barry Evans, Dr Bryony Butland, Dr Elaine Gadd, Dr Ben Goldacre, colleagues at the Faculty of Public Health of the Royal Colleges of Physicians of the United Kingdom, Hermine Kelly-Hall, John Graham, Professor Mark Johnson, Professor Ron Bayer, Sarah Clark, Stephen Peckham and Professor Trevor Sheldon. Finally, we thank Anais Rameau, an intern with the Council, for her valuable work.

Members of the Working Group

Lord Krebs Kt FRS FMedSci (Chair)
Principal, Jesus College, University of Oxford

Dr Raghib Ali
Clinical Lecturer, Department of Clinical Pharmacology, Green College, University of Oxford

Professor Tom Baldwin
Professor of Philosophy, Department of Philosophy, University of York

Professor Roger Brownsword
Professor of Law, Centre for Medical Law and Ethics, King's College London

Professor Sir Kenneth Calman KCB FRCS DL FRSE
Chancellor, University of Glasgow

Professor Christine Godfrey
Professor of Health Economics, Department of Health Sciences, University of York

Professor Trisha Greenhalgh OBE
Professor of Primary Healthcare, Department of Primary Care and Population Sciences, Whittington Hospital, London

Professor Anne Johnson FMedSci
Head, Department of Primary Care and Population Sciences, Hampstead Campus, Royal Free and University College Medical School

Professor Sally Macintyre FRSE CBE
Director, MRC Social and Public Health Sciences Unit

Professor Jonathan Montgomery
Professor of Health Care Law, University of Southampton, and Chair, Hampshire Primary Care Trust

Ms Julia Unwin CBE
Director, Joseph Rowntree Foundation, York

Terms of reference

1. To identify and consider ethical, legal and social issues arising when designing measures to improve public health.

2. To consider, by means of case studies:

   a. the variety of aims for such measures, such as informing individual choices and protecting the wider community, and their relative priorities;

   b. the role of autonomy, consent and solidarity;

   c. issues raised by decisions about, and perceptions of, risk;

   d. the special situation of children and those who are poor or socially excluded.

3. To examine the implications of the above for the development of frameworks for policy making in public health.

Table of contents

Chapter 6: Case study – Alcohol and tobacco **99**

Chapter 7: Case Study – Fluoridation of water **119**

Executive summary

Introduction

In this Report we consider some of the ethical issues that arise from efforts to improve health at the population level, and we examine the roles and responsibilities of the different parties involved. Although some might see personal behaviour as the primary factor determining the health of the population, we consider that to be too simplistic. Individual behaviour certainly plays a role, but health is influenced by many factors, such as clean air, the built and work environment, socio-economic and genetic background, and access to healthcare. Industries such as those producing, selling and marketing food, drink and tobacco also play an important role, and the impact of almost all these factors is influenced directly or indirectly by government policy.

The political, regulatory and economic environments in which people live establish a setting that has a considerable influence on the extent to which they are able to lead healthy lives (paragraphs 1.4, 3.20–3.21). The term 'public health' is generally used to refer to efforts made to improve that setting, and in this Report we understand public health as the "science and art of preventing disease, prolonging life and promoting health through organised efforts of society".[1] Public health measures focus on stopping the healthy becoming sick, rather than treating the sick, either by implementing preventative measures or by trying to reduce unhealthy behaviour. We note that 'public health' can also be used to refer to the collective state of health of members of a population. To avoid confusion or ambiguity, we use the term 'population health' for this latter meaning throughout this Report. Thus, public health measures are designed to improve population health (see paragraph 1.6 and Box 1.4).

Historical background to public health

Historically, many of the most substantial advances in improving population health have been made through non-medical developments. These include improved housing and sanitation, which considerably reduced morbidity and mortality in western European countries in the 19th and 20th Centuries. Law and regulation also played a crucial role, and a wide range of highly prescriptive health and safety regulations helped reduce ill health and premature death. Measures derived from medical advances, such as vaccination programmes, have also made a significant contribution. However, although, overall, health has improved and life expectancy has increased in the UK and other western European countries in the 20th Century, considerable inequalities in health persist, and in some cases these have widened, especially between socio-economic groups (see paragraphs 1.3, 3.23–3.27).[2]

Ethical issues

The context of the debate

Public health measures raise complex questions about the relationship between the state and the individuals and organisations that are affected by its policies. They also raise questions about the duties that individuals have towards each other. A substantial body of literature in political philosophy examines these relationships of duties and entitlements, and we provide an overview in Chapter 2. The younger academic field of bioethics has also generated an influential body of

---

[1] See Royal Colleges of Physicians of the United Kingdom, *What is Public Health*, available at:
http://www.fphm.org.uk/about_faculty/what_public_health/default.asp.

[2] Acheson D (1998) *Independent Inquiry into Inequalities in Health* (Norwich: The Stationery Office), available at:
http://www.archive.official-documents.co.uk/document/doh/ih/ih.htm.

literature and much of this work takes an individual-centred approach. Public health, however, is not generally concerned with the *individual* level, but with the population level, and it is not always easy or appropriate to apply concepts such as autonomy, which carry considerable weight in the traditional bioethics literature, to the area of public health (see paragraphs 2.22–2.25, 7.38–7.31, 8.10–8.12).

The Working Party's approach

In Chapter 2 we set out an ethical framework which builds on existing literature and provides a general structure for the consideration of ethical issues arising in public health. We consider the basic parameters of a liberal framework for public health policy and its relationship to different theories of the state (paragraphs 2.3–2.9). John Stuart Mill's 'harm principle', to which we refer as the 'classical harm principle', suggests that state intervention is primarily warranted where an individual's actions affect others (paragraphs 2.13–2.15). This forms a crucial constituent part of our proposed framework and sometimes is sufficient on its own to justify a public health policy.

Building on this principle we identify several further issues that are important to public health. We highlight especially the limitations of individual consent and the importance of reducing health inequalities. We comment on different types of inequality, different groups between which inequalities may exist and different ways of reducing them (paragraphs 2.27–2.32). We argue that the focus in reducing health inequalities should be on 'prioritarian' strategies that aim to improve health opportunities and outcomes in the most disadvantaged groups.

On consent, we differentiate between interventions where explicit individual consent is required, those where preventing harm to others outweighs its requirement, and those where the degree of interference with a person's liberty or preferences may obviate the need for consent. Public health interventions sometimes fall into the latter category, and democratic decision-making procedures may be appropriate to give an 'authorisation' or 'mandate' to implement a certain measure. The procedures should be transparent, fair and inclusive (paragraphs 2.22–2.26, also paragraphs 4.58–4.62).

Acting, and failing to act, to improve population health

The central issue in public health is the extent to which it is acceptable for the state to establish policies that will influence population health. Some take the view that 'doing nothing' is the morally most acceptable or 'neutral' option, as it gives the greatest scope for individuals to act freely, guided by their own preferences and choices. However, many policies that constrain liberties at some level, such as compulsory primary and secondary education, play an important role in assisting people in developing the ability to act autonomously in the first place. Moreover, **it would be wrong to require justification only for active intervention. Any policy, including a policy to 'do nothing', implies value judgements about what is or is not good for people, and requires justification** (see paragraphs 2.27–2.38, 3.37–3.38, 8.17).

The stewardship model

We discuss the question of what degree of intervention might be acceptable to improve population health (paragraphs 2.34–2.40), and we present what we call the stewardship model.

The concept of 'stewardship' is intended to convey that liberal states have a duty to look after important needs of people individually and collectively.[3] It emphasises the obligation of states to

---

[3] See World Health Organization (2000) *World Health Report 2000* (Geneva, Switzerland: WHO); "Stewardship is the overarching function that determines the success or failure of all other functions of the health system. It places the responsibility back on government and calls for the strengthening of ministries of health. However, it does not call for necessarily a hierarchical and controlling role of government but more of that of overseeing and steering of the health system. It calls for vision, setting of regulations and implementing them, and the capacity to assess and monitor performance over time. A strong stewardship should in fact permit a more efficient use of the private sector to meet the needs of the health system."

provide conditions that allow people to be healthy and, in particular, to take measures to reduce health inequalities. The stewardship-guided state recognises that a primary asset of a nation is its health: higher levels of health are associated with greater overall well-being and productivity. Box 1 and paragraphs 2.41–2.44 describe in more detail the goals and constraints of the stewardship model.

Box 1: The stewardship model (see paragraph 2.44)

Core characteristics of public health programmes carried out by a stewardship-guided state can be summarised as follows:

Concerning goals, public health programmes should:

■ aim to reduce the risks of ill health that people might impose on each other;

■ aim to reduce causes of ill health by regulations that ensure environmental conditions that sustain good health, such as the provision of clean air and water, safe food and appropriate housing;

■ pay special attention to the health of children and other vulnerable people;

■ promote health not only by providing information and advice, but also by programmes to help people overcome addictions and other unhealthy behaviours;

■ aim to ensure that it is easy for people to lead a healthy life, for example by providing convenient and safe opportunities for exercise;

■ ensure that people have appropriate access to medical services; and

■ aim to reduce health inequalities.

In terms of constraints, such programmes should:

■ not attempt to coerce adults to lead healthy lives;

■ minimise interventions that are introduced without the individual consent of those affected, or without procedural justice arrangements (such as democratic decision-making procedures) which provide adequate mandate;

■ seek to minimise interventions that are perceived as unduly intrusive and in conflict with important personal values.

Note that the positive goals and negative constraints are not listed in any hierarchical order. The implementation of these principles may, in theory, lead to conflicting policies. However, in each particular case, it should be possible to resolve these conflicts by applying those policies or strategies that, in the circumstances, enable the desired social goals to be achieved while minimising significant limitations on individual freedom (see Box 2). We illustrate the role of particular components in the discussion of the case studies considered in Chapters 4–7.

Role of third parties

Although the state should be guided in its public health policies by the concept of stewardship, this does not absolve other parties, in particular the corporate sector, from their responsibilities. We discuss the concept of corporate social responsibility, and note that while companies may have different motivations for pursuing social responsibility strategies, they increasingly recognise that they have obligations beyond simply complying with relevant laws and regulations. If industry fails to meet these obligations and the health of the population is significantly at risk, the market fails to act responsibly. In such cases, we argue, it is acceptable for the state to intervene (paragraphs 2.47–2.50, 5.26, 5.16–5.25, 6.18–6.31, 8.24).

The stewardship model and the principles we set out in Chapter 2 do not provide a fixed set of rules or a hierarchy of principles. Rather, the framework suggests what should be taken into account when developing policy (paragraphs 2.44, 2.52, 8.3–8.12).

Policy issues

Evidence

Evidence about, first, causes of ill health and, secondly, the efficacy and effectiveness of interventions is important to public health policy (paragraphs 3.3–3.4). Ideally, evidence should be based on peer-reviewed research, and not on preliminary results or unpublished reports. Selective use of evidence or 'policy-based evidence'[4] that has been commissioned or interpreted to support

---

[4] House of Commons Science and Technology Committee (2006) *Scientific Advice, Risk and Evidence Based Policy Making*, available at: http://www.publications.parliament.uk/pa/cm200506/cmselect/cmsctech/900/900-i.pdf.

existing or planned policies is unhelpful and can lead to confusion. In practice, evidence is often incomplete, or it may be ambiguous, and usually it will be contested. Although scientific experts may sometimes be tempted or pressured into offering precise answers to policy makers, the honest answer will often be "we don't know" or "we can only estimate the risk to within certain, sometimes wide, limits". Claims of absolute safety or certainty should therefore generally be treated with great caution (see paragraphs 3.7–3.12, 8.19–8.23).

The media, stakeholders and campaigning groups have particular roles in relation to the presentation of evidence for or against particular health risks and we emphasise the crucial importance of accuracy and fairness in presenting evidence (see paragraphs 3.7–3.9, 4.33–4.35, 7.47).

Risk

We contrast two different views about what risk assessments should entail. According to the 'statistical view', risk is defined in terms of the probability of an event occurring, multiplied by the severity of its impact. On the 'social construct view', risk is framed by personal biases that result in certain kinds of risks being more relevant than others, and by what is accepted in particular social groups or society as a whole. **We take the view that the assessment of risk in the development of policy should be based on the 'statistical view'; however, we recognise that acceptability of risk to the public may also depend on subjective perceptions** (paragraphs 3.13–3.14).

Precaution and proportionality

The 'precautionary principle' is often invoked where there is some evidence of a serious threat to health, safety or the environment. The precise meaning of the principle has been the subject of much debate and it would be wrong to see it as a simple rule. This is why we prefer the term precautionary *approach*, rather than precautionary *principle* (paragraphs 3.15–3.16).

A Communication by the European Commission on the matter[5] helpfully suggests that five main elements can be distinguished: (a) scientific assessment of risk, acknowledging uncertainties and updated in light of new evidence; (b) fairness and consistency; (c) consideration of costs and benefits of actions; (d) transparency; and (e) proportionality.

Whether an intervention is proportionate depends largely on: whether the public health objectives are sufficiently important to warrant particular laws, policies or interventions; how likely the intervention is to achieve certain ends; and whether the means chosen are the least intrusive and costly whilst still achieving their aims (paragraphs 3.16–3.19). The concept of proportionality is closely linked to what we call the 'intervention ladder'.

The intrusiveness of different policies: the intervention ladder

Our proposed 'intervention ladder' suggests a way of thinking about the acceptability and justification of different public health policies (Box 2). The least intrusive step is generally 'to do nothing', or at most monitor the situation. The most intrusive is to legislate in such a way as to restrict the liberties of individuals, the population as a whole, or specific industries. In general, the higher the rung on the ladder at which the policy maker intervenes, the stronger the justification has to be. A more intrusive policy initiative is likely to be publicly acceptable only if there is a clear indication that it will produce the desired effect, and that this can be weighed favourably against any loss of liberty that may result (paragraphs 3.37–3.38).

---

[5] *European Commission (2000) Communication from the Commission on the Precautionary Principle* COM(2000). Note that the Communication uses the term 'precautionary principle' rather than 'precautionary approach' used by us. In one sense it may be unimportant which term is used. However, we think that the term 'approach' conveys more immediately that there is not just one, but several principles or considerations that need to be considered.

Box 2: The intervention ladder (paragraphs 3.37–3.38, Box 3.2)

The ladder of possible government actions is as follows:

Eliminate choice. Regulate in such a way as to entirely eliminate choice, for example through compulsory isolation of patients with infectious diseases.

Restrict choice. Regulate in such a way as to restrict the options available to people with the aim of protecting them, for example removing unhealthy ingredients from foods, or unhealthy foods from shops or restaurants.

Guide choice through disincentives. Fiscal and other disincentives can be put in place to influence people not to pursue certain activities, for example through taxes on cigarettes, or by discouraging the use of cars in inner cities through charging schemes or limitations of parking spaces.

Guide choices through incentives. Regulations can be offered that guide choices by fiscal and other incentives, for example offering tax-breaks for the purchase of bicycles that are used as a means of travelling to work.

Guide choices through changing the default policy. For example, in a restaurant, instead of providing chips as a standard side dish (with healthier options available), menus could be changed to provide a more healthy option as standard (with chips as an option available).

Enable choice. Enable individuals to change their behaviours, for example by offering participation in a NHS 'stop smoking' programme, building cycle lanes, or providing free fruit in schools.

Provide information. Inform and educate the public, for example as part of campaigns to encourage people to walk more or eat five portions of fruit and vegetables per day.

Do nothing or simply monitor the current situation.

Public health measures are frequently viewed as infringements of liberties, especially where they become more coercive. Yet, comparable measures are often accepted in general health and safety policies, for example, in relation to protective clothing or use of seat belts (see Chapter 3, Box 3.3, paragraph 8.17, Box 8.1). However, as the latter example illustrates, initial resistance often turns into acceptance, and even approval, if the interventions are seen to be successful.

Targeting versus universal approaches

There are clear correlations between health and socio-economic status: in general, poorer health and less healthy behaviours are associated with lower socio-economic position (see paragraphs 3.23–3.27). The stewardship model includes an obligation to reduce health inequalities and to pay special attention to the health of children and other vulnerable people. Different strategies that may be pursued include targeting the disadvantaged (paragraphs 3.29–3.30) or at-risk groups (paragraph 3.30). Some object to any targeting approach on the basis that it may lead to stigmatisation (paragraphs 4.45, 5.12, 5.30–5.31, 5.34, 5.38, 5.42, 6.16 and 8.27–8.28), and instead favour universal approaches. However, different people may respond differently to universal measures. For example, better food labelling may benefit some more than others, as not everyone will read the labels or use the information provided to change their behaviour. In general those most able to benefit from information-based strategies are better educated and from higher socio-economic status groups. Universal measures can therefore increase health inequalities, and **systematic monitoring is therefore a crucial component of universal as well as targeted measures** (see paragraphs 3.23–3.24, 8.29).

The implications of our discussions of ethical and policy issues are illustrated in the following case studies on infectious diseases, obesity, smoking and alcohol, and fluoridation of water.

Infectious disease

The main ethical issues in the surveillance, control and prevention of infectious disease concern how to reconcile individual consent and civil liberty with community benefit, including the prevention of harm to others. In addition, infectious diseases require consideration of health inequalities at a national and global level. We also discuss issues arising from international programmes for the surveillance and control of pandemics.

Prevention of infectious diseases through vaccination

Vaccination strategies often seek not only to protect individuals against infection, but also to bring about 'population immunity'[6] (see paragraphs 4.9–4.10). It is sometimes claimed that all those who refuse to receive vaccinations (or to have their children vaccinated) are 'free-riders', in the sense that they may be avoiding taking on their 'share' of the burden for the benefit of the community while nevertheless benefiting from population immunity. However, the situation is more complicated than this, as people may object to vaccinations for many reasons (paragraph 4.17).

Population immunity can confer a substantial collective benefit, but achieving it requires the organised efforts of society in establishing vaccination schemes, and collective action and cooperation by the population in taking part to achieve high levels of vaccination coverage. We consider three broad approaches to vaccination policy: voluntary, incentivised and quasi-mandatory.[7] In all cases, education and information campaigns are generally used to improve uptake (paragraphs 4.20–4.29). **In general, public health policies should use the least intrusive means to achieve the required public health benefit. Directive vaccination approaches that go further than simply providing information and encouragement to take up the vaccine may, however, be justified on the basis of minimising risks of harm to others, or protecting the health of children and other vulnerable people. A case-by-case assessment will always be required. When assessing whether more directive policies are acceptable, the following factors should be taken into account: the risks associated with the vaccination and with the disease itself, and the seriousness of the threat of the disease to the population. In the case of incentivised policies, the size of the incentive involved should be appropriate so that it would not unduly compromise the voluntariness of consent** (paragraph 4.26).

We identified two circumstances in which quasi-mandatory vaccination measures are more likely to be justified. First, for highly contagious and serious diseases, for example with characteristics similar to smallpox. Secondly, for disease eradication if the disease is serious and if eradication is within reach (paragraph 4.27).

There also needs to be consideration of whether a directive measure will be more effective than voluntary ones. The evidence on this for routine childhood vaccinations is complex and limited. **At present, there is not sufficient justification in the UK for moving beyond the current voluntary system and implementing incentivised or quasi-mandatory policies for routine childhood vaccinations** (paragraph 4.32).

When a disease causes serious harm only in certain groups in the population, high vaccination levels might still be sought across the whole population in order to achieve population immunity. Vaccinating boys against rubella or against a virus that causes cervical cancer, or vaccinating girls against mumps would be examples (paragraphs 4.18–4.19, 4.28). **On the basis of the value of community and stewardship considerations, it is in principle ethically justified to encourage individuals to take part in vaccination programmes when there is no, or only a small, personal**

---

[6] Population immunity is also commonly known as 'herd-immunity'.

[7] By quasi-mandatory we refer to schemes that require individuals to be vaccinated unless they qualify for an exemption and where there are penalties for those who do not comply.

benefit, but significant benefits for others. **However, consent is essential, and there should be careful assessments of the benefits to be gained for the population and the possible harm that may result for the people who receive the vaccination** (paragraph 4.29).

Surveillance of infectious disease

We discuss two types of infectious disease surveillance. First, population surveillance of infectious disease trends, which involves the systematic collection, analysis and interpretation of data about disease incidence and prevalence. With this type of surveillance, data are generally collected anonymously (paragraphs 4.36–4.38). Secondly, notifiable disease surveillance, in which individual cases of particular diseases must be notified to the relevant authorities for the purpose of monitoring and disease control (paragraphs 4.41–4.42, also Box 4.5).

The collection of anonymised surveillance data on trends in infectious disease ranks low on the intervention ladder. Without sufficient data, it may not be possible to assess and predict trends and risks in infectious diseases. **It is acceptable to collect and use anonymised data for assessing and predicting trends in infectious disease without consent, as long as any invasion of privacy is reduced as far as possible** (paragraph 4.39).

Legislation on notifiable diseases requires the collection of data about individuals with particular infections which includes identifying information. One of the main aims of such measures is to prevent harm to others from the spread of disease, which means that they can be justified under the classical harm principle (paragraphs 2.13–2.14). **The avoidance of significant harm to others who are at risk from a serious communicable disease may outweigh the consideration of personal privacy or confidentiality, and on this basis it can be ethically justified to collect non-anonymised data about individuals for the purposes of implementing control measures. However, any overriding of privacy or confidentiality must be to the minimum extent possible to achieve the desired aim** (paragraph 4.43).

Surveillance on an international level is also important, particularly for diseases that could lead to large-scale epidemics or pandemics. International disease surveillance is compromised where countries do not have the capacity to undertake effective disease surveillance or where they decide not to fully cooperate with international surveillance efforts (paragraphs 4.47–4.49). **Based on an application of the stewardship model at the global level, countries have an ethical obligation to reduce the risk of ill health that people might impose on each other across borders. Therefore countries should notify other relevant countries and bodies about outbreaks of serious diseases at the earliest stage, following the relevant procedures laid out by WHO (the World Health Organization)** (paragraph 4.50).

Early detection of outbreaks requires an efficient surveillance system, and different countries have different capacities for surveillance, monitoring and reporting of infectious disease. We note that both WHO and a Foresight report have identified a need for greater investment in surveillance capacity in poorer countries,[8] which is compatible with applying the stewardship model at the global level.

Recommendation 1: **Countries such as the UK should seek to enhance the capacities of developing countries to conduct effective surveillance of infectious diseases. The UK health departments, in liaison with the Department for International Development, should work to take this forward with international partners such as WHO, the European Centre for Disease Prevention and Control (ECDC) and the Centers for Disease Prevention and Control (CDC) in the USA.** (Paragraph 4.50)

---

[8] Foresight (2006) *Infectious Diseases: Preparing for the future. Executive Summary* (London: Office of Science and Innovation); World Health Organization (2006) *Strengthening pandemic-influenza preparedness and response, including application of the International Health Regulations (2005),* available at: http://www.who.int/gb/ebwha/pdf_files/WHA59/A59_5-en.pdf.

A case of lack of cooperation with global surveillance has recently been seen with Indonesia, which, for a period in 2006/7, ceased to provide influenza viral isolates to the WHO-managed international surveillance system because of concerns that the country would not have reasonable access to the benefits produced with the aid of these viral isolates. The Indonesian case is made more complex by the involvement of a pharmaceutical company, with which a deal was allegedly made, although the full details of this are unclear (paragraphs 4.51–4.53).

Further to our observations on corporate social responsibility (paragraphs 2.47–2.50), the effect of commercial interests and intellectual property rights on public health surveillance measures requires careful consideration. **WHO is in a unique position to enable centralised and transparent determination that a novel virus has emerged, to evaluate pandemic-related evidence, and to develop response strategies, as acknowledged in the *International Health Regulations 2005*. This capacity must be sustained.**

Recommendation 2: **We urge pharmaceutical companies not to enter into agreements with countries in a way that would potentially undermine the work of the WHO Global Influenza Surveillance Network.** (Paragraph 4.54)

Virus isolates should not be treated like any ordinary commodity, as adequate access and use is required to allow surveillance systems to function effectively, and so that timely vaccine production is not unduly hindered. Access is therefore of the greatest importance for public health, both on a national and global level.

Recommendation 3: **We urge WHO to explore, in liaison with governments and relevant industries, the notion of viewing virus isolates as a form of 'public good', and to take a flexible approach to patenting and intellectual property protection.** (Paragraph 4.55)

Recommendation 4: **WHO should not merely facilitate access to virus isolates for commercial companies, leaving the question of availability of vaccines to market forces. It should use its authority to impress on pharmaceutical companies their social responsibilities.** (Paragraph 4.55)

Control of infectious diseases

Quarantine and isolation of individuals known or suspected to have a particular infection are some of the most liberty-infringing measures available to policy makers.[9] These measures may be considered either on a larger scale in the case of an epidemic, or, more often, on a smaller scale, for individual cases of a serious disease (such as patients with multi-drug-resistant tuberculosis, or chronic typhoid carriers; see paragraphs 4.58–4.61). **Liberty-infringing measures to control disease, such as compulsory quarantine and isolation, rank towards the top of the intervention ladder. The ethical justification for such measures involves weighing the classical harm principle on the one hand, and individual consent and the importance of avoiding intrusive interventions on the other. Where risk of harm to others can be significantly reduced, these considerations can be outweighed** (paragraph 4.62).

Information and communication

Infectious disease surveillance, prevention and control measures raise important issues about the need to communicate with individuals, populations and organisations (paragraphs 4.69–4.71). **Where a potentially serious infectious disease outbreak or incident occurs, the relevant authorities should ensure that they neither downplay the risks, which may lead to higher rates of preventable infections, nor overstate the risks, as this may result in panic or a lack of public trust that could be long-lasting.**

[9] We note that there is the potential for these types of measures could be implemented inappropriately or abused, or that people may be suspicious of potential abuses, particularly for example, in countries with totalitarian regimes.

Recommendation 5: **The UK health departments and health protection agencies,**[10] **in particular, have a responsibility to ensure the timely provision of adequate and appropriate information about the nature of an infectious disease outbreak or incident, the type of interventions to be implemented and the rationale for their use.** (Paragraph 4.72)

The coverage of doubts about the MMR (measles, mumps and rubella) vaccine in the media provides an example of how inaccurate or poor reporting of evidence and risk can have a highly damaging effect on population health, in this case through a loss of public confidence in the vaccine (paragraphs 4.33–4.35, Box 4.3). **We consider that researchers, journalists and others who report research have a duty to communicate findings in a responsible manner.**

Recommendation 6: **Those who report research should take account of the *Guidelines on Science and Health Communication* published by the Social Issues Research Centre, the Royal Society and the Royal Institution of Great Britain.**[11] **In particular we emphasise that the source and the status of scientific evidence alluded to should be identified (including, for example, whether it is preliminary or based on a conference presentation, and whether it has been peer reviewed). We also encourage initiatives that provide independent information that is accessible to the public on the accuracy and reliability of medical stories reported in the media. An example of such an initiative is the National Library for Health's 'Hitting the Headlines' resource,**[12] **which provides summaries relating to media reports within two days of their publication.** (Paragraphs 4.34–4.35)

Obesity

Becoming overweight or obese is a risk factor for several serious health conditions (paragraphs 5.2–5.4). The prevalence of obesity in children and adults has increased dramatically over the past decade in the UK and many other countries. Reversing this trend is likely to take many years because food and physical activity habits are deeply ingrained in social and individual patterns of behaviour. Policies with potential long-term benefits are sometimes difficult to reconcile with government priorities in the short term. As the prevalence of obesity appears to be the result of many different factors, reducing obesity in the population is likely to require multifaceted measures taken by many different agents (paragraphs 5.5–5.11).

Children are especially vulnerable, and evidence shows that children's early diet has a long-term impact on health, including obesity and its related health risks. Additionally, children are more susceptible to external influences, including marketing by industry, and they have limited control and ability to make genuine choices.

Role of industry: corporate social responsibility

Many people's diets include food that has been prepared or processed by others, and therefore consumers' choices are at least partly influenced by the products available and the way they are promoted, priced and distributed. We focus on two particular examples of the responsibilities of corporations: the promotion of foods and drinks high in fat, salt and sugar to children; and the labelling and composition of food. Our recommendations are based on our observations on corporate social responsibility (paragraphs 2.47–2.50) and the stewardship model's emphasis on conditions that make it easy for people to lead healthy lives, paying special attention to vulnerable people, and reducing causes of ill health through appropriate regulations (paragraph 2.44). **Businesses, including the food industry, have an ethical duty to help individuals to make**

---

[10] By this we refer to the Health Protection Agency, Health Protection Scotland, the National Public Health Service for Wales and the Communicable Disease Surveillance Centre (Northern Ireland).

[11] Social Issues Research Centre, the Royal Society and the Royal Institution of Great Britain (2001) *Guidelines on Science and Health Communication*, available at: http://www.sirc.org/publik/revised_guidelines.pdf.

[12] See: http://www.library.nhs.uk/hth/ and http://www.library.nhs.uk/rss/newsAndRssArchive.aspx?storyCategory=0.

healthier choices. The food and drink industries should therefore review both the composition of products that they manufacture and the way they are marketed and sold. Where the market fails to uphold its responsibility, for instance in failing to provide universal, readily understandable front-of-pack nutrition labelling or in the marketing of food more generally, regulation by the government is ethically justifiable (paragraph 5.25).

Several different models of providing labelling information have been introduced since 2000. It is premature to judge which of these is most effective in enabling consumers to make appropriately informed decisions (paragraph 5.24, Box 5.3). We note that the Food Standards Agency has commissioned a study[13] to investigate whether front-of-pack labels contribute to healthier choices being made and, if so, which elements of the various schemes are the most effective.

Recommendation 7: **When the Food Standards Agency (FSA) has reviewed its commissioned study on the effectiveness of labelling schemes, and the findings have been peer reviewed, they should form the basis for adoption by the food industry of the most effective scheme. If, however, the food industry does not accept the scheme, it would be appropriate for the UK Government to pursue legislation (if appropriate, at the European level). As we have noted elsewhere, such information-based schemes could increase health inequalities, and this should be monitored.** (Paragraph 5.25)

Parental influence is a key factor in preventing childhood obesity, but other parties have an ethical duty to support parents. Given the special vulnerability of children, it would be desirable, for example, not to advertise foods high in fat, salt and sugar to children by any medium, including on the Internet. The stewardship-guided state should aim to protect children from harm and provide an environment in which they can lead healthy lives. An example of the way in which the state might intervene includes regulation of the promotion of unhealthy foods and drinks to children, if industry fails to adequately regulate itself. A study in Australia published in 2006 suggests that this may be a particularly cost-effective way of reducing obesity in children (paragraphs 5.19–5.22).[14]

In May 2007, the European Commission published a White Paper entitled *A Strategy for Europe on Nutrition, Overweight and Obesity-related Health Issues,*[15] which included details of a best-practice model for self-regulation of food advertising for children. The Commission plans a review in 2010 of the extent to which agents across the EU are contributing to the achievement of the objectives in the Strategy.

Recommendation 8: **Following the planned review of the EU Strategy on obesity in 2010, the European Commission should consider whether there are cases in which self-regulation of food advertising for children has proved unsatisfactory and whether more binding regulation across the EU is required.** (Paragraph 5.23)

Role of government and public services

Education of children

Education plays a central role in providing individuals with the capacity to lead a healthy life. It is therefore appropriate for schools to seek to influence positively the food and exercise habits of children. **The stewardship model's emphasis on circumstances that help people to lead healthy lives, especially if they are in vulnerable positions, leads to an ethical justification for the state**

---

[13] Food Standards Agency (2007) Press release: *Front of pack labelling research project moves forward,* 9 July, available at: http://www.food.gov.uk/news/pressreleases/2007/jul/frontpackresearchpress.

[14] Victorian Department of Human Services (2006) *ACE-Obesity Assessing Cost-effectiveness of obesity interventions in children and adolescents* Summary of Results (Victorian Government Department of Human Services), available at: http://www.health.vic.gov.au/healthpromotion/quality/ace_obesity.htm.

[15] Available at: http://ec.europa.eu/health/ph_determinants/life_style/nutrition/documents/nutrition_wp_en.pdf.

to intervene in schools to achieve a more positive culture towards food, cooking and physical activity (paragraph 5.36).

As in many other areas of public health policy, the only way of establishing whether a new policy is likely to lead to improved health is by trialling it. **Because the need being addressed is an important one, it is desirable to explore the potential of promising policies, even if evidence for their effectiveness is incomplete.** In addition, changes in attitudes and culture towards food and physical activity are likely to take a long time. For example, the effectiveness of recent initiatives to introduce healthier meals and free fruit and vegetables in schools needs to be evaluated over many years (paragraph 5.36).

Recommendation 9: **The UK Government departments responsible for food, health and education should develop long-term strategies for schools with the aim of preventing obesity, and changing food and exercise culture, accompanied by monitoring and follow up.** (Paragraph 5.36)

The Department of Health for England and Scottish health authorities currently collect data on height and weight of children in schools both to inform local planning and to track progress against the public service agreement target to reduce obesity (paragraph 5.37). **Data on the prevalence of obesity are a crucial part of understanding trends and the impact of interventions. Weighing and measuring young children is ethically justifiable, provided the data are anonymised and collected in a sensitive way.**

Recommendation 10: **The collection of the data on obesity in children should be managed in a way that minimises the risks of stigmatisation, for instance by encompassing it within a broader programme of health checks. The UK health departments should give consideration to how this could be best realised in practice.** (Paragraph 5.38)

Protecting children from harm in the home

The classical harm principle could be invoked to justify interventions by the appropriate authorities where children become obese as a direct result of their parents' preferences for food and exercise. However, determining when intervening in the home would be appropriate involves a balancing of competing values. **In general, direct regulation of food provided to children in the home would be disproportionate, as any health benefits achieved would be outweighed by the value of private and family life** (see also paragraph 6.15). **However, where severe obesity is caused by overfeeding by parents or guardians, child protection issues would be raised if the child was at risk of significant harm to health.**[16]

Recommendation 11: **The Secretary of State for Children, Schools and Families, with the advice of the Office of the Children's Commissioner, should develop criteria for deciding when interventions, such as removing a child from their home, would be appropriate under the Government's *Every Child Matters* approach.**[17] (Paragraph 5.39)

Provision of healthcare

Obesity-related illnesses account for considerable NHS expenditure and this is likely to increase with the rising prevalence of obesity. However, the question of whether or not to make treatment for obese people conditional on behaviour change does not fall within the remit of public health, but rather in the realm of clinical decision-making.

---

[16] The fact that state intervention in home life is generally considered a last resort in a liberal state may in part explain why the focus of much government action (whether on eating or exercise habits) is often directed towards the school rather than home environment.

[17] *Every Child Matters* is the Government's approach to the well-being of children and young people from birth to age 19.

Obesity has complex causes. It is usually not easy to determine to what extent a person's weight is under their own control, and to what extent it is influenced by environmental factors that make it difficult to exercise or eat healthily. There is a significant risk of stigmatisation and unfair 'victim-blaming', where already-disadvantaged people are held unduly responsible for their poor health state. Any policies that single out obese people could also substantially undermine the concept of solidarity and the value of community. **It would not generally be appropriate for NHS treatment of health problems associated with obesity to be denied to people simply on the basis of their obesity. However, appeals to change behaviour before or subsequent to an intervention could be justified, provided that the change would enhance the effectiveness of the medical intervention, and people were offered help to do this** (paragraph 5.42).

On the whole, the focus of efforts should be on avoiding the need for treatment in the first place. This is a fairer approach, and it seems likely that it would cost less.

The built environment

The design of urban environments and buildings can help to improve opportunities for people to increase their energy expenditure with ease. A focus on the built environment might help to compensate for the low levels of effectiveness of health education strategies or policies aiming to help individuals to increase their physical activity by taking up sport (paragraph 5.29).

Recommendation 12: **Planning decisions by central and local government should include the objective of encouraging people to be physically active. This may entail some restrictions of people's freedoms, for instance to drive anywhere they wish to, but these restrictions would be justified in terms of public health benefits.** (Paragraph 5.32)

Recommendation 13: **The training of architects and town planners should include measures for increasing people's physical activity through the design of buildings and public spaces. This can be viewed as analogous to the recent incorporation of the study of energy efficiency and sustainability of buildings. The recommendation is directed to those who design training programmes, including the Architects Registration Board, the Royal Institute of British Architects and the Royal Town Planning Institute. Planning regulations by local planning authorities should set requirements in this area.** (Paragraph 5.33)

Alcohol and tobacco

Alcohol and tobacco are enjoyed legally by many people in the UK and other countries. Low to moderate intake of alcohol does not cause demonstrable harm and has even been suggested to have some health benefits. Excessive alcohol consumption[18] is extremely harmful to the health of consumers themselves and is often linked to problems of public safety that impact upon third parties. For tobacco, regular smoking of even a small number of cigarettes is harmful to the health of the smoker and people around them. Drinking alcohol and smoking are among the highest risk factors for mortality and morbidity (paragraphs 6.4–6.7). Given these and other similarities, we consider alcohol and tobacco together in this case study.

People in socio-economic groups with fewer resources are disproportionately affected by the harms caused by alcohol and tobacco and, therefore, under the stewardship model, public health policies in this area should aim to reduce these health inequalities (see paragraphs 2.27–2.32). They should also aim to pay special attention to the health of children and other vulnerable groups.

---

[18] In this Report we use 'excessive' alcohol consumption to refer to drinking that leads to alcohol use disorders as defined in the Alcohol Needs Assessment Research Project (ANARP). This Report used the World Health Organization categorisation of alcohol use disorders which specifies three categories: 'hazardous drinking', people drinking above recognised 'sensible' levels but not yet experiencing harm; 'harmful drinking', people drinking above 'sensible' levels and experiencing harm; and 'alcohol dependence', people drinking above 'sensible' levels and experiencing harm and symptoms of dependence.

Role of government and public services

Considerable harm to others is caused by people who have consumed excessive amounts of alcohol (paragraphs 6.10–6.11), and governments have acted to reduce this harm by implementing certain coercive measures, such as prohibiting driving or operating machinery with a blood-alcohol level over prescribed limits. These measures are publicly accepted and appropriate authorities enforce them. Further measures could be implemented that reduce harms to individuals themselves as well as to other people. **The stewardship model provides justification for the UK Government to introduce measures that are more coercive than those which currently feature in the National Alcohol Strategy (2004 and 2007).**

Recommendation 14: **We recommend that evidence-based measures judged effective in the WHO-sponsored analysis** *Alcohol: No ordinary commodity*[19] **are implemented by the UK Government. These include coercive strategies to manage alcohol consumption, specifically in the areas of price, marketing and availability. For example, taxes on alcoholic beverages could be increased, which has been shown to be an effective strategy for reducing consumption. We also recommend that the Home Office, the UK health departments and the Department of Culture, Media and Sport analyse the effect of extended opening hours of licensed premises on levels of consumption, as well as on anti-social behaviour.** (Paragraph 6.31)

As with alcohol, the harm to others caused by tobacco smoking justifies the implementation of coercive measures. The introduction in the UK of legislation to prohibit smoking in enclosed public places is therefore justified. (Paragraph 6.13)

Smoking within the home impacts negatively upon the health of non-smoking members of the household, especially children. **In principle, the general ethical and scientific arguments that apply to banning smoking in enclosed public spaces also apply to banning smoking in homes (and other places) where children are exposed to environmental tobacco smoke. However, this would be extremely difficult to enforce without compromising privacy.**

Recommendation 15: **We recommend that the Department for Children, Schools and Families should communicate to local authority children's services that there may be exceptional cases where children, for example, those with a serious respiratory condition, would be at risk of such a substantial level of harm from passive smoking that intervention to prevent such harm may be ethically acceptable. This would usually need to be decided in the courts.** (Paragraph 6.15; see also Recommendation 11)

Provision of healthcare for people who smoke and/or drink excessively

Questions about the extent to which a person's behaviour has contributed to their requirement for NHS treatment fall primarily in the domain of clinical medicine, rather than public health, as with obesity. **It might be justified for doctors to appeal to patients to change their behaviour in relation to alcohol and tobacco before or subsequent to an intervention provided by the NHS, provided that the change would enhance the effectiveness of the intervention, and people were offered help to do this. For example, alcohol treatment programmes might be offered in advance of performing a liver transplant as the cessation of excessive drinking would be likely to increase its clinical effectiveness, or could even make the transplant unnecessary.**

As with obesity, the focus of efforts should be on avoiding the need for treatment in the first place (paragraph 6.17, see also paragraphs 5.41–5.42).

Recommendation 16: **The UK health departments should further liaise with employers about how best to offer assistance with behaviour change programmes, such as smoking cessation, which could benefit the employer as well as employees.** (Paragraph 6.17)

---

[19] Babor T, Caetano R, Casswell S *et al.* (2003) *Alcohol: No ordinary commodity – Research and public policy* (Oxford: Oxford University Press).

xxvii

Role of industry

Large and profitable companies are involved in the alcohol and tobacco industries, and almost all of these have established 'corporate social responsibility' policies, which often include so-called 'harm-reduction strategies'. In the case of the tobacco industries, a stringent harm-reduction strategy is difficult to imagine as this would ultimately require them simply not to sell their products. In principle, if government wanted to pursue more aggressively its ethical objective of reducing health inequalities, it might ban the sale of tobacco products altogether, given that in developed countries, smoking is the leading single risk factor for mortality and is closely associated with socio-economic inequalities (paragraph 6.4). However, at present, the introduction of such a measure would be highly unlikely, which illustrates the complex set of interests of stakeholders that influence public health. Our recommendations therefore focus on what is achievable in the current situation (paragraphs 6.18–6.27).

A recent initiative of the industry to reduce harms has been to develop a form of smokeless tobacco known as snus. Snus, which is placed underneath the lip, has been used legally in Sweden and some other countries for many years although it is banned in all other Member States of the European Union. It is addictive to the consumer but eliminates the risk of harm to third parties. The industry argues that there is epidemiological evidence that this form of tobacco presents considerably lower health risks than cigarette smoking.[20] However, although there may be lower health risks compared with cigarette smoking, it is still associated with harm and addiction.[21]

Recommendation 17: In view of the health risks and the possibility that consumers may be led to believe they are using a relatively harmless product, we are not persuaded that permitting snus or conducting further research on the health risks is a helpful approach. Allowing snus might also carry the risk of increasing health inequalities in the UK as members of certain ethnic groups who already have a culture of chewing stimulants, such as betel nut, might more easily take up snus. (Paragraph 6.25)

Although, generally, we focus in this Report on the situation in the UK, in the case of tobacco and alcohol it is also relevant to consider the international context. **It is ethically inconsistent for tobacco and alcohol companies advertising and selling their products in developed countries to claim corporate social responsibility, and yet apply different standards for protecting consumers in different countries, depending on local laws. Acting ethically exceeds simply complying with relevant laws and regulations.**

Recommendation 18: Policies on selling and advertising tobacco and alcohol that afford the greatest protection to consumers should be adopted worldwide. The members of the UK Tobacco Manufacturers' Association and other companies that produce or market tobacco products should implement a voluntary code of practice that universalises best practice in terms of consumer protection. One example would be worldwide adherence to standards in advertising that have been developed and agreed by the industry in the EU, and particularly the UK. (Paragraph 6.27)

Alcohol and tobacco use in children

Drinking alcohol and smoking are associated with dependence and harms, and the levels of consumption and use in children and adolescents raise concerns. **We welcome the raising of the minimum age for the purchase of tobacco from 16 to 18 years that has taken place throughout the UK as part of a strategy to protect vulnerable people. Although thought needs to be given to the way in which this measure can be implemented most effectively, it is an appropriate**

[20] See, for example, British American Tobacco *Smokeless Snus and Health*, available at: http://www.bat.com/OneWeb/sites/uk__3mnfen.nsf/vwPagesWebLive/8C2FF319B8EFFB63C125700B00334456?opendocument&DTC=&SID.

[21] For a review article, see Gray N (2005) Mixed feelings on snus *Lancet* **366**: 966–7.

initiative in the context of the stewardship model, as the market has largely failed to self-regulate in this area.

Recommendation 19: Producers, advertisers and vendors of alcohol and tobacco need to recognise more fully the vulnerability of children and young people, and take clearer responsibility for preventing harms to health. This would include refraining from understating risks, and from exploiting the apparent desirability of drinking alcohol and smoking, particularly in ways that appeal to children and young people. Furthermore, it would appear that whatever the legal position, these products are widely available to underage children, and existing law and policy need to be implemented more stringently. (Paragraph 6.33)

Fluoridation of water

Fluoride occurs naturally in the water supply in some regions, and it has been suggested that adding fluoride to the water supply more generally may reduce tooth decay. Water fluoridation schemes have been in place for over 50 years in parts of the UK and elsewhere. A major literature review published in 2000, the 'York review', found that there was evidence that water fluoridation improved the health of teeth although this benefit is difficult to quantify. The review also found evidence that ingesting fluoridated water could be associated with harms, in particular fluorosis. Overall, however, the evidence both for benefits and for harms was found to be weak (paragraphs 7.4–7.7, 7.31). This is somewhat surprising, given that fluoridation has been implemented as a policy option for several decades.

Three elements of the stewardship model could, in principle, be used to justify water fluoridation: the reduction of health inequalities; the reduction of ill health; and concern for children, who constitute a vulnerable group. Water fluoridation has the potential to contribute to these goals, particularly where the health need of a particular locality is high. However, three further ethical principles need also to be considered: minimising interventions that affect important areas of personal life; not coercing ordinary adults to lead healthy lives; and consent. **The principles of avoiding coercive interventions and minimising interventions in personal life could be used to argue against the addition of any substance to the water supply. However, we do not accept that the addition of potentially beneficial substances to the water supply should always be prohibited. Rather, we seek to identify the situations in which this may be appropriate** (paragraph 7.25). **The acceptability of any public health policy involving the water supply should be considered in relation to: (i) the balance of risks and benefits; (ii) the potential for alternatives that rank lower on the intervention ladder to achieve the same intended goals; and (iii) the role of consent where there are potential harms** (paragraph 7.26).

Alternative fluoride-based interventions are in use in other parts of the world, including fluoride supplements and fluoridation of salt or milk, which rank lower than water fluoridation on the 'intervention ladder' (see paragraph 7.13, Box 7.4 and paragraphs 3.37–3.38). Their relative costs and benefits both to population health and individual liberty should be assessed when considering water fluoridation.

With water fluoridation, a whole area either receives fluoridated water or does not. Populations do not remain static, as people move to and from an area. In practical terms it would therefore not be feasible to seek individual consent. In this situation it could be suggested either that the intervention never be implemented because individual consent cannot be obtained, or that an alternative approach to obtain mandate is used (paragraphs 2.22–2.25).

Both action (adding fluoride) and inaction (not adding it) might disadvantage some groups of people, either through limiting personal choice or through preventing individuals from receiving any health benefits of the measure. Overall the prevalence of caries has reduced considerably over recent decades, but inequalities between regions persist. Therefore, the extent to which people might be affected by these two options varies. **The most appropriate way of deciding whether fluoride should be added to water supplies is to rely on democratic decision-making procedures. These should be implemented at the local and regional, rather than national level,[22] because the need for, and perception of, water fluoridation varies in different areas. Account should be taken of relevant evidence, and of alternative ways of achieving the intended benefit in the area concerned. Whatever policy is adopted, dental health and any adverse effects of fluoridation should be monitored** (paragraph 7.40).

Recommendation 20: **The UK health departments should monitor the effects of water fluoridation, including the incidence and severity of fluorosis and other possible harms. Water fluoridation policy should be objectively reviewed by the UK health departments on a regular basis in light of the findings of ongoing monitoring and further research studies. Furthermore, the conclusions and their basis should routinely be published.** (Paragraph 7.42)

Information about the evidence is important in policy decisions, particularly where people are asked to vote or contribute to policy decisions. **Neither the public nor policy makers are helped by information that makes it difficult for the non-expert to obtain a good understanding of current evidence** (paragraphs 7.43–7.47).

Recommendation 21: **All the groups involved in the fluoridation debate should ensure that the information they produce presents a balanced account of risks and benefits, and indicates accurately the strengths and weaknesses of the evidence base.** (Paragraph 7.47)

For contentious issues such as fluoridation, the media have a responsibility to report research findings accurately. In this context, we reiterate the earlier recommendation, made in relation to vaccination, about the reporting of research and how this should be conducted (see Recommendation 6 and paragraphs 4.33–4.35, 7.47).

---

[22] Within the constraints of the water supply network.

Chapter 1
Introduction

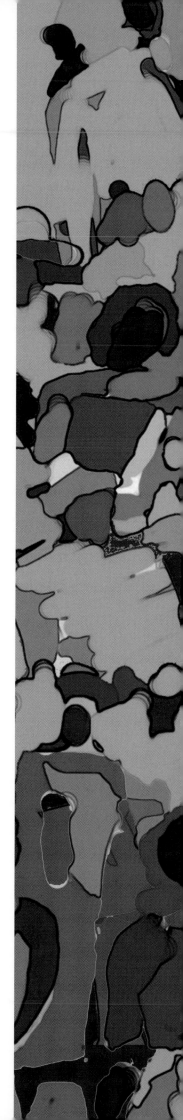

Introduction

1.1 Health matters to everyone: to ourselves, our families and our communities. Many people like to be healthy as part of their idea of what constitutes a 'good life'. As well as the efforts that individuals make, many states have in place policies, aimed at a range of stakeholders, that seek to promote health through a variety of strategies and programmes. State-directed initiatives that concern very personal behaviour, or that involve powerful industries, can give rise to many different types of tension. This Report deals with some of the ethical issues that arise from efforts to improve health at the population level. In Box 1.1 we set out the key definitions that we will be using for 'public health'.

> **Box 1.1: Public health and population health**
> The term 'public health' is often used in many different senses. In this Report, we distinguish it from the term 'population health' as follows:
> *Public health* refers to "the science and art of preventing disease, prolonging life and promoting health through organised efforts of society" (see paragraph 1.6 and Box 1.4).
> *Population health* is used to refer to the state of health of the members of a certain population.

1.2 Over the past 20 years or so, a comprehensive body of bioethical literature has evolved that addresses ethical conflicts at the *individual* level, for example in relation to end-of-life decisions, abortion or medical research. However, many of the established frameworks and principles in bioethics are of somewhat limited use when applied at the *population* level (see paragraphs 2.3, 2.10, 2.22–2.26). This Report seeks to contribute to the emerging field of 'population-level bioethics'.[1] It does not aim to formulate guidance on, for example, how to allocate resources in particular areas of public health, nor is it concerned with the organisational structure of public health services. Rather, we seek to offer in this Report an ethical framework for the scrutiny of public health policies. In this Chapter we introduce different factors that influence population health, comment on different ways in which the concept of 'public health' is used and how we understand it, and describe the overall structure of the Report.

Background

1.3 Over the years, improvements in the health of the population have been achieved by a wide range of measures. These have included those delivered within a healthcare context, such as vaccination programmes, and those delivered in other ways, such as in the workplace, home and general environment (see Box 1.2).[2] Historically, many of the most substantial advances in improving population health have been made through non-medical developments (see Figure 1.1). Clean air legislation and improved housing and sanitation considerably reduced morbidity and mortality in western European countries in the 19th and 20th Centuries. Similarly, a wide range of highly prescriptive health and safety regulations for public places, and especially the workplace, have helped reduce ill health and premature death.

---

[1] Wikler D and Brock D (2007) Population-level bioethics: mapping a new agenda, in *Ethics, Prevention, and Public Health*, Dawson A and Verweij M (Editors) (Oxford: Oxford University Press).

[2] Royal Institute of Public Health (2006) *150 years of public health milestones*, available at: http://www.riph.org.uk/pdf/celebrating_150yrs_june06.pdf.

> **Box 1.2: Some examples of health improvement measures introduced in the UK**
>
> ■ The first Clean Air Act was passed in 1956, following the London smog of 1952, in which 4,000 people died.[3] This was the first piece of legislation to seek to control domestic, as well as industrial, sources of air pollution, and it is said to have contributed to improvements in air quality over subsequent decades.
>
> ■ Britain has one of the best records on road safety in the world, with the number of deaths per person per kilometre travelled lower than in any other country. The number of road accident casualties peaked in the mid-1960s and has fallen gradually since. This decrease is attributed in no small part to road safety measures, such as laws prohibiting drink driving and requiring the use of seat belts.[4]
>
> ■ The Industrial Revolution of the Victorian era saw a huge increase in the numbers of people living in urban areas. This created significant population health problems due to overcrowded living conditions and lack of running water.[5] The Sanitary Act of 1866 forced local authorities to supply running water, provide for disposal of sewage and waste, made overcrowding illegal, and set up special hospitals for infectious diseases. Two further Public Health Acts were passed in 1872 and 1875.
>
> ■ Coal-mining is a good example of a hazardous occupation that has been made safer by health and safety measures. A century ago, around one miner in a thousand would die each year as a result of a mining-related accident. In recent years, this has been less than one per year in total in Great Britain, with more than 5,500 people working as miners.[6] Improvements in health have also been seen more recently in the quarry industry, in which the number of reportable injuries was reduced by 52% between 2000 and 2005, following a new health and safety campaign.[7]

Figure 1.1 Tuberculosis death rates in England and Wales, 1838–1970*

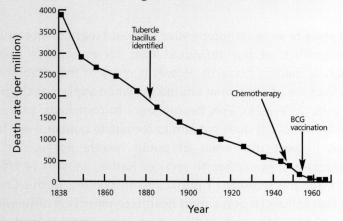

Deaths attributable to tuberculosis have declined over time. It is notable that the decline began before the agent responsible for the disease had been identified and before medical interventions were initiated. The reasons for the decline are disputed, but it is clear that factors other than medical interventions, for example, social and economic changes, played a role.

*Source: McKeown T (1979) *The Role of Medicine: Dream, mirage, or nemesis?* (Oxford: Basil Blackwell). Reproduced with permission.

Factors affecting population health

1.4 Many of the issues discussed in the context of public health arise from what some commentators call 'lifestyle diseases', such as obesity- and smoking-related conditions. Implicit in the use of this term is the idea that a disease is simply a result of individuals' choices about how to live their lives. Such a view is problematic as a person's health is influenced by a very wide range of factors. Attributing poor or good states of health simply to different 'lifestyle choices' (whether for specific individuals or particular social or ethnic subgroups of the population) ignores the role of several other important factors that have a substantial influence on health. These include: genetic background, social and economic living standards, the built environment, the availability of, and

[3] Jochelson K (2005) *Nanny or Steward? The role of government in public health* (London: King's Fund); Giussani V, *The Clean Air Act 1956: An empirical investigation*, available at: http://www.uea.ac.uk/env/cserge/pub/wp/gec/gec_1994_20.pdf.

[4] Jochelson K (2005) *Nanny or Steward? The role of government in public health* (London: King's Fund).

[5] Baggott R (2000) *Public Health: Policy and politics* (Basingstoke: Palgrave Macmillan); Royal Institute of Public Health (2006) 150 years of public health milestones, available at: http://www.riph.org.uk/pdf/celebrating_150yrs_june06.pdf.

[6] Health and Safety Executive, *Mining*, available at: http://www.hse.gov.uk/mining/index.htm.

[7] Health and Safety Executive, *Quarries – Programme of work*, available at: http://www.hse.gov.uk/quarries/programme.htm.

access to, preventative and curative health services, and the influence of commercial organisations such as the food and drink industries. In this Report, we have adopted the term 'personal behaviour' rather than 'lifestyle choice'. Personal behaviour indisputably plays an important role, but is itself affected by external factors that are equally important in ethical and policy discussions.

1.5 The many factors affecting health create problems for public health professionals and policy makers, as it is often difficult to identify a single causal factor for a specific population health problem. Furthermore, some of the contributory factors may interact in complex ways, and one factor may modify others. Thus, it may be possible to establish that certain industry emissions can cause respiratory problems, but the exact effect on an individual's health may vary, depending on proximity of work or home to the emission source, genetic predisposition, or personal behaviours, such as smoking (see Box 1.3).

Box 1.3: The main determinants of health*

A schematic overview, by Dahlgren and Whitehead, of the range of factors that can contribute causally, or in modifying form, to the variation in people's health:[8]

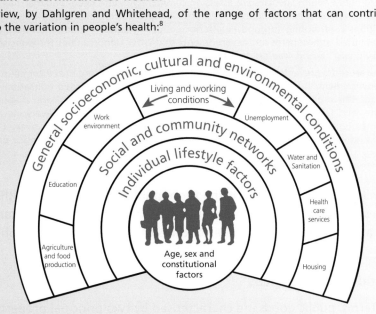

*Originally published in: Dahlgren G and Whitehead M (1991) *Policies and Strategies to Promote Social Equity in Health* (Stockholm: Institute of Futures Studies); Reproduced from: Acheson D (1998) *Independent Inquiry into Inequalities in Health Report*, available at: http://www.archive.official-documents.co.uk/document/doh/ih/ih.htm. Reproduced with permission.

The concept of 'public health'

1.6 Given the various contexts of, and approaches to, public health action, and the many factors affecting health that could be targeted, defining 'public health'[9] is not straightforward (see Box 1.4). The Faculty of Public Health of the Royal Colleges of Physicians of the United Kingdom defines it as: "The science and art of preventing disease, prolonging life and promoting health through organised efforts of society".[10] We use the concept in a similar way. In our interpretation

---

[8] Note that the differing sizes of the sections in the diagram are not intended to represent their importance or other meaning, but a case-by-case assessment is needed of the relative weight of the different factors and the role of interactions between them. Note also that whereas the diagram uses the term 'lifestyle factors', in this Report, we have chosen to use instead the term 'personal behaviour' (see paragraph 1.4).

[9] Similarly the concept of 'health' is far from clear: for example not everyone agrees with the World Health Organization's concept of health as "a state of complete physical, mental and social well-being and not merely the absence of disease or infirmity"; see: Preamble to the Constitution of the World Health Organization as adopted by the International Health Conference, New York, 19–22 June 1946; signed on 22 July 1946 by the representatives of 61 States (Official Records of the World Health Organization, no. 2, p.100) and entered into force on 7 April 1948.

[10] See Faculty of Public Health of the Royal Colleges of Physicians of the United Kingdom *What is Public Health?*, available at: http://www.fphm.org.uk/about_faculty/what_public_health/default.asp.

of the term, two notions are of special importance: first, the *preventative*[11] *nature* of public health interventions, and secondly, that these are to be achieved through *collective efforts*. In our view, this characterisation has clear implications for the state to enable, sustain and lead on such efforts (see paragraphs 1.11, 2.41–2.44).

Box 1.4: Public health: definitions

There are several different definitions of public health, including the following:

"The science and art of preventing disease, prolonging life and promoting health through organised efforts of society." *Faculty of Public Health of the Royal Colleges of Physicians of the United Kingdom*[12]

"The mission of public health is to 'fulfil society's interest in assuring conditions in which people can be healthy'." *Institute of Medicine, USA*[13]

"Public Health is the science of protecting and improving the health of communities through education, promotion of healthy lifestyles, and research for disease and injury prevention" *Association of Schools of Public Health, USA*[14]

"An art and a science; and also a movement dedicated to the equitable improvement of health and well-being (of communities with their full participation)." *World Federation of Public Health Associations*[15]

"The key functions of public health agencies are assessing community health needs and marshalling the resources for responding to them, developing health policy in response to specific community and national health needs, and assuring that conditions contributing to good health, including high-quality medical services, safe water supplies, good nutrition, unpolluted atmospheres and environments that offer opportunities for exercise and recreation are available to the individuals." *World Medical Association*[16]

"The science and the art of (1) preventing disease, (2) prolonging life, and (3) organized community efforts for (a) the sanitation of the environment, (b) the control of communicable infections, (c) the education of the individual in personal hygiene, (d) the organization of medical and nursing services for the early diagnosis and preventive treatment of disease, and (e) the development of the social machinery to ensure everyone a standard of living adequate for the maintenance of health, so organizing these benefits as to enable every citizen to realize his birthright of health and longevity." *CEA Winslow, former Chair of Department and Professor of Public Health, Yale University*[17]

1.7 There are similarities in the way that the term 'public health' is used with the use of other common terms such as 'public education', 'public highways' and 'public libraries'. As we discuss below, these are all underpinned by the concepts of 'public good' and 'public services'.

Public goods and public services

1.8 In economic terms, public goods are characterised by two principal properties: they are *non-rival* and *non-excludable*. So, for example, fresh air might be considered a public good because one person breathing it outdoors does not affect other people's ability to do so (non-rivalness), and because it is practically impossible to prevent everyone from doing so (non-excludability)[18]. Other examples are infrastructural arrangements such as cycle lanes or parks.[19] The term 'public good' is also often used to denote what is better described as 'public services': resources or institutions that respond to important needs of members of the population, and that are managed by the state in a way that ensures that the needs are

---

[11] While 'preventing diseases' may be understood as suggesting a somewhat one-sided focus on prevention, we also recognise that preventing disease progression is an integral part of public health strategies, as are efficient curative services. However, in our view, the overall emphasis of public health initiatives is on preventative measures. It is worth pointing out that improved curative systems are often seen as more acceptable by the public than attempts at preventing poor health, which are more frequently seen as unnecessarily intrusive or paternalistic.

[12] See: http://www.fphm.org.uk/about_faculty/what_public_health/default.asp.

[13] Institute of Medicine, Committee for the Study of the Future of Public Health, Division of Health Care Services (1988) *The Future of Public Health* (Washington, DC: National Academy Press).

[14] See: http://www.whatispublichealth.org/what/index.html.

[15] See: http://www.wfpha.org/.

[16] World Medical Association (1995) *World Medical Association Statement on Health Promotion*, available at: http://www.wma.net/e/policy/h7.htm.

[17] Winslow CEA (1920) The untilled field of public health *Modern Medicine* **2**: 183–91.

[18] Varian HR (1994) *Microeconomic Analysis* (New York: Norton).

[19] It is widely agreed that the criteria of non-rivalness and non-excludability are not as clear-cut as they seem, and different goods may fulfil the criteria to different degrees. Thus, although there may be rivalry between different users of cycle lanes

addressed in a fair and effective manner. In this sense, public services are a facility or resource that is valuable to all citizens, although its availability is not necessarily unlimited or free of charge.

1.9 There are different reasons as to why certain public goods or services should be considered worthy of protection.[20] One is based on fairness considerations. For example, in the case of air, individuals (or, more often, industries) may not be too concerned about polluting it, perhaps thinking that their particular actions are of a small or unimportant nature. However, taking advantage of a good, while not contributing to its maintenance, can be a form of 'free-riding' (see also paragraph 4.17) that, if more widely adopted, would adversely affect the sustainability of the good in question. Moreover, the 'costs' of the unfair action may be incurred by people other than those who initiated it; economists often call such costs 'externalities'. The period of rapid industrial expansion and associated uncurbed air-pollution that began in the first half of the 20th Century provides a clear illustration of this. Air pollution harmed many people who had no relationship with the industries that were the main cause, incurring significant health costs, but gaining no benefits (see Box 1.2).

1.10 Then there are services that society provides in order to ensure that everyone receives the benefits of them, such as education for children. Here, individuals may be able to meet the need, but there is no guarantee that they will do so. In recognition of the vulnerable status of children, and the importance of basic knowledge, most developed countries have in place a public education system. Such systems are often centred on a core curriculum and require education up to a certain age. Once such systems are in place they are usually monitored to ensure that they assist in furthering goals such as equality of opportunity and a sense of community.

1.11 An important part of the UK's public health system is the National Health Service (NHS). The main reason for seeing such a system as a public service is that, like children's education, the need it addresses is considered too important to be left to private suppliers alone:

■ First, focusing on equity and fairness considerations, there is a risk that a fully privatised approach would increase inequalities. Although part-payment is required for some services, currently a wide range of core NHS services are provided 'free at the point of need' to all,[21] irrespective of sex, age, risk-assessments or socio-economic status. Experiences from other countries indicate that highly privatised systems result in unequal access to healthcare services and increased health inequalities.[22] As we set out in the next chapter (see paragraphs 2.27–2.32), the reduction of health inequalities must be one of the principal aims of public health policy. The provision of some form of public healthcare system – though not necessarily organised in the same way as the NHS – is therefore a public service of exceptional

and parks, and although it may be possible to exclude some users from access through, for example, entrance fees to parks, in principle it can make sense to see such goods as part of the package of non-rival, non-excludable public health goods.

[20] Public goods need not necessarily be provided only through public providers, such as governments: many private organisations play important roles in their delivery. In addition the voluntary sector, including churches and charities, contributes considerably to the recognition and maintenance of public goods. This variety in methods of organisation need not undermine the fact that the end result remains a public good that is available to all at a reasonable cost and there is in place an appropriate form of public accountability.

[21] Note, however, that NHS services are not necessarily free for people who do not normally live in the country, including failed asylum seekers (although there are some situations in which their treatment would be free, for example emergency treatments and treatments of certain infectious diseases in order to protect the health of the wider population). Note also that NHS prescriptions and dental care are not free to everyone. Department of Health (1999) *HSC 1999/018 Overseas visitors' eligibility to receive free primary care*, available at: http://www.dh.gov.uk/en/PublicationsAndStatistics/LettersAndCirculars/HealthServiceCirculars/DH_4004148; Department of Health (2004) *Implementing the overseas visitors hospital charging regulations: Guidance for NHS trust hospitals in England*, available at: http://www.dh.gov.uk/en/Publicationsandstatistics/Publications/PublicationsPolicyAndGuidance/DH_4080313.

[22] Mackintosh M (2003) *Health Care Commercialisation and the Embedding of Inequality* (RUIG/UNRISD Health Project Synthesis Paper), available at: http://www.unrisd.org/80256B3C005BCCF9/(httpAuxPages)/4023556AA730F778C1256DE500649E48/$file/mackinto.pdf.

value, complementing other strands of public health initiatives, such as provision of clean water, social housing and environmental protection. We also note that in ratifying the European Social Charter, the United Kingdom has recognised a 'right to health'. This, in effect, obliges states to provide effective healthcare structures for the population and to implement policies for the prevention of illness.[23] The Charter also requires states to ensure "that any person who is without adequate resources and who is unable to secure such resources either by his own efforts or from other sources be granted adequate assistance, and, in the case of sickness, the care necessitated by his condition".[24]

■ Secondly, a system such as the NHS may help to protect people from making bad choices for themselves over their healthcare. Were the healthcare system privatised, people might take 'health gambles' by buying insufficient or no health insurance, either to save money or because they are unable to afford it. Under the current system, the state collects mandatory contributions to the NHS through general taxation.[25] In this sense, the state might be said to 'force its citizens to be free',[26] stipulating that access to healthcare is an essential part of enjoying freedom, and some perceive this as an unjustified act of paternalism (see paragraphs 2.35–2.40). However, we start in this Report with the assumption that in maintaining the NHS as a publicly accountable system that provides resources and expertise to meet the basic health needs of all members of the public, the state fulfils an important part of its *stewardship* function.[27] The implications of the notion of *stewardship* will be expanded later in the Report (paragraphs 2.41–2.44, see also paragraph 2.39).

1.12 In summary, the collective efforts of all parts of society, including individuals, healthcare professionals, industries, urban planners, health policy and other policy makers and politicians, should contribute to generating and supporting measures that improve the health of all. The role of the government is to provide certain key services that should not be left to the market alone, and to establish the rules under which the different agents operate in a way that is compatible with promoting population health and reducing inequalities. The stewardship role of the state also implies, among other things, that it has good reasons to intervene where there is a risk that some agents will free-ride on important goods at the expense of others, or where only regulation can ensure that desirable goods or services are available. At the same time, the stewardship responsibility of the state does not absolve other parties, such as the commercial sector, from their responsibilities. We outline the implications of this web of responsibilities for public health in more detail in Chapters 2–7.

Outline of the Report

1.13 We begin by setting out in Chapter 2 a general structure for the consideration of ethical issues arising in public health by explaining the guiding principles that feature in what we

[23] Hunt P (2006) *Report of the Special Rapporteur of the Commission on Human Rights on the right of everyone to the enjoyment of the highest attainable standard of physical and mental health* Sixty-second session of the United Nations Human Rights Commission, Agenda item 10, E/CN.4/2006/48, paragraph 4, available at: http://daccess-ods.un.org/TMP/4598173.html.

[24] *European Social Charter*, revised 1996, Part I Article 13, available at: http://conventions.coe.int/treaty/en/Treaties/Html/163.htm.

[25] Statistics collated by the Organisation for Economic Co-operation and Development (OECD) show that, in 2004, the amount of UK health expenditure that was publicly funded, either from taxation or from national insurance contributions, equated to US$2,164 per person (in purchasing power parities), compared with an OECD average of US$1,833 per person (note that the OECD only includes developed countries), OECD (2007) *OECD Factbook 2007: Economic, environmental and social statistics*, available at: http://titania.sourceoecd.org/vl=2896985/cl=31/nw=1/rpsv/factbook/.

[26] Rousseau famously argued that the Social Contract he proposed enabled the people of a state to be secured "against all personal dependence"; Rousseau JJ (1762) *Social Contract*, Book I, part 7, translated by Cole GDH; text available at: http://www.constitution.org/jjr/socon.htm.

[27] Saltman RB and Ferroussier-Davis O (2000) The concept of stewardship in health policy *Bulletin of the World Health Organization* **78**(6): 732–9; Jochelson K (2005) *Nanny or Steward? The role of government in public health* (London: King's Fund).

call the 'stewardship model'. We develop this framework from discussions about different conceptions of the role of the state, and about the 'harm principle', established by the philosopher John Stuart Mill. We go on to identify a range of positive goals that public health programmes should seek to achieve under the stewardship model, as well as negative constraints that need to be considered. In establishing this framework we consider, among other things: conceptual and normative questions arising from seeking to reduce health inequalities; the concept of consent in population-level bioethics as opposed to individual-centred bioethics; issues raised by the recent emergence of corporate social responsibility; and the question of whether it is useful to establish an exhaustive list of principles that should feature in the stewardship model.

1.14 Chapter 3 concerns the policy process. In it we consider how certain elements of the ethical framework play out in a policy context. We first discuss conceptual and practical problems in relation to assessments of 'evidence', 'risk' and 'choice', and highlight the need for clarity of these concepts. We then return to the observations on health inequalities made in Chapter 2, and illustrate their bearing on policy and practice. We describe what we call the 'intervention ladder', a device for comparing different policy options according to their degree of intrusiveness. In the second part of the chapter we examine more closely which parties are, and should be, involved in the policy process, ranging from professional groups to the media.

1.15 There follow four chapters of case studies that aim to illustrate in more detail the stewardship model and other concepts introduced in Chapters 2 and 3. Chapter 4 concerns infectious diseases; obesity is considered in Chapter 5; alcohol and smoking in Chapter 6; and fluoridation of water in Chapter 7. In each chapter, we provide a brief outline of the scientific evidence relating to health impacts, referring the reader elsewhere for more comprehensive analyses of previous scientific or policy discussion.[28] In each chapter we comment on options for intervention, and on specific ethical and policy-related issues. Several conclusions and recommendations are made, aimed at various agencies, including industry and the government.

1.16 As many respondents to our consultation[29] observed, a range of other public health issues could have been included as case studies. Examples include mental health, breast-feeding, environmental pollution, radiation, additives in foods, or complementary therapies. The Working Party decided to focus on the specific cases mentioned above because they illustrate the ethical and policy-relevant tensions that arise in public health but have not always been explicitly recognised in government or other policy documents.[30]

1.17 Finally, Chapter 8 draws together the central themes of the Report. We comment on a range of important over-arching and cross-cutting issues and reassess some of the principal assumptions made in Chapters 2 and 3.

---

[28] See Appendix 7 for a list of major recent reports.

[29] See Appendix 2 for a list of respondents and a summary of responses.

[30] For example, the White Paper *Choosing Health* emphasised individual choice, with little discussion of the range of factors that can enhance or reduce options for people, see paragraph 1.4 and paragraphs 3.20–3.21.

Chapter 2

An ethical framework

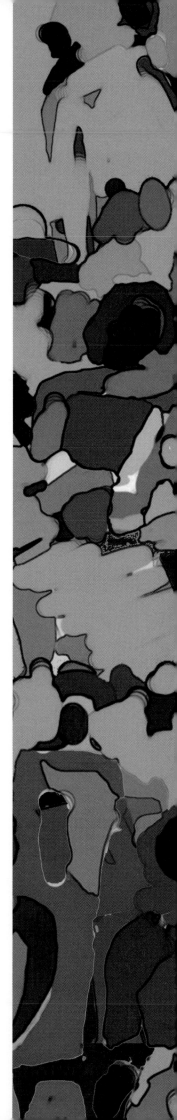

An ethical framework

Introduction: an ethical framework for policy

2.1 A great deal of bioethical literature focuses on the way the individual can be protected in the medical context, for example in relation to research. Public health programmes, by contrast, extend beyond the clinical context and focus on the population level, affecting the lives of the whole population, or large subgroups of the population. Many of these measures focus on prevention and may have implications for those who would not consider themselves to be ill. As a result they raise issues about the responsibilities and authority of the state and other agents whose policies and actions shape or affect people's lives. Much depends on the kind of intervention, the situation of those most directly affected by it, and the seriousness of the risks involved by implementing, or not implementing, a certain programme. Our aim in this chapter is to develop an ethical framework that identifies the most important values to guide public policy in this area. There is a complex network of interests, rights and ideals to consider, and it is not possible to prescribe a mechanistic formula that would dictate how these values should be applied. However, we aim to show how our ethical framework provides a coherent approach to the difficult issues raised by public health policies.

2.2 We begin by briefly reviewing the role of the state and then sketching an initial framework for a public health policy, based on a classical liberal conception of the state's role. Although this framework is suitable to address some of the principal issues arising in the context of public health, it also has certain limitations. We therefore propose a revised and extended version of the initial framework, which we call the stewardship model. This model is developed further in the next chapter on policy and it is then assessed in light of the issues raised by the case studies in Chapters 4–7. In Chapter 8 we return to this framework and draw some overarching conclusions.

The state and the citizen

Libertarians versus collectivists

2.3 A question that is fundamental to our inquiry is the relationship between the state's authority and the position of individual people and intermediate bodies such as institutions, schools and companies that are governed by its rules.[1] This issue is central to political philosophy, and attracts a wide range of points of view. We present here an overview of salient ethical theories that seek to describe the state–individual relationship. We locate these theories along a spectrum ranging from those that give priority to the individual, to those that prioritise the collective interests of the population as a whole.

2.4 At one end of the spectrum is the libertarian perspective, which affirms what are classically regarded as the 'natural' rights of man: life, liberty and property. The authority of the state in these rights is limited to ensuring that members of the population are able to enjoy these rights without interference from others. This radically individualist point of view allows only a minimal state. Apart from the ability to defend itself from external aggression, the state's legitimate activities comprise only: political institutions which provide authoritative statements of individual rights; judicial institutions which determine when these rights have been violated; and penal institutions to punish those who are found to have committed such violations. Beyond these institutions the libertarian state does not see the promotion of the welfare of its population as its proper role; so it provides little support for the establishment

---

[1] Clearly, the laws of a state affect not only people individually, but also other agents, such as charitable organisations or commercial companies. We address the role of companies in paragraphs 2.47–2.50.

of public health programmes, except for those that are essential in a practical way to the enjoyment of the rights it recognises.

2.5 At the other end of the spectrum there is what can be called a collectivist point of view. There are several forms, and we focus here on utilitarian and social contract approaches.[2]

2.6 In utilitarian traditions the primary aim is to maximise utility by focusing on achieving the greatest possible collective benefit. This means that actions or rules are generally measured by the degree to which they reduce pain and suffering, and promote overall happiness, well-being, or what might be called 'good health'. Hence, in the context of public health, when choosing between several competing interventions or programmes, states and policy makers ought to opt for those that are likely to produce the greatest aggregate benefit. For example, in the case of an epidemic, a utilitarian approach would usually favour isolation and quarantining, whereas such measures would be likely to lead to considerable tensions in the libertarian framework sketched above. As this example illustrates, one of the reasons why utilitarian approaches are controversial is that, in principle, they may allow the welfare or interests of some people to be 'sacrificed' if this were to lead to an increase in overall welfare.

2.7 An alternative collectivist approach is found in social contract theory. Here, the state's authority is based on the collective will of a community (for example, as expressed in a democratic vote) to live together as an enduring nation state. The rights of individual citizens are dependent upon this shared will of their community, and not antecedent to it. On this view, these rights do not constitute a limit to the state's authority to intervene in the lives of its citizens; instead the state's authority is properly exercised in that it realises the collective will of the community. This position will typically favour measures to promote the welfare of its citizens, including public goods and services of all kinds.

The liberal state

2.8 There are, of course, a range of positions in between these two ends of the spectrum. These intermediate positions hold that although it is the state's business to uphold and defend certain fundamental individual rights,[3] it is also the state's responsibility to care for the welfare of all citizens. These welfare considerations may include ensuring that all have a fair opportunity to make a decent life for themselves, and that efforts are made to level out unfair inequalities affecting disadvantaged groups or individuals.

2.9 Positions of this kind are thought of as liberal, and they place emphasis on equality between citizens, both in the personal and political spheres of life. The liberal agrees with the libertarian that the protection of individual freedoms constrains the state's authority. Nonetheless, the liberal rejects the libertarian thesis that legitimate state power is restricted to protection of these freedoms, and agrees with the social contract version of collectivism that the state's power may rightly be used to advance the welfare of its citizens. The liberal will generally reject the utilitarian claim that it is acceptable, without further argument, to pursue beneficial interventions, even if these significantly affect the liberty of some individuals. Thus, for the liberal state, some interventions to promote the interests of the population may be acceptable without providing further justification (such as ensuring opportunities for health for the

---

[2] We recognise that there are other theoretical frameworks that are collectivist (such as social democracy, which may be based on religious and ethical ideas), and that neither utilitarianism nor social contract theory by necessity has to lead to collectivism.

[3] Most notably those central to the life of a free citizen who shapes their own life in accordance with their own values and plays a part in democratic public affairs.

disadvantaged and vulnerable), whereas other interventions require explicit justification, or may simply not be acceptable at all.[4]

Autonomy

2.10 The liberal's emphasis on the importance of the individual's ability to determine the course of their own life reflects the value of personal autonomy. It is important to recognise that autonomy is not just a 'negative' freedom from interference. Literally, autonomy means 'self-governance'. Its realisation requires, among other things, knowledge of the possibilities available, and the basic capabilities necessary to take advantage of them. Thus the liberal state attaches great importance to the universal provision of education. It is content to put in place policies that make education mandatory, while recognising that this infringement of individual freedom may not be acceptable to some libertarians. These infringements are seen as justifiable as they enable people to develop basic capacities that allow them to make full use of the opportunities available in a society that values equality of opportunity. Recognising autonomy requires, in addition to universal provision of education, other policies that enable individuals to make their own way in the world and pursue their own personal goals. While the state cannot guarantee this, a liberal state will seek to promote it through policies aimed, for example, at minimising ill health, since this is an important obstacle to the achievement of independence and personal autonomy.

Health as a value

2.11 A reasonable level of health is generally regarded to be an essential ingredient of a good life. The World Health Organization (WHO) defines health as "a state of complete physical, mental and social well-being and not merely the absence of disease or infirmity".[5] Although this may be too wide-ranging, as hardly anyone might be considered fully healthy under the definition,[6] WHO's concept does illustrate that assessments of well-being can include value-judgements. This means there may be disagreement about the justification of specific policies. States should therefore be cautious about imposing paradigms of health on those who might reject them, especially where it might entail some intrusion into their personal life. In view of this, liberal states will typically see it as their responsibility to provide frameworks that reduce the risks its citizens pose to each other's health, but also to promote the health of those, such as children, who cannot take full responsibility for themselves.

2.12 Most modern Western states are liberal under this classification, and the question is how far it is proper for the state to introduce programmes that interfere to different degrees (see paragraphs 1.3, 3.37–3.38) in the lives of its population, in order to reduce the risks to the health of all or some of them. This illustrates the tension inherent in the liberal state, as a political community that seeks both to protect personal autonomy and promote the welfare of all people.[7]

---

[4] The relationship between the liberal state and the libertarian and collectivist framework could also be clarified by focusing on the rights of individual people. Collectivists might argue that rights provide a constraint upon society through the codification of the collective will into human rights declarations, which then limit the choices that governments can make. In this sense, the collective will of society is exercised at two levels: first, by establishing a level of agreed fundamental principles in the form of rights which cannot be breached without special procedures such as constitutional change; and secondly, through democratic government and processes which assess current opinion on what is desirable. These principles are not limited to negative constraints on state power; they could also make obligatory some state intervention.

[5] Preamble to the Constitution of the World Health Organization as adopted by the International Health Conference, New York, 19–22 June 1946; signed on 22 July 1946 by the representatives of 61 States (Official Records of the World Health Organization, no. 2, p.100) and entered into force on 7 April 1948.

[6] See also: Saracci R (1997) The World Health Organization needs to reconsider its definition of health Br Med J **314**: 1409.

[7] Note that there is no necessary exclusivity between either respecting individual autonomy or promoting the welfare of all. In many cases measures aimed at protecting autonomy may well lead to an increase in overall welfare at the same time. However, public health also gives rise to a range of competing scenarios, as we explore in Chapters 4–7.

A liberal proposal

Mill's harm principle

2.13 One way to start thinking about resolving the tension between the promotion of public health and the protection of individual freedoms is provided by the famous 'harm principle' advanced by John Stuart Mill in his essay *On Liberty*:

> "The object of this Essay is to assert one very simple principle, as entitled to govern absolutely the dealings of society with the individual in the way of compulsion and control, whether the means used be physical force in the form of legal penalties, or the moral coercion of public opinion. That principle is, that the sole end for which mankind are warranted, individually or collectively in interfering with the liberty of action of any of their number, is self-protection. That the only purpose for which power can be rightfully exercised over any member of a civilized community, against his will, is to prevent harm to others. His own good, either physical or moral, is not a sufficient warrant. He cannot rightfully be compelled to do or forbear because it will be better for him to do so, because it will make him happier, because, in the opinions of others, to do so would be wise, or even right. These are good reasons for remonstrating with him, or reasoning with him, or persuading him, or entreating him, but not for compelling him, or visiting him with any evil, in case he do otherwise. To justify that, the conduct from which it is desired to deter him must be calculated to produce evil to someone else. The only part of the conduct of any one, for which he is amenable to society, is that which concerns others. Over himself, over his own body and mind, the individual is sovereign."[8]

Public health and the harm principle

2.14 To introduce Mill's principle in this way is not to suggest that it provides a satisfactory answer to all the questions that arise in the context of public health. Nor does it commit us to the wider theoretical framework in which it was set out, or to claim that harm to third parties is always a sufficient legitimisation of coercion.[9] Rather, we use it to illustrate that, even in an approach that seeks to ensure the greatest possible degree of individual liberty and the least possible degree of state interference, there is a core principle according to which coercive, liberty-infringing state intervention is acceptable: where the purpose is to prevent harm to others.[10] Throughout this Report, we refer to this version of the harm principle as the *classical harm principle*.

2.15 Several of Mill's observations are often overlooked, and we will use these to establish an initial framework for public health ethics that extends beyond merely preventing harms to others. We note, first, his comments about the type of people to which his principle applies; secondly, the type of goods that should be promoted by society; thirdly, his observations about means other than coercion that could be used to suggest behaviour change to people; and fourthly, his emphasis on individual liberty.

---

[8] Mill JS (1859) On liberty, in *On Liberty and Other Essays* (1989) Collini S (Editor) (Cambridge: Cambridge University Press), p.13.

[9] Therefore, harm to others is in most cases a necessary, but not by itself a sufficient, reason for coercive intervention. For example, there may be cases in which harm to others is caused, but it is preferable not to intervene in coercive ways, as the costs of intervention, whether these are financial or social, are too high. Considerations about proportionality will therefore usually become relevant in determining how to proceed in cases of harm to others, see paragraphs 3.17–3.18 and the discussion in Chapters 4–7.

[10] The assessment of what should count as harm, and to what extent a given harm should justify infringing liberties is however not always straightforward. See, for example, Feinberg J (1984) *Harm to Others* (Oxford: Oxford University Press). We provide examples of cases in which the classical harm principle is relevant in the Chapters 4–7.

Care of the vulnerable

2.16 Mill stated that his principle was to apply only to "human beings in the maturity of their faculties", and he goes on to say:

> "We are not speaking of children, or of young persons below the age which the law may fix as that of manhood or womanhood. Those who are still in a state to require being taken care of by others, must be protected against their own actions as well as against external injury."[11]

So Mill recognises that the state can rightfully intervene to protect children,[12] and other similar vulnerable people who require protection, from, for example, damaging their own health.

Public services

2.17 Secondly, Mill makes it clear that his defence of individual liberty is founded on his commitment to advancing 'utility', which can be understood as general welfare. Hence his principle is to be interpreted to allow the state to support "joint work necessary to the interest of society",[13] including, for example, the provision of clean water and regulations that limit working hours.[14] In the context of public health policy this provision is especially important as such policy is often directed at public goods and services.

Educating the public

2.18 The third point is Mill's view on the importance of educating and informing people so that they can make up their own minds about important questions concerning both the public affairs of the state, and their own personal decisions as to how to lead their lives. Hence, although Mill's discussion of the harm principle shows that he would strongly oppose public health programmes which simply aim to coerce people to lead healthy lives, he would be likely to support programmes which seek to "advise, instruct and persuade"[15] them so that they can make informed decisions about, for example, what to eat and how to exercise.

Protecting individuality

2.19 Finally, it is important to bear in mind the central theme in Mill's essay, the fundamental importance of what he calls 'individuality': the exercise of freedom in the construction of one's personal life. This value implies that interventions in personal life, even when they are intended to reduce health risks to others, carry a significant ethical cost. So far as it can be managed, the less intrusive and directive an intervention can be, the better (see paragraphs 3.37–3.38).

An initial liberal framework

2.20 In light of these points it is possible to construct an initial ethical framework for public health programmes. In this framework, such programmes have certain goals and constraints.[16]

Concerning goals, public health programmes should:

- aim to reduce the risks of ill health that people might impose upon each other;

[11] Mill JS (1859) On liberty, in *On Liberty and Other Essays* (1989) Collini S (Editor) (Cambridge: Cambridge University Press), p.13.
[12] The quote may also raise the question of whether it is useful to think of homogeneous classes such as children who, categorically, differ in their ability to make judgements from "human beings in the maturity of their faculties". The important point here is that the reasoning behind the harm principle does not mean that groups with less developed capacities should be neglected.
[13] Mill JS (1859) On liberty, in *On Liberty and Other Essays* (1989) Collini S (Editor) (Cambridge: Cambridge University Press), p.14.
[14] *Ibid.* p.95.
[15] *Ibid.* p.94.
[16] The different goals and constraints should not be understood as being ranked in a hierarchical order.

■ pay special attention to the health of children and other vulnerable people;

■ aim to reduce ill health by regulations that ensure environmental conditions that sustain good health, such as the provision of clean air and water, safe food and decent housing; and

■ aim to make it easy for people to lead healthy lives by the provision of advice and information.

In terms of constraints, such programmes should:

■ not attempt to coerce adults to lead healthy lives; and

■ seek to minimise interventions that affect important areas of personal life.

2.21 This provides a coherent starting point for a framework for policy, although there are potential conflicts between some of the goals and constraints, for example, between the duty to care for children and the aim of minimising interventions in personal life. However, apart from such internal problems that are likely to occur in any framework to some extent, is this framework really satisfactory? Critics may feel that despite the acknowledgement here of the importance of public goods and services, this framework remains too strongly committed to individual autonomy. So we turn to consider some ways in which this criticism might be addressed.

Broadening the debate

Individual consent and its limitations

2.22 The liberal's stress on the importance of individual autonomy implies that the concept of consent plays a key role. Much of the bioethical discussion of the past two decades or so has sought to establish autonomy and consent as the cornerstones of biomedical ethics. However, we noted above that many of the issues raised by public health differ from those usually addressed in bioethics. The question of what weight consent can carry in public health, and when it is, and is not, required is a case in point as its relevance and usefulness is often overestimated in this context.

2.23 The core notion underlying the concept of consent that currently features in the bioethical literature and much healthcare law and policy can be traced back to the 1947 Nuremberg Trials of German physicians,[17] and it was later incorporated into the *Declaration of Helsinki* of the World Medical Association (WMA), and other ethical codes and laws. These codes thus established consent as a powerful and indispensable condition: any intervention that may expose someone to significant risk is morally unacceptable unless the person concerned agrees to being exposed to the risks, and, in legal terms, waives the corresponding rights.[18] Within the clinical context, the feasibility of consent, the degree to which it is, or should be, informed, genuine, specific or explicit, and the general conditions required for it to be ethically acceptable, have continued to be the subject of intense debate.[19]

---

[17] The court proceedings were initiated because physicians and researchers in Nazi Germany systematically forced concentration camp prisoners and others to take part in medical experiments. Almost all of the experiments were exceptionally cruel and harmful, and few of those involved survived them. To prevent any repetition of such abuses, Directives for Human Experimentation in the form of the *Nuremberg Code* were produced. The Code sought to ensure the absence of force, coercion or duress in the research context and began by stating unambiguously that "The voluntary consent of the human subject is absolutely essential". (See: *Directives for Human Experimentation – Nuremberg Code*, available at: http://ohsr.od.nih.gov/guidelines/nuremberg.html.)

[18] This is so, irrespective of whether the intervention is aimed at benefiting the person concerned, for example, by performing invasive medical treatment, or whether it is aimed primarily at benefiting a third party, for example where someone is involved in a medical research study.

[19] See: Beyleveld D and Brownsword R (2007) *Consent in the Law* (Oxford: Hart); Manson N and O'Neill O (2007) *Rethinking Informed Consent in Bioethics* (Cambridge: Cambridge University Press); Nuffield Council on Bioethics (1995) *Human Tissue: Ethical and legal issues* (London: Nuffield Council on Bioethics).

2.24 The concept of consent is rightly at the centre of clinical medicine. Although some of the issues addressed in the sphere of public health concern medical interventions, such as vaccinations, many others, such as the provision of health-conducive environments, occupational health and safety regulations or measures aimed at preventing excessive consumption of tobacco and alcohol, do not. The question is therefore to what extent consent is morally relevant in these areas.[20] Public health interventions may interfere to different degrees with people's choices or liberties. For example, in the case of quarantine and isolation the degree of intrusion is considerable, but restricting the movement of people suspected of having a severe infectious disease, whether or not they agree with it, can be justified on the basis of the classical harm principle. Many other interventions do not concern this degree of intrusion, and it is important to recognise the difference between consent requirements that are relevant in the context of clinical medicine and research, and those for infringements of people's choices or liberties in the non-clinical context of public health. Often, requiring each person to consent individually to non-intrusive public health measures is almost impossible and certainly impractical. More importantly, the possible harms and restriction of liberties that are entailed by a range of public health measures may not be severe. The essential point is that a greater, more explicit justification is needed for the state to interfere in a situation where individual consent would otherwise be required due to the considerable health or other risks involved. In contrast, such justification may not be needed where an interference merely limits certain choices.

2.25 Therefore, although in the case of potentially harmful medical interventions individual consent is required to authorise the implementation of the procedure, a 'procedural justice' approach that uses conventional democratic decision-making processes may be sufficient to authorise measures where there are no substantial health risks. Key elements of such an approach, which has also been described under the concept of 'accountability for reasonableness',[21] are: transparency of decision-making processes (in terms of the evidence, reasons and rationales cited in favour of an intervention that reduces some choice of individuals or otherwise inconveniences them); a focus on rationales that those affected recognise as being helpful in meeting health needs fairly; and involvement of individuals and stakeholder groups in decision-making processes, with opportunities to challenge interventions in preparation and in practice.[22]

2.26 The implication of this discussion for our initial framework (paragraph 2.20) is therefore that it needs to be expanded, as the constraint that concerns minimising interventions affecting "important areas of personal life", if strictly interpreted, could be too far-reaching, making impossible a range of important public health measures.

Health inequalities

2.27 Two of the key positive goals of public health programmes in the initial liberal framework are a reduction in the causes of ill health, and the provision of facilities that make it easy for

---

[20] Especially as an argument might be made that certain measures should not be implemented unless all those who would be affected consent to them.

[21] Daniels N and Sabin J (1997) Limits to health care: fair procedures, democratic deliberation, and the legitimacy problem for insurers *Philosophy and Public Affairs* **26**: 303–50; Daniels N (2000) Accountability for reasonableness *Br Med J* **321**: 1300–1.

[22] In Chapter 7, for the example of fluoridation of water, we discuss how procedural justice arrangements may be appropriate to justify certain liberty-infringing policies, even if they do not meet with everyone's individual approval. Another important example, considered in Chapter 4, concerns the use of patients' healthcare data for public health surveillance and research. Although some might argue that this should not be done without individual consent, it can also be argued that arrangements such as anonymising data can ensure that values such as privacy or confidentiality are protected, without jeopardising epidemiological research and public health policy that depends on having access to data from a sufficient number of people; see paragraphs 4.37–4.39).

people to lead healthy lives. In devising such programmes it is important to avoid a 'one size fits all' approach, as particular groups of people may differ in their health status, have varying health needs and respond differently to particular programmes. The uneven burden of ill health among different groups raises not only practical issues, but also the question of whether public health programmes should seek to reduce health inequalities. In Chapter 1 we answered this in the affirmative (paragraph 1.11), and noted that we viewed the reduction of health inequalities as central to any public health programme. Here, we clarify our reasoning behind this, which leads to a further important revision to the initial liberal framework. First, we consider in what sense inequalities in health might differ from other kinds of inequality. Next, we turn to a range of more detailed issues raised by seeking to reduce health inequalities: what kinds of inequality should be reduced? Between which kinds of group are we concerned about inequalities? And what strategies are the most appropriate, ethically, to promote equality?

Health inequalities versus income inequalities

2.28 Many liberal societies accept that there are inequalities, for example, in income, so why should inequalities in health be less acceptable?[23] Those defending the special status of health inequalities make an argument along the following lines. Inequalities in wealth are acceptable within a liberal framework only in cases where higher financial rewards for the best off have the implication that their performance contributes to improving the situation of the worst off (for example because of a resulting increase in welfare through the availability of cheaper goods and services for all).[24] Additionally, inequalities in income concern a good that has primarily instrumental value: more money enables people to do more. By contrast, health has both an instrumental value, and an intrinsic value. Good health is an instrumental prerequisite to do things because it concerns people's normal functioning and capabilities. However, health is also constitutive of people's overall well-being and, in a more direct sense, affects their quality of life. In other words, good health is central to making use of opportunities that are available in societies, and policies that do not provide people with fair and equal starting positions in the pursuit of such opportunities must be judged unjust. Formulated positively, "the moral function of [public health programmes] must be to help guarantee fair equality of opportunity".[25] Since fair equality of opportunity approaches[26] are central to the kind of democratic states we considered above (paragraph 2.9), it is clear that 'eliminating or reducing unfair health inequalities' is a feature that needs to be added explicitly to our initial list of positive goals of public health programmes.

[23] See Daniels (1985) *Just Health Care* (Cambridge: Cambridge University Press); Anand S (2004) The concern for equity in health, in *Public Health, Ethics, and Equity*, Anand S, Peter F and Sen A (Editors) (Oxford: Oxford University Press), pp.15–20; Sen A (2004) Why health equity?, in *Public Health, Ethics, and Equity*, Anand S, Peter F and Sen A (Editors) (Oxford: Oxford University Press), pp.21–34.

[24] See Rawls J (1971) *A Theory of Justice* (Cambridge, Massachusetts: Harvard University Press).

[25] Daniels N (1985) *Just Health Care* (Cambridge: Cambridge University Press). Note that, by extending Rawls' 'justice as fairness', Daniels initially presented such a framework in relation to the more narrowly defined context of healthcare only. However, more recently he revised the approach and used Rawls' principle of fair equality of opportunity to address the wider range of determinants of health: see Daniels N, Kennedy B and Kawachi I (2004) Health and inequality, or, why justice is good for our health, in *Public Health, Ethics, and Equity*, Anand S, Peter F and Sen A (Editors) (Oxford: Oxford University Press), pp.63–92; see also Anand S (2004) The concern for equity in health, in *Public Health, Ethics, and Equity*, Anand S, Peter F and Sen A (Editors) (Oxford: Oxford University Press), pp.15–20; Sen A (2004) Why health equity?, in *Public Health, Ethics, and Equity*, Anand S, Peter F and Sen A (Editors) (Oxford: Oxford University Press), pp. 21–34.

[26] Note that Daniels emphasises the distinction between two different types of equality of opportunity: in a *negative* version it "requires only that society refrains from imposing certain barriers to equal opportunity, such as ... racial or sexual quotas on hiring". In the positive version, it consists of correcting "all the influences which interfere with equality of opportunity ... [through measures such as] compensatory education programs, ... or 'affirmative action' hiring procedures. This positive

Equality of what?

2.29 However, important questions remain about what exactly is required to 'reduce unfair health inequalities' and 'promote health of people equally'. Two principal strategies, which are not mutually exclusive, are:

■ *Equality of health outcomes*. It could be argued that equality is achieved only where objectively measurable data such as life expectancy, body mass index (BMI) or blood pressure are the same among the groups or individuals under comparison.[27] One of the practical advantages of outcome-focused approaches is that, in principle, it is possible to measure degrees of equality in a relatively straightforward manner.[28]

■ *Equality of opportunity and access (to health services and health-conducive environments)*. An alternative approach is to focus on equality of access. By this, one might include access both to health services and to health-conducive environments, such as cycle paths, parks, sports facilities, or safe working and living environments. In practice, many equality-of-outcome approaches are likely to give some weight to access issues.[29] One problem of access-based approaches is that people may have different capacities to make use of the provisions of access. Consequently, although access may be equal, outcomes may not.[30]

Equality among whom? Inequalities of status

2.30 As well as the 'equality of what?' dimension, two further questions need to be asked. The first is 'equality among whom?'. Health outcomes often differ across sub-groups of a given population. In seeking to create equality among these groups, one may focus on a range of different criteria that include age, gender, socio-economic status, racial or ethnic background, disability and geographical location. Analysing inequalities of status between such groups allows us, first, to identify those groups that suffer, or are at particular risk of suffering, poor health. Secondly, it allows us to focus on those inequalities that are

---

conception is called *fair* equality of opportunity." Instead of an exhaustive discussion of the justification of *fair* equality of opportunity, Daniels notes that for his purposes it is sufficient to settle for a weaker, conditional, claim, and that healthcare institutions and, by our extension, public health programmes (see previous footnote) "should be governed by a principle of fair equal opportunity provided two conditions obtain: (1) an acceptable general theory of justice includes a principle which requires basic institutions of society to guarantee fair equality of opportunity, and (2) the fair equality of opportunity principle acts as a constraint on permissible economic inequalities" (Daniels (1985) *Just Health Care* (Cambridge: Cambridge University Press)). Because these conditions are met by the kinds of state we considered here, Daniels' qualification applies equally in our case, and we do not use the term 'equality of opportunity' (or fair opportunity) to mean an uncompensated form of meritocracy, where equality is exhausted in simply ensuring equal access to key positions in society (without regard to the different chances people have in making use of these opportunities).

[27] Note that such an approach might commit one to hold that, for example, differences in life expectancy between men and women should be compensated for. However, the primary point of outcome-focused approaches in public health is to identify those outcomes that are modified by factors that are regarded as unfair and that can be changed through appropriate policy.

[28] The collection of data on life expectancy, BMI or blood pressure is straightforward in the sense that the measures make no controversial methodological assumptions. However, measures such as disability-adjusted life years (DALYs), proposed to capture, among other things, the quantity of ill health among particular groups, are more problematic, see Brock DW (2004) Ethical issues in the use of cost effectiveness analysis for the prioritisation of health care resources, pp.201–24; Kamm FM (2004) Deciding whom to help, health-adjusted life years, pp.225–42; Broome J (2004) The value of living longer, pp.243–60; Anand S and Hanson K (2004) Disability-adjusted life years: a critical review, pp.183–200, all in *Public Health, Ethics, and Equity*, Anand S, Peter F and Sen A (Editors) (Oxford: Oxford University Press).

[29] Although the argument from equality of access can also be made independently.

[30] Within both options, a sub-set of equality issues arises. Firstly, the infrastructure put in place to ensure access can differ in quality in different regions, for example, because of political priorities. Secondly, the services and environments used to realise equality of outcome or access can be divided into those that could directly extend or save lives, and others that merely improve quality of life (Daniels N (1985) *Just Health Care* (Cambridge: Cambridge University Press)). Hence, an argument could be made that some services or outcomes are more important, and more central to equality, than others. Consequently health equality might be said to exist as long as there is access to a 'decent minimum', such as, for example, a health service that is free at the point of need. Equality might, on the other hand, require a far more extensive scenario, where all citizens (or those residing in a state) have equal access to equally health-conducive work or living environments. We therefore need to ask: "equality of access to what degree of which health-conducive services or environments?".

particularly unjust and thus inequitable.[31] For example, certain poorer health outcomes associated with living in big cities may be considered less unjust than say, differences in health outcomes between different ethnic groups.

Ways of reducing inequalities

2.31 Lastly, the question arises of 'how should inequalities be reduced?'. There are several different strategies that might be pursued. In principle, it would be possible to achieve equality either by lifting the level of welfare or opportunities of those who are worst off to the level of those who enjoy the highest standards, or by lowering the welfare of those at the top. Regarding the latter option, in order to avoid the problem of the 'levelling down objection' to egalitarian approaches that seek to even out inequalities,[32] some commentators have set out a prioritarian strategy: instead of relative health status one should focus on the absolute position of the worst off and raise it.[33] Such an approach may have different consequences in practice, and the implications need to monitored closely.[34]

2.32 Clearly, "health equality has many aspects, and is best seen as a multidimensional concept".[35] We do not seek here to prioritise particular health outcomes. Nor do we attempt to specify inequalities that are more unacceptable in some groups rather than others. However, the framework should provide a useful reference tool for establishing whether or not inequalities exist, and if so, in what sense health outcomes or opportunities are distributed unevenly, whether this distribution is unfair,[36] and if so, how it should be corrected.

Changing habits and the limits of information-only approaches

2.33 As noted earlier (paragraphs 2.10, 2.18), public education and information have a key role in the liberal framework, since they are non-coercive ways of bringing about improvements in health. Their success is dependent upon the ability to motivate people to change their attitude, and ultimately their behaviour, by information that they find persuasive. However, sustainable behaviour change is a major challenge even for those who have changed their attitude, and would like to act differently. It is even more difficult for those who are only partly persuaded. The latter group may additionally find requests for behaviour change, even if provided only in the form of information, a nuisance. The limited success of information strategies is illustrated by the example of seatbelts (see also Box 8.1). Although people were exhorted to wear seatbelts through information campaigns, the outcome was

---

[31] Equality considerations come into play where inequalities of a certain kind raise issues of justice and fairness. Inequality is therefore generally not particularly relevant in cases such as differences in life expectancy between men and women.

[32] Parfit D (2000) Equality or priority? in *The ideal of equality*, Clayton M and Williams A (Editors) (Basingstoke: Macmillan), pp.81–125; Dahlgren G and Whitehead M (2006) *Levelling up (part 1): A discussion paper on European strategies for tackling social inequities in health* (Copenhagen: WHO, Regional Office for Europe).

[33] Arneson R (2002) Egalitarianism, in *Stanford Encyclopedia of Philosophy*, available at: http://plato.stanford.edu/entries/egalitarianism/.

[34] There are three principal conceptual ways in which such a strategy might work in practice. In the best case, it will bring the lowest level at par with the highest (whether this is the highest attainable in principle, or the highest level feasible in certain given circumstances occurring in a state). However, sometimes, those who are better off may also benefit from the intervention that was initiated with the aim of benefiting the least well off. Therefore, in the second case, although the lowest group benefits and improves, groups enjoying higher levels may move up as well, to what may be a lesser, an equal, or even a greater degree, thereby reducing inequalities only moderately, or perhaps maintaining or even increasing them. In the third case, although the aim may be to lift the lowest levels, they may actually remain the same or decrease in relation to all other levels, perhaps because certain interventions or initiatives have not been taken up at all by the intended groups.

[35] Sen A (2004) Why health equity?, in *Public Health, Ethics, and Equity*, Anand S, Peter F and Sen A (Editors) (Oxford: Oxford University Press), pp.21–34.

[36] See footnote 34. Note also that an assessment of the fairness of the distribution of outcomes or opportunities must not be limited to comparing simply the levels of the best and worst off. Such an approach may ignore the possibility that often a gradient approach may be required which also considers the various levels between the best and worst position, since here, too, inequalities may be unfair and require responses in policy. From a policy perspective another issue to be considered is whether the overall curve of health distribution can be shifted most effectively by focusing on improving the situation of those at the lowest levels, or by focusing on particular groups who are slightly better off but still considerably worse than those enjoying the highest levels.

only achieved, with use becoming nearly universal, when it was made a legal requirement. As this illustrates, strategies that focus overly on the 'negative constraints' of the liberal framework may prove less effective than the liberal might hope. This is not to say that it should not be pursued in the first instance, but rather that when such an approach fails, a more invasive public policy may be needed, especially if it is to significantly reduce health inequalities (see paragraphs 3.18, 3.37–3.38).[37]

Adding a social dimension

The value of community

2.34 The discussions about consent, health inequalities and changing habits indicate that the initial liberal framework proposed above (paragraph 2.20) is too individualistic. An ethical framework for public health needs to include values that bring the framework closer to social contract theory (paragraph 2.7). What is required is a value that expresses the way that we each benefit simply from being members of a society in which the health needs of others are addressed. There is no settled term for this value: some speak of 'fraternity', others of 'solidarity'. We prefer the term 'community', which is the value of belonging to a society in which each person's welfare, and that of the whole community, matters to everyone. This value is central in the justification of both the goal of reducing health inequalities (paragraphs 2.27–2.28) and the limitation on individual consent when it obstructs important general benefits. Public health often depends on universal programmes which need to be endorsed collectively if they are to be successfully implemented. Although the initial liberal framework supports the promotion of public goods and services, it presents these primarily as ways of promoting individual welfare. Hence, it does not adequately express the shared commitment to collective ends, which is a key ingredient in public support for programmes aimed at securing goods that are essentially collective.

Paternalism

2.35 The initial liberal framework therefore needs to be revised, to make it less individualistic, and accommodate better the value of the community. Does this mean that we need to advocate paternalism, usually understood as the "interference of a state or an individual with another person, against their will, and justified by a claim that the person interfered with will be better off or protected from harm"?[38] We suggest that it does not.

2.36 Ideally, coercive policies should not be implemented without political *mandate* or *authorisation*. Lack of such legitimisation would render the interventions incompatible with the democratic nature of modern liberal states. They would also be undesirable from a more technical public health perspective, as opposition to the measures is likely to be strong, especially in personal areas such as food or sexual behaviour. The justification and feasibility of public health policies therefore depends heavily on their having a mandate. At the same time, there may be questions about which policies adequately address people's will, desire, individuality or autonomy, and how conflicts should be resolved where there is a mismatch. Are only those policies acceptable that people agree with entirely? For example, many individuals have a strong desire to eat, drink and smoke. However, the structure of desires is

---

[37] Public acceptance of the health-outcome-focused approach that made the wearing of seat belts mandatory can be explained by the fact that this is a relatively minor restriction of people's liberty, and there is an obvious benefit in terms of diminished risk of personal injury. The situation is different, for example, in the case of the wearing of cycle helmets by cyclists: despite the diminished risk of personal injury after an accident, a requirement to wear a helmet would be a nuisance and not cost-free, see also Box 8.1.

[38] Dworkin R (2002) Paternalism, in *Stanford Encyclopedia of Philosophy*, available at: http://plato.stanford.edu/entries/paternalism/.

complex, and individuals may have desires at a higher level,[39] to the effect that, actually, they would overall prefer to lose weight, stop smoking or drink less alcohol. In the case of smoking, raising taxes is an effective way of reducing consumption (see Chapter 6). Although such a policy may be against the 'will' or first-order desires, of many smokers, it is not clear that imposing taxes is necessarily an unacceptable form of paternalism. Indeed, in seeking to establish an environment where it is easy for people to be healthy, it may be an acceptable response to higher-order desires.[40]

2.37 Some suggest that, to reconcile the importance of individuality with the obligations of the state to guide us towards prudent behaviour, we should consider modified versions of paternalism.[41] For example, with regard to pension arrangements, a libertarian might argue that whether or not people wish to make contributions should be up to them, and that no-one should be forced to accept regular deductions from their income. A paternalist, on the other hand, might argue the opposite and view compulsory deductions as justified, because they concern important future needs. 'Libertarian paternalism' would suggest that the baseline option of policies should express value judgements about what is good for one's life, although individuals should be able to opt out at relative ease and low cost.[42] So, in the case of pensions, deductions should be made, but where people decide that they would prefer to make alternative arrangements, they should be free to do so. Another example closer to the sphere of public health that is considered by the proponents of this approach is to reorganise food at a buffet in such a way that the most healthy option is most likely to be chosen.[43]

2.38 Among the ideas underlying this approach is the recognition that environments in which people make choices are not value free. Whatever form an environment takes, it is likely to make certain behaviours easier than others. Additionally, different people may have different capacities in benefiting from specific environments. Strictly speaking, the libertarian's emphasis on individual choice can only be fair if all people have the same abilities and capacities to make decisions – where they do not, those who are less capable, or have less opportunity to compare and assess different options, are at a disadvantage. Often, people with less time or capacity will therefore just accept the default policy – the 'normal practice'. We acknowledge the difficulties associated with behaviour change (see paragraphs 2.33, 3.20, 5.11, 5.35, 6.9), and the framework set out in this Report emphasises that, in principle, it is acceptable for the state to bring about policies that have a clear aim of

[39] Frankfurt H (1971) Freedom of will and the concept of person *J Philos* **68**: 5–20.

[40] The principal problem with paternalism is thus that it may impose a value, without mandate against people's will. However, as the example shows, the will-test is often complicated by the complex structure of human desire, and it is questionable therefore whether such policies should be seen as paternalistic.

[41] Broadly, an advocate of *soft* paternalism would see state interference as justified if it helped determine whether the person interfered with is acting truly voluntarily and knowledgeably (a *hard* paternalist might argue that there can be occasions where interference is acceptable, even if the conditions of voluntariness and knowledge are satisfied). A distinction between *weak* and *strong* paternalism concerns peoples' assessments of achieving certain ends. Weak paternalism states that interference may be acceptable if people are mistaken about the fact that certain means will achieve desired ends. Strong paternalism argues that some ends people chose may be wrong in themselves, and that state intervention is acceptable to prevent people from achieving those ends. See: Dworkin R (2002) Paternalism, in *Stanford Encyclopedia of Philosophy*, available at: http://plato.stanford.edu/entries/paternalism/.

[42] Sunstein C R and Thaler R H (2003) Libertarian paternalism is not an oxymoron *University of Chicago Law Review* **70**: 1159–1202.

[43] Sunstein C R and Thaler R H (2003) Libertarian paternalism *American Economic Review* **93**: 175–9. Note that Sunstein and Thaler do not apply their approach directly to the context of public health. Transposing the principle to a somewhat fictitious example, a possible extension might be to permit free and ubiquitous sale only of cigarettes that are non-addictive and do not cause harm to health (such as certain herbal cigarettes), but permit, for example, sale of the currently marketed cigarettes only through channels such as mail ordering or similar, where more effort needs to be put into pursuing the less healthy option. The point is that, in principle, an approach such as libertarian paternalism might be developed to address a range of public health problems; however, as we discuss below, we do not think such an attempt would be useful for our purpose here, mainly because in some occasions the possibility of opting out is too risky and not helpful in reducing health inequalities (paragraph 2.40).

furthering some social good, such as reducing health inequalities. So, should we subscribe to a version of 'libertarian paternalism' as a basis of our revised liberal framework?

2.39 Although full-blown paternalism would be an inappropriate basis because it is insufficiently sensitive to the need for a mandate, libertarian paternalism is not suitable as it may allow too much choice, and it might also absolve the state from some important responsibilities. For example, in the UK, the state collects mandatory contributions to the NHS from all taxpayers as part of the taxes levied. In this way, the state establishes an important default option of having access to healthcare, ideally free at the point of need. This arrangement forms an important part of public health efforts more generally. While some perceive this as an unjustified act of paternalism, we are not persuaded that the language of paternalism is useful here, as it would be wrong to view a system such as the NHS as a policy that constitutes "interference of a state or an individual with another person, against their will"[44] (see paragraph 2.35). Some people might prefer to opt out of the NHS, but it is far from clear that many, the majority, or everybody would prefer to do so. So, the question is whether respect for the wishes of a particular group (or possibly even one single person) should be sufficient to counter arrangements that benefit a larger group of people, and, importantly, where these benefits can only be sustainably achieved through collective efforts.

2.40 Therefore, although paternalism goes too far, libertarian paternalism does not go far enough. Below, in what we call the stewardship model, we set out a proposal that we consider appropriate to capture the best of both approaches, and suitable to underpin a revised version of our initial liberal framework (paragraph 2.20).

A revised liberal framework: the stewardship model

2.41 The concept of stewardship means that liberal states have responsibilities to look after important needs of people both individually and collectively. Therefore, they are stewards both to individual people, taking account of different needs arising from factors such as age, gender, ethnic background or socio-economic status, and to the population as whole, including both citizens of the state, and those that do not have citizen status, but fall under its jurisdiction.[45] In our view, the notion of stewardship gives expression to the obligation on states to seek to provide conditions that allow people to be healthy, especially in relation to reducing health inequalities.[46]

2.42 The state needs to take a more active role in promoting the health of the public than was envisaged in our initial liberal framework (see paragraph 2.20). In addition to the goals specified therein, public policies should actively promote health, for example, by providing appropriate access to medical services, establishing programmes to help people combat addictions, and supporting the conditions under which people enjoy good health, such as through the provision of opportunities for exercise. Equally, concern for the needs of the population as a whole means that very demanding interpretations of individual consent as an expression of individuality and autonomy should be viewed with caution. Instead,

---

[44] Dworkin R (2002) Paternalism, in *Stanford Encyclopedia of Philosophy*, available at: http://plato.stanford.edu/entries/paternalism/.

[45] See World Health Organization (2000) *World Health Report 2000* (Geneva, Switzerland: WHO): "Stewardship is the overarching function that determines the success or failure of all other functions of the health system. It places the responsibility back on government and calls for the strengthening of ministries of health. However, it does not call for necessarily a hierarchical and controlling role of government but more of that of overseeing and steering of the health system. It calls for vision, setting of regulations and implementing them, and the capacity to assess and monitor performance over time. A strong stewardship should in fact permit a more efficient use of the private sector to meet the needs of the health system." See also Jochelson K (2005) *Nanny or Steward? The role of government in public health* (London: King's Fund).

[46] The maintenance of a service such as the NHS is one way of exercising this responsibility.

democratic, transparent decision-making procedures can often ensure an appropriate balancing of the interest of individuals and those of society (see paragraph 2.25).

2.43 The difference between paternalism and our stewardship model is that the latter is less likely to support highly coercive universal measures. Instead, the stewardship model is more sensitive to the need to respect individuality, by seeking the least intrusive way of achieving policy goals, taking into account also the criteria of effectiveness and proportionality (see paragraphs 3.18, 3.37–3.38). The stewardship approach is also more sensitive than paternalism to the concept of mandate, and the need for policies to be adequately justified. It recognises the importance of open and transparent participatory processes as a necessary condition for public health policy making, but it is also clear that these are not sufficient by themselves. Stewardship is not exercised simply by following the public vote, especially where issues involve complex scientific evidence. Under the stewardship model, public health policy should be compatible with the views of the public, and the government should create conditions that allow the public to scrutinise and judge the appropriateness of proposed polices.

2.44 The result of this discussion is a revised framework for public health, which we call the *stewardship model*. The model still incorporates the classical harm principle (paragraphs 2.13–2.14), which is a central part of the approach and which usually provides the strongest justification for public health interventions. Several important issues in public health can be addressed by reference to the classical harm principle alone. However, there is also a range of cases where the classical harm principle is of limited use, and this is where the stewardship model as a whole provides a particularly suitable reference framework. Revising the initial liberal framework, then, we summarise below the core characteristics that public health programmes carried out by a stewardship-guided state should have.

Concerning goals, public health programmes should:

- aim to reduce the risks of ill health that people might impose on each other;
- aim to reduce causes of ill health by regulations that ensure environmental conditions that sustain good health, such as the provision of clean air and water, safe food and decent housing;
- pay special attention to the health of children and other vulnerable people;
- promote health not only by providing information and advice, but also with programmes to help people to overcome addictions and other unhealthy behaviours;
- aim to ensure that it is easy for people to lead a healthy life, for example by providing convenient and safe opportunities for exercise;
- ensure that people have appropriate access to medical services; and
- aim to reduce unfair health inequalities.

In terms of constraints, such programmes should:

- not attempt to coerce adults to lead healthy lives;
- minimise interventions that are introduced without the individual consent of those affected, or without procedural justice arrangements (such as democratic decision-making procedures) which provide adequate mandate; and
- seek to minimise interventions that are perceived as unduly intrusive and in conflict with important personal values.

These positive goals and negative constraints are not listed in any hierarchical order. The implementation of these principles may, of course, lead to conflicting policies. However, in each particular case, it should be possible to resolve these conflicts by applying those policies or strategies that achieve the desired social goals while minimising significant limitations on individual freedom (see paragraphs 3.37–3.38).

Discouragement and assistance

2.45 The revised position above remains opposed to coercive interventions whose aim is simply to force people to be healthy. In this way, it respects Mill's anti-paternalist injunction that, "his own good, either physical or moral, is not a sufficient warrant" for the state to impose an intervention to make a person healthier.[47] However, whereas our initial liberal framework (paragraph 2.20) merely encouraged programmes to 'advise, instruct and persuade' people with addictions and other potentially unhealthy habits, the revised stewardship framework (paragraphs 2.41–2.44) encourages the provision of services through which risks are minimised and people are helped to change their behaviour.

Third parties

2.46 So far, the discussion has been directed at the way in which the state can legitimately introduce effective public health programmes in the light of the ethical relationship between the state and those under its jurisdiction. However, various third parties also have a role in the delivery of public health. These may be medical institutions, charities, businesses, local authorities, schools and so on. Where publicly funded, these institutions can be thought of as agents of the state and thus share the obligation to implement public health policies. On the other hand, many are not publicly funded, and may have agendas and particular goals of their own – such as charities that work with those whose health is damaged by addictions, and whose motivation may include particular cultural, religious or other values. This does not necessarily mean that their role is inconsistent with the ethical framework for public policy. Nor does it mean that they have no obligation to reflect on their role in public health.

Business

2.47 Corporate agents that are independent of government but whose activities affect public health include businesses such as food, drink, tobacco, water and pharmaceutical companies, owners of pubs and restaurants, and others whose products and services can either contribute to public health problems or help to alleviate them. There are two principal ways in which one might approach the responsibilities of corporate agents.

2.48 First, the view could be taken that, as long as companies adhere to the law, and fulfil their primary function, which usually is to satisfy their customers or shareholders, they have discharged their duties. Certainly, many companies operate in this way.[48]

2.49 An alternative view would be to argue that as actors within the public sphere, corporate agents have more extensive responsibilities, both towards their employees and the society within which they operate. Recent years have seen a significant rise in corporate social responsibility initiatives, and many large companies publish annually the results of their corporate social responsibility activities alongside their financial reports. The extent to which such initiatives are driven by marketing strategies rather than genuine social concern is difficult to assess. The emergence of corporate social responsibility is noteworthy nonetheless: if it is not driven by companies actively reflecting on their social responsibilities it seems more than likely that consumer expectations have played an active role and created a new kind of 'ethical' demand.[49]

---

[47] Mill JS (1859) On liberty, in *On Liberty and Other Essays* (1989) Collini S (Editor), (Cambridge: Cambridge University Press), p.13.

[48] Friedman M (1970) The social responsibility of business is to increase its profits *New York Times Magazine* 13 September.

[49] A recent Report by the Department for Constitutional Affairs views growing demand for corporate social responsibility as one of the principal drivers of the future of citizenship, suggesting that businesses will increasingly be expected to fulfil civic duties and contribute to the public good; Department for Constitutional Affairs (2007) *The Future of Citizenship*, available at: http://www.dca.gov.uk/elections/pdfs/future-of-citizenship.pdf.

2.50 For our discussion, two points follow. First, in the same way that we would not judge the ethical acceptability of actions of individuals by merely assessing whether or not they have broken the law, it is reasonable to argue that commercial companies have responsibilities beyond merely complying with legal and regulatory requirements. Secondly, although most liberal states strive to ensure a free market, there are numerous cases where the state intervenes to protect important goods, such as the health of workers, the environment, or the health of consumers, for example by banning certain types of ingredient. We commented earlier that such measures are part of the stewardship function of the state. However, if corporate social responsibility were taken seriously, some of these interventions might not be necessary. Furthermore, regulation need not always be to the detriment of industry, but can be a driver of innovation. Recent trends have shown that the potential of health-orientated products is far from exhausted.[50] This potential can be explored proactively through initiatives by the industry, or reactively, where the industry responds to regulation. We emphasised in Chapter 1 that there is a complex web of responsibility for public health, by highlighting the importance of 'organised efforts of society' in preventing disease, prolonging life and promoting health (paragraph 1.6). Genuine corporate social responsibility clearly has a role to play in this respect. Likewise, if there is lack of corporate responsibility, or a 'market failure', it is acceptable for the state to intervene, where the health of the population is significantly at risk.

Summary

2.51 We set out in this chapter an initial liberal framework and explained its relationship to libertarian and collectivist conceptions of the state. Starting with a discussion of the 'classical harm principle', we identified several further principles that are important in considering public health issues. We recognised the importance of reducing health inequalities and noted that in seeking to reduce inequalities a range of different dimensions need to be considered, as there may be different types of inequality (outcome versus opportunity), different ways of reducing them (egalitarian and prioritarian strategies) and different groups between which inequalities may exist. In the discussion about consent we clarified the notions of individual consent and procedural justice arrangements, emphasising that it would be wrong to seek to address public health issues by reference to individual consent only.

2.52 With reflections about other principles, the considerations of health inequalities and consent illustrated that our initial liberal framework needed to be revised. We therefore presented a framework for public health policy with further goals and constraints, which we called the stewardship model. The revised framework was nevertheless incomplete, and we made some further observations, in particular on the role of corporate agents in the complex web of stakeholders whose actions determine public health. We also recognise that there are other values that might be brought into the discussion. We need, therefore, to keep our discussion open-ended at this stage, and we will return to it in Chapter 8, after the discussion of policy process and practice in Chapter 3, and the four case studies of Chapters 4–7. Next, we consider how some of the themes emerging from this chapter feature in policy and practice.

---

[50] Unwin J (2006) A responsibility for health – the role of business in determining what we eat, in *Whose Responsibility? The role of business in delivering social and environmental change* (London: Smith Institute), pp.16–23.

Chapter 3

Policy process and practice

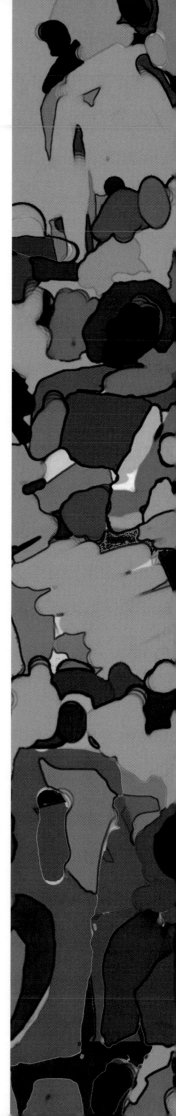

Policy process and practice

Introduction

3.1 At first sight, achieving an ethical public health policy seems straightforward: data on a particular public health problem need to be assessed, and an evidence-based strategy that can be justified in ethical terms needs to be adopted. However, while an evidence-based approach should be central to public health strategies, it is only part of what is required. Several other factors are important for successfully identifying, planning and implementing public health policies.

3.2 In the first part of this chapter we outline the main elements that need to be considered in any public health policy. We will comment on: the nature of evidence; the perception of risk; and the notion of a precautionary approach. All of these are often, if not invariably, invoked in discussions of state intervention in relation to public health. We then explore the objectives of public health policy and set out the processes of policy development. The objectives of policy have several dimensions, in theory and in practice. We highlight issues of individual choice, preservation of autonomy, reduction of inequalities, protection of vulnerable groups and targeting of at-risk groups. The challenge for public health measures at the population level is to achieve the right balance when several of these goals have simultaneously to be met. We also comment on factors that influence the acceptability of different types of policy and offer a model for comparison of different types of intervention, which we call the 'intervention ladder' (see paragraphs 3.37–3.38).

Evidence

3.3 According to one definition, evidence-based healthcare is:

"the conscientious use of current best evidence in making decisions about the care of individual patients or the delivery of health services. Current best evidence is up-to-date information from relevant, valid research about the effects of different forms of health care, the potential for harm from exposure to particular agents, the accuracy of diagnostic tests, and the predictive power of prognostic factors."[1]

3.4 In the context of public health, there are two areas where consideration of relevant research findings is especially important: first, evidence about causes of ill health; and secondly, evidence about the efficacy and effectiveness of interventions.

■ Evidence about causes: Sufficiently robust evidence is required to establish a causal link between a suggested risk factor and an illness or otherwise undesirable health outcome, for example between smoking and lung cancer. For some diseases, many factors may contribute and, for various reasons, the strength of the causal link between a risk factor and the harm is impossible to estimate accurately. For example, how much domestic violence is directly 'caused by' alcohol, and how much obesity is 'caused by' advertising of processed foods? It is often a question of using the most robust data available to aim for the best possible decision in the face of residual uncertainty.

■ Evidence about effective interventions: In seeking to bring about a change in health policy, evidence is required about the potential of different paths of action to promote health or reduce harm, for example to determine the effect of pricing on tobacco consumption. This has also been called the 'Can it work?' question.[2] Because many interventions bring

---

[1] First Annual Nordic Workshop on how to critically appraise and use evidence in decisions about healthcare, National Institute of Public Health, Oslo, Norway, 1996, see: http://www.shef.ac.uk/scharr/ir/def.html.
[2] Haynes B (1999) Can it work? Does it work? Is it worth it? *Br Med J* **319**: 652–3.

potential harms as well as benefits, and the potential for both benefits and harms may be unevenly distributed in the population, this question must be answered by assessing the overall balance between risks and benefits, and how these are distributed among different members of the population. A further question is whether an intervention that is efficacious in a research setting will have a similar degree of effectiveness in a particular real-world context. This has been called the *'Does it work?'* question.[3]

3.5 Public health interventions such as education and behaviour change programmes are not invasive and might be viewed as unlikely to cause any harm. However, there is evidence that some may do so. For example, training children in bicycle safety has been shown in some instances to have increased accident rates among children who cycle (probably because they or their parents became more confident after the training and they were then exposed to more risks). The 'Bike ed'[4] programme in Australia, designed to reduce cycle injuries, actually increased the risk of injury overall, doubling it in boys. Furthermore, the most adverse effects were observed among younger children, children from families with lower parental education, and children who lacked other family members who cycled, hence increasing socio-economic and gender inequalities which are particularly marked in any case for childhood injuries.[5] The implications of this observation are that well-intentioned and plausible interventions, even of a non-invasive kind involving only education, can do unanticipated harm.[6] This suggests that there is a duty on those introducing such measures to monitor their actual impact over appropriate timeframes, rather than simply assuming they are beneficial.

3.6 Moreover, the design of such interventions, where the exact weight and role of different factors may not be clear-cut from the outset, often requires a different kind of approach to evidence gathering. The assessment of both evidence about causes and evidence of effective interventions needs to be sensitive to the specific issues raised in that particular area of public health.

3.7 The adoption of an evidence-based approach brings with it certain assumptions as to what constitutes good evidence, and it is important to scrutinise carefully any source of evidence. For example, media stories often turn out to be based on anecdotes, unpublished reports or preliminary results, or they overstate, misrepresent or misunderstand the claims of the researcher.[7] The minimum hurdle for evidence to be reported (or to be considered in public health policy more generally) is that it should be published in the peer-reviewed literature, or have been subject to an equivalent scrutiny by expert peers. This hurdle by no means guarantees that the evidence is irrefutable as, for example, the quality of papers accepted varies greatly between scientific journals. However, peer review suggests a certain robustness as findings are scrutinised by experts in the field and research is open to repeat investigation.[8]

3.8 One further important aspect of evidence gathering is the selective use of evidence. Perhaps only some of the literature will be cited, or explanations rely on a particular strand of scientific evidence, ignoring or excluding other evidence. All groups, politicians, the media, single

[3] *Ibid.*

[4] A school-based education programme for developing cycle safety skills and knowledge; see: www.bikeed.com.au.

[5] Carlin J, Taylor P and Nolan P (1998) School based bicycle safety education and bicycle injuries in children: a case control study *Injury Prevention* **4**: 22–7.

[6] Macintyre S and Petticrew M (2000) Good intentions and received wisdom are not enough *J Epidemiol Community Health* **54**: 802–3.

[7] The Bad Science column of the *Guardian* newspaper provides many telling examples, see http://www.badscience.net; as does the National Library for Health's 'Hitting the Headlines' resource, see http://www.library.nhs.uk/rss/newsAndRssArchive.aspx?storyCategory=0.

[8] Science Media Centre (2003) *Peer Review in a Nutshell*, available at: http://www.sciencemediacentre.org/downloads/peer_review_in_a_nutshell.pdf; Sense About Science (2005) *"I Don't Know What to Believe ..." Making Sense of Science Stories*, available at: http://www.senseaboutscience.org.uk/index.php/site/project/30.

interest groups and scientists are capable of this. An example that we cover in a later chapter concerns inadequate presentations of the evidence on fluoridation (see paragraphs 7.42–7.47). We also note that the UK House of Commons Science and Technology Committee's Report *Scientific Advice, Risk and Evidence Based Policy Making* describes cases where research has been commissioned or interpreted to support existing or planned policies. The authors coin the term 'policy-based evidence' for using evidence in this way.[9]

3.9 A related issue is the status of views that are not considered to be 'mainstream' or typical of the scientific community. Such heterodox views sometimes turn out to be correct, so it is important that they are not ignored. At the same time, they need to be seen in context. Science progresses by challenging and testing current ideas and explanations of whatever phenomenon is under scrutiny. Therefore when scientists 'disagree with one another', this merely reflects the normal process of scientific enquiry. Often, there is a 'centre of gravity' of scientific opinion, with a distribution of views around it. Sometimes this polarises into competing hypotheses or interpretations of data. These kinds of disagreement, however, are rather different from the case where only one or a few individuals hold an unrepresentative view against the overwhelming body of current scientific evidence. The best approach to the issue of scientific disagreement, as recommended in the Chief Scientific Advisor's Guidelines in 2000,[10] is to acknowledge openly where there is disagreement and take into account a wide range of views.

3.10 A further challenge for an evidence-based approach is dealing with the question of proving a negative finding. The statement 'there is no evidence that *x* is harmful to human health' prompts the question 'is absence of evidence of harm the same as evidence of absence?' It is generally accepted that it is difficult or impossible to prove a negative, because further investigation may eventually reveal a positive instance. Therefore, the 'no evidence' proposition should always be accompanied by both a summary of what has been done to look for a risk and the qualification that there can be no absolute certainty.

3.11 As we will see below (paragraphs 3.14, 3.39–3.44) and in the case studies in the following chapters, even where every reasonable step has been taken to ensure that evidence is robust, in practice it is often incomplete or ambiguous, and usually will be contested. Thus scientific evidence does not necessarily lead to a clear policy that is likely to be the most effective. Choices between competing policy options often need to be made under extreme time pressure, allowing little time for reassessment of evidence or more information gathering. Although scientific experts may sometimes be tempted, or pressured, in these circumstances into offering precise answers to policy makers, the honest answer will often be "we don't know" or "we can only estimate the risk to within certain, sometimes wide, limits". It follows that claims of absolute safety or certainty should be treated with great caution.

3.12 While an evidence-based approach to public health policy can be fraught with difficulty, it is worth emphasising that in the UK and in many other countries (as well as at European Union (EU) level) there are established structures of independent scientific advisory committees. These committees seek to thoroughly and impartially assess the available evidence underpinning public health and other policies.[11] Increasingly these committees meet in public, so that their work is transparent and open to challenge.

---

[9] House of Commons Science and Technology Committee (2006) *Scientific Advice, Risk and Evidence Based Policy Making*, available at: http://www.publications.parliament.uk/pa/cm200506/cmselect/cmsctech/900/900-i.pdf.

[10] See May R (2000) *Guidelines 2000: Scientific Advice and Policy Making*, available at http://www.berr.gov.uk/science/page15432.html; see also: HM Government (2000) *Guidelines on scientific analysis in policy making*, available at: http://www.berr.gov.uk/files/file9767.pdf.

[11] These include the following: Advisory Committee on Novel Foods and Processes, Committee on the Medical Effects of Air Pollutants, Advisory Committee on Dangerous Pathogens and European Commission Scientific Committee for Food.

Risk

3.13 Part of the answer to the question of whether or not the state should intervene to protect and promote health depends on the nature and extent of the risk involved, including the degree to which it is potentially under the control of the individual. However, there is disagreement on how risk should be defined. For example:[12]

■ According to what might be termed the statistical view, health risk is defined primarily in terms of the probability of an event occurring in relation to the severity of the impact of the event.[13] The focus is therefore mainly on estimating the magnitude of the risk by means of scientific and technical assessment. This is the usual basis of risk assessment for policy formulation. Sometimes health risks, assessed by scientific evidence, are expressed in terms of frequency of deaths. For instance the risk from smoking could be expressed as premature deaths per thousand people. One development of this idea is to present scales of relative risk with which to compare different health factors, for example one disease causing a higher morbidity rate than another.[14]

■ Some commentators reject views such as the statistical one, and in particular those approaches that are presented as 'absolute', 'objective' or 'pure' measures of risk, arguing that perceptions of risk always vary with people's value judgements. In what might be termed the social construct view, risk is framed both by inbuilt personal biases that result in certain kinds of risks being more relevant than others, and by what is accepted in particular social groups, or society as a whole. Some factors that influence the way that people perceive risks are summarised in Box 3.1.

Box 3.1: Factors that may influence people's perception of risk

Familiarity with risk: Some risks (such as lung cancer from smoking) are often viewed as more acceptable than others (such as damage from a vaccine), even when the actual likelihood of harm is in the other direction. Where hazards are familiar; are perceived as being under the individual's control; are natural rather than man-made; or the consequences are only seen much later, they are often considered to be more acceptable.[15] Two particularly important factors are the possible scale of harm, for example where consequences are perceived as 'catastrophic', and 'unknowable risks', where people feel insufficiently qualified to judge the likelihood of the occurrence of a bad event.

The base-rate fallacy: Risks are often misinterpreted when presented as percentages or probabilities. One such error is the so-called base-rate fallacy. For instance: if a cancer-screening programme is reported to reduce the risk of dying from breast cancer by 25%, how many lives are saved? Is it 25 out of every 100 women? It is not; the correct answer depends on the overall frequency of deaths from breast cancer in the female population (the base rate). If, for example, the overall mortality rate is four in 1,000, the 25% reduction in risk from screening is from four to three per 1,000 women, or 0.1%.[16]

Focus on benefits or harms: A glass can be described as either 'half empty' or 'half full': the problem is the same but it is framed differently. This can have a direct and powerful impact on decisions of lay people and professionals alike.[17] A specific instance is 'prospect theory' according to which losses loom larger than gains to most people making risk assessments.[18]

---

[12] See The Royal Society (1992) *Risk: Analysis, Perception and Management, Report of a Royal Society Study Group* (London: The Royal Society); The Royal Society (1997) *Science, Policy and Risk* (London: The Royal Society).

[13] See: Hansson SO (2007) Risk, in *Stanford Encyclopedia of Philosophy*, available at: http://plato.stanford.edu/archives/sum2007/entries/risk/.

[14] Calman K and Royston GHD (1997) Risk language and dialects *Br Med J* **315**: 939–42; Calman K (1996) Cancer: science and society and the communication of risk *Br Med J* **313**: 799–802; House of Commons Science and Technology Committee (2006) *Scientific Advice, Risk and Evidence Based Policy Making*, available at: http://www.publications.parliament.uk/pa/cm200506/cmselect/cmsctech/900/900-i.pdf.

[15] House of Commons Science and Technology Committee (2006) *Scientific Advice, Risk and Evidence Based Policy Making*, available at: http://www.publications.parliament.uk/pa/cm200506/cmselect/cmsctech/900/900-i.pdf, p.95; Hampson SE, Severson HH, Burns WJ, Slovic P and Fisher KJ (2001) Risk perception, personality factors and alcohol use among adolescents *Personality and Individual Differences* **30**: 167–81.

[16] Gigerenzer G (2002) *Reckoning with Risk* (London: Penguin Books), pp.59–60.

[17] Tversky A and Kahneman D (1981) The framing of decisions and the psychology of choice *Science* **211**: 453–8; McNeil BJ, Pauker SG, Sox HC and Tversky A (1982) On the elicitation of preferences for alternative therapies *New Engl J Med* **306**: 1259–62.

[18] Kahneman D and Tversky A (1979) Prospect theory: an analysis of decision under risk *Econometrica* **47**: 263–91.

3.14 We take the view that the assessment of health risks in the development of policy should be based on what we have termed the 'statistical approach'. In other words, policy should be based on the best available scientific evidence, using generally accepted criteria for evaluating the quality and implications of the evidence. We recognise that people's perceptions of risk are shaped by many factors (see Box 3.1), as well as by the way in which the media presents the 'facts', and may not coincide with the scientific evaluation. So in drawing on a statistical or scientific evaluation of risk, it is important to spell out the assumptions and uncertainties so that people are as fully aware as possible of what lies behind the assessment. Policy makers might nevertheless include in their decision making not only the scientific assessment of risk, but also people's perceptions, which influence the acceptability of a particular risk. For instance, rail travel is safer than road travel, but it would be politically difficult to regulate road safety (for instance by lower speed limits and stricter enforcement) to a level equivalent to rail, because most people are willing to accept a higher risk in a car than in a train. Travelling by train may be safer in the statistical sense, but the factors that make risk less acceptable, such as lack of individual control and the potential catastrophic nature of an accident, mean that the acceptable level of risk for rail travel is lower than that for road travel.

Precaution and proportion

3.15 The 'precautionary principle' is often invoked in discussions about public health. It is regarded by many as the key to responsible risk management where there is some evidence of a serious threat to health, safety, or the environment. The principle exists in several different forms, one of which is set out in Principle 15 of the *Rio Declaration on Environment and Development*. This states that:

> "Where there are threats of serious or irreversible damage, lack of full scientific certainty shall not be used as a reason for postponing cost-effective measures to prevent environmental degradation."[19]

The precise meaning of the principle has been the subject of intense debates, and we make no attempt to repeat the discussion here.[20] However, in applying the precautionary principle it is important to recognise that it is not a single inflexible rule, but a way of applying a set of interacting criteria to a given situation. For this reason we prefer the term precautionary *approach*, rather than precautionary *principle*.

3.16 The central feature of the precautionary approach is that it is *dynamic*. Drawing on a Communication by the European Commission,[21] five main elements can be distinguished: (a) scientific assessment of risk, acknowledging uncertainties and updated in light of new evidence; (b) fairness and consistency; (c) consideration of costs and benefits of actions; (d) transparency; and (e) proportionality. Stated this way, the approach seems so sound as to be unexceptionable, but of course the challenge arises in making judgements when applying it. To justify precautionary action, the nature or degree of acceptable uncertainty needs to be

---

[19] Rio Declaration on Environment and Development (1992) *The United Nations Conference on Environment and Development*, Rio de Janeiro, 3–14 June 1992; available at: http://habitat.igc.org/agenda21/rio-dec.htm.

[20] For a summary see House of Commons Science and Technology Committee (2006) *Scientific Advice, Risk and Evidence Based Policy Making*, available at: http://www.publications.parliament.uk/pa/cm200506/cmselect/cmsctech/900/900-i.pdf; and Nuffield Council on Bioethics (2003) *The Use of Genetically Modified Crops in Developing Countries* (London: NCOB), pp.57–9.

[21] European Commission (2000) *Communication from the Commission on the Precautionary Principle*, available at: http://ec.europa.eu/dgs/health_consumer/library/pub/pub07_en.pdf. Note that the Communication uses the term 'precautionary principle' rather than 'precautionary approach', used by us. In one sense it may be unimportant which term is used; however, we think that the term 'approach' conveys more immediately that there is not just one, but several principles or considerations that need to be considered.

assessed on a case-by-case basis, as do the risks of 'doing nothing', and the risks of other alternatives.[22]

3.17 In any policy decision, it is furthermore important to consider the seriousness of the problem and the urgency with which it should be addressed. Policy makers have limited time and resources, and issues that pose severe and urgent threats to the health of many people are rightly prioritised over those that are only 'possible threats', affect health in a relatively minor way or involve fewer people. The need for a public health intervention may be dictated by urgency, most obviously with the emergence of an epidemic of a serious infectious disease (see paragraphs 4.47–4.55, 4.57–4.72). However, a problem may be severe without being 'urgent', as in the case of chronic behaviour-related conditions such as obesity, which affect large numbers of people and put increasing pressure on the healthcare budget (see paragraphs 5.40–5.42).[23] In practice, an estimate of 'severity' and 'level of urgency' may be difficult to make and potentially contestable, for the kinds of reasons discussed above (paragraphs 3.3–3.12).

3.18 As this discussion illustrates, one of the most difficult decisions that policy makers need to take relates to identifying which policy response is appropriate in each particular case. A central criterion for judging appropriateness is highlighted in the European Commission's Communication on the precautionary approach: that of proportionality. There are several different aspects to the concept. First, in the form of a *balancing* test, it enjoins us to assess whether the aims of public health goals are sufficiently important to permit consideration of particular means, such as laws, policies or specific interventions. Secondly, a *suitability* test concerns an assessment of the degree to which a certain means will achieve the desired end. Thirdly, a *necessity* test requires that if a particular objective can be achieved by more than one means, then the means should be chosen that causes the least intrusion in the lives of the individuals or communities concerned while still achieving adequate effectiveness. We illustrate these different dimensions further in paragraphs 3.37–3.38.

3.19 In summary, application of the precautionary approach and of proportionality comes down, not simply to applying a formula, but to a judgement that takes into account the particular circumstances of the problem to be addressed. The different dimensions we have highlighted above help guide our scrutiny of justifications given for particular polices or interventions.

Choice

3.20 We concluded in Chapter 2 that liberal societies respect individuals' autonomy by enabling them to make responsible choices for themselves. Current UK Government policy in relation to public health has a clear focus on this approach, as expressed, for example, in the 2004 White Paper *Choosing Health*.[24] However, choice and autonomy are not straightforward concepts in relation to public health (see also paragraph 1.4). First, many apparent choices are not actually available to certain sectors of society. This may be because of constraints of affordability, accessibility, information, education and social or cultural background, or, as for

---

[22] See also: Better Regulation Task Force (2003) *Five Principles of Good Regulation*, available at: http://www.brc.gov.uk/upload/assets/www.brc.gov.uk/principlesleaflet.pdf. The five principles are proportionality, accountability, transparency, consistency and targeting. A proportionate approach requires that any action to protect public health must be judged not only in relation to the risks to the public, but also in relation to the costs, both economic and social to those who might be affected by a specific action. The Better Regulation Task Force was set up by the UK Government in 1997, and is now the Better Regulation Commission.

[23] Wanless D (2002) *Securing our Future Health: Taking a long-term view*, available at: http://www.hm-treasury.gov.uk/consultations_and_legislation/wanless/consult_wanless_final.cfm.

[24] Department of Health (2004) *Choosing Health: Making Healthy Choices Easier*, available at: http://www.dh.gov.uk/en/Publicationsandstatistics/Publications/PublicationsPolicyAndGuidance/DH_4094550.

children, because choices are made for them by others. Secondly, many activities that appear to be voluntary choices are often an expression of rather unreflective habitual behaviour, such as the types of food we buy, what we eat for breakfast or how we spend our leisure time. These deeply engrained habits are often difficult to change. Thirdly, choices are frequently predetermined to some extent by the industries that manufacture the products people buy, the planners who design their built and work environments, and the advertisers who promote certain options over others. In this context the government has an important facilitatory role, for example through regulations on the types of product that may be marketed, to whom, and in which form (see paragraphs 2.41–2.44, 2.47–2.50). Fourthly, even for those with the means and knowledge to make choices, the abundance of options available means that making an optimal choice is difficult.[25] In many of these situations, people often adopt the 'coping strategy' of making a choice that is satisfactory rather than the best possible.

3.21 From an ethical and practical standpoint, an important dimension of public health policy is therefore to balance the liberal emphasis on choice and autonomy, with the imperative to support those who do not have the opportunities to choose, because of, for instance, poverty or dependency (see paragraphs 2.27–2.32). So strategies could aim either to change external circumstances, so that healthy choices are easier to make, or, to leave those circumstances unchanged, but improve people's capacities, so that they are better able to make healthy choices.

Vulnerable groups, health inequalities and targeted interventions

3.22 Few people would disagree that societies should put in place measures to protect vulnerable individuals and groups. However, what is less clear is who counts as vulnerable and the extent to which particular freedoms may be curtailed to ensure their protection. A child whose parents feed her a diet of biscuits and chips is 'vulnerable' but does society have the right to interfere with parents' choices and the 'sanctity' of the home? Clearly both 'vulnerability' and 'protection' require careful assessment in the context of any particular decision. At the same time there are legally established notions of abuse that constitute unacceptable forms of behaviour towards the vulnerable (see paragraphs 5.39, 6.14, 6.32–6.33).[26]

Social inequalities in health

3.23 There is great variation between social groups in health risks, health-related behaviours, physical and mental health, and life expectancy.[27] Variation often depends on socio-economic status, gender, race or ethnicity, migration history, degree of urbanisation, and religion or caste. Influences on social inequalities in health include: genetics; prenatal and postnatal environments; personal and family dispositions, resources and habits; local environments; and political and economic forces.

3.24 There is clear evidence to link low socio-economic status (usually measured by occupation, education, income or ownership of assets such as homes or cars) to poorer health (see Boxes 5.5, 6.2, 6.4).[28] It is especially striking that the link appears to be one with relative poverty rather

---

[25] Schwartz B (2004) *The Paradox of Choice* (New York: Harper Collins).

[26] For example, the Children Act 1989 (section 31) establishes the threshold for intervention in terms of (a) risk of significant harm to the child, (b) this harm being attributable to parenting failures and (c) intervention being to the child's benefit.

[27] Acheson D (1998) *Independent Inquiry into Inequalities in Health* (Norwich: The Stationery Office), available at: http://www.archive.official-documents.co.uk/document/doh/ih/ih.htm.

[28] Health and health behaviours usually display a gradient by socio-economic status, so that successively more advantaged groups show longer life expectancy, better health and more health-promoting behaviours. For example, in 1997–1999 in England and Wales, life expectancy at birth was 78.5, 77.5, 76.2, 74.7, 72.7 and 71.1 years, respectively, among men in the six occupational classes ranked from the most to the least socially advantaged. See: Donkin A, Goldblatt P and Lynch K (2002) Inequalities in life expectancy by social class, 1972–1999 *Health Statistics Quarterly* 15: 5–15. There is a steady gradient all the way up the social scale, rather than a threshold between the low-income groups and the rest of society. This means it is difficult to define one segment of the population as 'deprived' or 'disadvantaged', and other segments as 'non-deprived' or 'advantaged'.

than the absolute level of income.[29] Absolute levels of income rose considerably throughout the 20th Century, and life expectancy for both the lowest and highest socio-economic groups has increased.[30] However, the association between poor health (and less healthy behaviours) and belonging to the lowest socio-economic group in one's society has remained almost constant, although the forms of ill health have changed. For example, higher rates of heart disease, smoking and obesity are more common among poorer sections of society in developed countries.

3.25 Gender differences in health and life expectancy are partly biological and partly the result of different social roles, exposures and expectations.[31] These differences vary in different countries and regions, and are influenced by social, cultural, employment and economic factors, but often result in health inequalities between men and women within a population.

3.26 Many diseases and behaviours are patterned by ethnic group, but ethnic minority groups do not always have poorer health, and there is considerable variation among ethnic groups. For example, relative to the general population, the prevalence of hypertensive-related diseases is high in African-origin populations but that of coronary heart disease is low.[32] Whereas the prevalence of diabetes tends to be consistently higher among ethnic minorities than the general population, this is not the case for obesity.[33] With the exception of those from Black Caribbean, Black African and Irish backgrounds, men from minority ethnic groups have markedly lower obesity prevalence rates than those in the general population (see Box 5.6). For almost all minority ethnic groups it has been shown that individuals are more likely than those in the general population to be non-drinkers, and less likely to be 'binge-drinkers' (see Box 6.2).[34]

3.27 The reduction of health inequalities is a crucial element of public health policy, and was chosen by the UK Government as a major topic for its presidency of the EU in 2005. Reducing health inequalities was, in 2006/7, included for the first time by the Department of Health for England as one of the top six priorities for the NHS, and since April 2007 it has been a mandatory target for local authorities through local area agreements.[35] In 2002 the

---

[29] Wilkinson RG (1997) Socioeconomic determinants of health: health inequalities: relative or absolute material standards *Br Med J* **314**: 591. There are several competing theories about the major factors that determine ill health and life expectancy. For example, according to some authorities inequalities per se can be source of ill health, see Marmot MG, Shipley MG and Rose G (1984) Inequalities in death: specific explanations of a general pattern *Lancet* i: 1003–6; Marmot MG, Davey Smith G, Stansfeld S *et al.* (1991) Health inequalities among British civil servants: the Whitehall II Study *Lancet* **337**: 1387–93.

[30] Although, generally, life expectancy, health and health-related behaviours have shown a steady improvement over the past 50 years, those in more advantaged social groups have often seen a faster improvement. Where this occurs, for example particularly for men, this means that the gap between those at the bottom and top of the social scale has been widening (although there are some indications that very recent years have seen a narrowing trend). For example, the difference in mortality between professional and unskilled manual men since the 1930s has increased more than twofold. In more recent years the difference in life expectancy between men in social group I and social group V has increased from 5.4 years in 1972–6 to 8.4 years in 1997–2001. For women, the difference has decreased from 5.3 to 4.5 years over the same period. Department of Health (2005) *Tackling Health Inequalities: Status report on the Programme for Action* (London: Department of Health), p.15.

[31] Macintyre S and Hunt K (1997) Socio-economic position, gender and health *J Health Psychol* **2**: 315–34; Macintyre S, Hunt K and Sweeting H (1996) Gender differences in health: are things really as simple as they seem? *Soc Sci Med* **42**: 617–24; Gender and Health Group at the Liverpool School of Tropical Medicine *Guidelines for the Analysis of Gender and Health*, available at: http://www.liv.ac.uk/lstm/hsr/GG-1.html.

[32] Becker E, Boreham R, Chaudhury M *et al.* (2006) *Health Survey for England 2004: The health of ethnic minorities* (Leeds: The Information Centre), available at: http://www.ic.nhs.uk/pubs/hlthsvyeng2004ethnic; Nazroo J (1997) *The Health of Britain's Minorities* (London: Policy Studies Institute); Harding S and Maxwell S (1998) Differences in mortality of migrants, in *Health Inequalities. ONS Decennial Supplement Series DS No 15*, Whitehead and Drever (Editors) (London: The Stationery Office); Harding S (2000) Examining the contribution of social class to high cardiovascular mortality among Indian, Pakistani and Bangladeshi male migrants living in England and Wales *Health Statistics Quarterly* **5**: 26–8, available at: http://www.statistics.gov.uk/articles/hsq/HSQ5migrant.pdf.

[33] Becker E, Boreham R, Chaudhury M *et al.* (2006) *Health Survey for England 2004: The health of ethnic minorities* (Leeds: The Information Centre), available at: http://www.ic.nhs.uk/pubs/hlthsvyeng2004ethnic.

[34] *Ibid*.

[35] Caroline Flint MP, *Hansard*, 5 December 2006, column 173.

Department of Health set a target for reducing inequalities in infant mortality and life expectancy at birth by 10% by 2010.[36] In 2004 further targets to reduce health inequalities were added, including: reducing adult smoking rates, with a particular emphasis on those among 'routine and manual groups'; halting the rise in obesity among children; and reducing the under-18 conception rate, all by 2010.[37] However, data for 2003–5 on infant mortality showed that the gap between the 'routine and manual groups' and the population as a whole had widened since the 1997–9 average. Additionally, data for 2003–5 show that nationally life expectancy had continued to increase although more slowly in areas with poorer health indicators.[38] For smoking, data for 2005 showed that the number of adults overall who smoked had fallen since 2001 from 27% to 24%, while for 'routine and manual groups' the figure reduced from 33% to 31%.[39]

3.28 Generally, we can distinguish between three policy approaches that play a significant role in avoiding health inequalities: those targeted at a particular disadvantaged group, those targeted at a particular at-risk group, and those offered universally, although in practice the distinctions can become somewhat unclear. Some people may benefit from all three, and many people who might benefit from strategies aimed at disadvantaged groups might also benefit from those aimed at at-risk groups. The following advantages and disadvantages of these three approaches are especially noteworthy.

Targeting disadvantaged groups

3.29 Targeted interventions typically aim to improve health outcomes or opportunities in a particular disadvantaged group (see paragraphs 2.27–2.32). Examples include free nicotine replacement for individuals on income support or the provision of additional resources for specific deprived areas (for example Health Action Zones or New Deal for Communities). Such interventions may be beneficial in reducing inequalities in health, although individuals in socially disadvantaged groups can find it difficult to change their behaviour because of lack of resources, lack of education, or co-existing social or health problems.[40] Where this is the case, such behaviour change programmes may produce relatively little aggregate health gain at comparatively high cost. However, targeted interventions should not be dismissed simply because of their comparatively higher costs. It has been observed we are "paying dearly – in higher crime rates, diverging mortality rates and widening levels of education achievement – for the soaring inequalities that began in the early 1980s."[41]

3.30 Several practical issues also need to be considered in targeted approaches. For example, interventions may fail to reach the intended recipients because of uncertainties about eligibility; and they may stigmatise already marginalised groups, or disadvantage those who fall just outside the eligibility criteria. Area-based targeting can raise questions of whether

---

[36] Department of Health, *Spending Review 2002 Public Service Agreement*, available at:
http://www.dh.gov.uk/en/Aboutus/HowDHworks/Servicestandardsandcommitments/DHPublicServiceAgreement/DH_074514.

[37] Department of Health, *Spending Review 2004 Public Service Agreement*, available at:
http://www.dh.gov.uk/en/Aboutus/HowDHworks/Servicestandardsandcommitments/DHPublicServiceAgreement/DH_4106188.

[38] Department of Health (2006) *Tackling health inequalities: 2003–05 data update for the national 2010 PSA target*, available at:
http://www.dh.gov.uk/en/Publicationsandstatistics/Publications/PublicationsStatistics/DH_063689. A three-year average for 2003–5 showed a slight narrowing of the gap between the 'routine and manual groups' and the population as a whole compared with the previous year.

[39] Department of Health (2006) *Autumn Performance Report 2006*, available at:
http://www.dh.gov.uk/en/Publicationsandstatistics/Publications/PublicationsPolicyAndGuidance/DH_062807.

[40] For example, smoking cessation services are least successful among those of lower socio-economic status, those smoking more than 31 cigarettes per day, those with health problems, and those with other smokers in the household. Judge K, Bauld L, Chesterman J and Ferguson J (2005) The English smoking treatment services; short term outcomes *Addiction* **100**: 46–58; Ferguson J, Bauld L, Chesterman J and Judge K (2005) The English smoking treatment services; one year outcomes *Addiction* **100**: 59–69.

[41] Lansley S (2006) *Rich Britain: The rise and rise of the new super-wealthy* (London: Politico's Publishing), p.202.

extra services are actually going to the areas where people have the lowest socio-economic status, or only to areas where local politicians or councillors have been highly influential or effective. Area-based approaches are often a combination of targeted and universal services, because although they select deprived areas, all local residents are eligible. As noted above, there is a continuous gradient of socio-economic and health disadvantage. Some targeted approaches seem to have most benefited the slightly better off among the target group, while even harming those lower down the scale. For example, Sure Start, an area-based programme aimed at tackling child poverty and social exclusion, is a universal area-based intervention for all families living in designated areas. The initial evaluation shows few significant differences between intervention and comparison areas, but some indication of adverse effects among the most deprived (those who were teenagers when their child was born, lone parents and workless households).[42]

Targeting at-risk groups

3.31 Although many strategies that target the disadvantaged face the problem of stigmatisation, this may matter less where interventions seek to help those who are at specific risk because of their general behaviour patterns. For example, where there are clear cause–effect relationships in relation to harm, the offer of an intervention may be more acceptable, such as when HIV screening is offered to groups who frequently engage in unprotected sex. However, there may still be a risk of stigmatisation, especially where those so targeted are also among the most socially marginalised, such as illicit drug users, prostitutes and homosexual men.

Universal provision

3.32 The universal provision of public health interventions might appear to be more neutral than the two alternative options of targeting, as it avoids stigmatisation, and simply relies on people taking up available opportunities. For example, there is evidence that structural changes such as Clean Air Acts, or banning smoking in public places, have positive effects on reducing health inequalities.[43] However, in the case of other interventions, especially those that are information based (such as nutrition labelling, anti-smoking adverts or drink-driving campaigns), strategies may actually increase social inequalities as more advantaged groups in society are more likely to avail themselves of health promotion advice.[44]

3.33 Therefore, although universal measures may not *aim* to target particular groups, they often have the *consequence* that some groups benefit more than others, and hence these groups might be targeted *indirectly*. For example, an intervention to provide better food labelling relies on people reading the labels, understanding the information and using the knowledge gained to buy appropriate healthy foods. In reality, the target population may be motivated

---

[42] Belsky J, Melhuish E, Barnes J, Leyland AH and Romaniuk H (2006) Effects of Sure Start local programmes on children and families: early findings from a quasi-experimental, cross sectional study *Br Med J* **332**: 1476–82; available at: http://www.nao.org.uk/pn/06-07/0607104.htm.

[43] The prevalence of smoking and exposure to passive smoking is highest in communities with the lowest socio-economic indicators. Therefore, a reduction in exposure to environmental smoke as a result of a ban in smoking in public places is expected to reduce health inequalities. Royal College of Physicians (2000) *Nicotine Addiction in Britain: A report of the Tobacco Advisory Group of the Royal College of Physicians* (London: RCP), available at: http://www.rcplondon.ac.uk/pubs/books/nicotine/.

[44] This appears to have happened in the case of some health education campaigns directed at the whole population, for example anti-smoking programmes or dietary advice. More socio-economically advantaged social groups have reduced smoking rates and moved towards dietary recommendations more quickly than their less-advantaged peers. Acheson D (1998) *Independent Inquiry into Inequalities in Health: Report* (London: The Stationery Office); Gepkens A and Gunning-Schepers LJ (1996) Interventions to reduce socioeconomic health differences: a review of the international literature *Eur J Public Health* **6**: 218–26. There is also evidence that they make more use of preventive services such as immunisation, dental check-ups and cervical screening.

by factors other than 'healthy' eating, such as convenience, palatability, price and availability or custom. They may hold an outdated model of 'healthy eating' that differs from that of policy makers, or they may simply be unable to read or understand the labels. This can lead to the argument that supports targeted approaches. If some groups are more likely than others to benefit from particular measures (by being targeted indirectly), it would be preferable for policy makers to consider from the outset who should benefit primarily.

3.34 Thus the two public health goals of improving population health and reducing health inequalities may sometimes be in conflict. Targeting the already advantaged may produce aggregate health gain at relatively little cost, whereas targeting the disadvantaged may produce less aggregate health gain and at greater cost. Providing universal services in order to avoid stigmatisation, or to provide equal access to improved services, may actually increase social inequalities in outcome. It is ultimately a political decision as to how the goals of improving aggregate health or reducing inequalities should be weighted, and monitoring that provides evidence about the effectiveness of particular strategies is of crucial importance in this context.

Behaviour change

3.35 Personal behaviours can have a significant effect on health, and therefore a common theme in public health policy is behaviour change. There are several different strategies aimed at individuals or communities, driven by numerous overlapping models of behaviour and behaviour change.[45] The types of measure that might be involved include regulation, taxes, subsidies and incentives, and provision of services and information. Such measures can be effective in bringing about behaviour change; however, again, these policies may actually increase health inequalities (see paragraphs 3.32–3.33).[46] They can also face difficulties such as cultural sensitivity and public acceptability.

3.36 One increasingly prominent approach is social marketing, which the National Social Marketing Centre defines as "the systematic application of marketing techniques and approaches to achieve specific behavioural goals, to improve health and reduce health inequalities".[47] Thus, social marketing uses many of the methods used by commercial companies to influence consumer behaviour including strategies such as consumer orientation, strategic planning, relationship building and stakeholder marketing. Social marketing has been used, for instance, in campaigns to persuade people not to smoke, not to drink excessively, especially when driving, to use condoms and to eat more healthily. Commentators have observed that there is a burgeoning evidence base to support the effectiveness of social marketing approaches.[48]

The intervention ladder

3.37 To assist in thinking about the acceptability and justification of different policy initiatives to improve public health we have devised what we call the 'intervention ladder' (Box 3.2). The first and least-intrusive step on the ladder is to do nothing, or at most monitor the situation. The most intrusive is to legislate in such a way as to restrict freedoms significantly, either for

---

[45] Halpern D, Bates C, Beales G and Heathfield A (2004) *Personal Responsibility and Changing Behaviour: The state of knowledge and its implications for public policy* (London: Prime Minister's Strategy Unit).

[46] *Ibid.*

[47] French J and Blair Stevens C (2005) *Social Marketing Pocket Guide*, 1st Edition (London: National Social Marketing Centre for Excellence).

[48] Gordon R, McDermott L, Stead M and Angus K (2006) The effectiveness of social marketing interventions for health improvement: what's the evidence? *Public Health* **120**: 1133–9.

some groups of the population or the population as a whole, in order to achieve gains in population health.[49] The higher the rung on the ladder at which the policy maker intervenes, the stronger the justification has to be. A more intrusive policy initiative is likely to be publicly acceptable only if it is clear that it will produce the desired effect and that this can be weighed against the loss of liberty that will result (see also Box 3.3).

Box 3.2: The intervention ladder

The range of options available to government and policy makers can be thought of as a ladder of interventions, with progressive steps from individual freedom and responsibility towards state intervention as one moves up the ladder. In considering which 'rung' is appropriate for a particular public health goal, the benefits to individuals and society should be weighed against the erosion of individual freedom. Economic costs and benefits would need be taken into account alongside health and societal benefits. The ladder of possible policy action is as follows:

Eliminate choice. Regulate in such a way as to entirely eliminate choice, for example through compulsory isolation of patients with infectious diseases.

Restrict choice. Regulate in such a way as to restrict the options available to people with the aim of protecting them, for example removing unhealthy ingredients from foods, or unhealthy foods from shops or restaurants.

Guide choice through disincentives. Fiscal and other disincentives can be put in place to influence people not to pursue certain activities, for example through taxes on cigarettes, or by discouraging the use of cars in inner cities through charging schemes or limitations of parking spaces.

Guide choices through incentives. Regulations can be offered that guide choices by fiscal and other incentives, for example offering tax-breaks for the purchase of bicycles that are used as a means of travelling to work.

Guide choices through changing the default policy. For example, in a restaurant, instead of providing chips as a standard side dish (with healthier options available), menus could be changed to provide a more healthy option as standard (with chips as an option available).

Enable choice. Enable individuals to change their behaviours, for example by offering participation in an NHS 'stop smoking' programme, building cycle lanes, or providing free fruit in schools.

Provide information. Inform and educate the public, for example as part of campaigns to encourage people to walk more or eat five portions of fruit and vegetables per day.

Do nothing or simply monitor the current situation.

3.38 The implications of the intervention ladder will be considered in more detail in the following chapters. For now we clarify that it is not the case that the option of 'doing nothing' requires no justification, as deciding to 'do nothing' is itself a value judgement and may have adverse consequences for some. For example, not regulating vehicle speed limits or blood-alcohol limits might result in deaths or injuries (see also paragraphs 3.15–3.19).[50] Primarily, the function of the ladder is to compare alternative approaches in terms of their intrusiveness and likely acceptability, and not a means of allowing judgements in absolute terms. The intervention ladder is, therefore, not a formulaic device, but, further to our observations on proportionality, a tool for bringing into sharper focus the issues at stake (see paragraph 3.18).

---

[49] And these benefits, again, might affect some groups of the population, or the population as a whole.

[50] In fact, the option of 'doing nothing' may require strong justification, for example in relation to rising levels of sexually transmitted infections.

> **Box 3.3: Coercive measures in place in the UK**
>
> There is a variety of coercive measures that the population in the UK is already familiar with, ranging from legislative measures to civil agreements. For example:
>
> - legal restrictions on owning a gun;
> - tenancy agreements that restrict the level of noise that can be made;
> - legislation that restricts the level of noise that companies can produce;
> - health and safety legislation on the wearing of protective clothing;
> - speed restrictions on roads;
> - pedestrianisation of some city centres;
> - restrictions on eating and drinking in public places (such as on buses or in 'alcohol control areas'); and
> - planning regulations and building standards.

Stakeholders and policy making

3.39 The success of public health interventions often depends on more than the cooperation of members of the population. Many different stakeholder groups, including health professionals, the corporate sector, non-governmental organisations (NGOs), institutions of civil society and the media, can have a crucial role to play.

3.40 Healthcare professionals may be the front line of giving advice to the public. At the same time they may have competing priorities, including providing treatment or engaging in research.

3.41 Commercial organisations have an important role in the case of obesity, alcohol and smoking (see Chapters 5 and 6), and we commented in paragraphs 2.47–2.50 on the emergence of the concept of 'corporate social responsibility'. In policy and practice, most industry-led initiatives aim to enable people to have a choice of more healthy, or less unhealthy, products. However, the fundamental tension for most industries is that their primary interest is in maximising profits, which is often in conflict with public health interests. This is perhaps most clear in the case of the tobacco industry (see also paragraphs 6.18–6.27). From a public health point of view, companies that take seriously the pursuit of 'harm reduction strategies', which feature prominently in most corporate responsibility approaches, should simply cease to offer their products. However, this is not a realistic option if they are to remain in business. One of the questions is thus to what extent it is necessary or appropriate for industries to be regulated by laws imposed by a stewardship-guided state (see also paragraphs 2.41–2.44, 2.50).

3.42 Other important stakeholders are the voluntary sector and NGOs. Many of these groups represent otherwise disadvantaged people whose interests might not ordinarily be heard in policy debates. For example, the Afiya Trust seeks to promote equality in health and social care for groups disadvantaged on ethnic grounds. Others include Action on Smoking and Health (ASH), which campaigns to reduce smoking, and Diabetes UK and Cancer Research UK, which combine research, advice and other support for individuals, with campaigning about particular health problems. By contributing to the policy process through responses to government consultations or more direct contact with officials, a wide range of groups challenge ongoing policy projects and aim to ensure that the interests of their constituencies are presented in an appropriate way to decision makers. Some of the campaigning organisations, such as Vaccination Awareness Network UK (VAN UK), are 'grass roots' groups that have been founded by an individual or group of individuals in relation to a particular cause or concern. Regardless of whether NGOs are 'grass roots' or established national or multinational organisations, they can have a valuable role to play in policy development.

3.43 Although NGOs are often perceived as acting 'for the good of the public' and therefore as more trustworthy than officialdom,[51] it should be borne in mind that NGOs may have a vested interest, a commercial imperative and a 'product' in a way that it not dissimilar to a business. Some may be sponsored by a commercial company with an interest or agenda in this area. An organisation that campaigns on behalf of a sector of the public with a particular kind of worry may even rely for its support on that worry being amplified and even distorted.

3.44 Views expressed through television, radio and print media, and increasingly the largely unrestricted information available on the Internet, have considerable influence on people's opinions. Concerning public health, two especially important areas relate to the concepts of 'risk' and 'evidence' (see paragraphs 3.3–3.14). Health and science programmes and features can assist people in forming their views about public health matters. At the same time, the media can also provoke or amplify public concerns by inaccurate, biased or unhelpful portrayal of risks and evidence. For example, it has been suggested that the media "did much to stoke fear and panic about MMR",[52] following the suggestion in a study published in the *Lancet* of a link between MMR vaccination, and Crohn's disease and autism.[53] The study was generally considered to be weak and considerable other evidence did not support its findings,[54] but it was widely reported in the media, causing misperceptions of the strength of the evidence.[55] We comment further on this case in Chapter 4 (see paragraphs 4.33–4.35, also paragraphs 8.20–8.24). There are also examples in which media stories dwell on disagreements among scientific experts, and there can be a tendency to champion the minority view, justified as 'representing a balance of different points of view'.[56] While we see it as a crucial part of scientific progress to ensure that dominant views are challenged, media stories are often driven by the notion of 'heroes and villains', with the lone scientist as the plucky outsider standing up to the establishment. Such formats can do far more harm than good in helping people to think through the issues for themselves, especially when the issues are complex.

3.45 The interpretation of all the various strands of opinion and its translation into policy is a matter that politicians and their advisors must consider. As representatives of the people, in the context of public health, politicians are expected to enact laws and implement policies that enable people to live healthy lives. At the same time, politicians can have personal or professional conflicts of interest, for example where an industry is a major employer in a Member of Parliament's constituency, or if he or she personally gains financially from a

---

[51] MORI (2003) *Trust in the Government Low*, available at: http://www.mori.com/polls/2002/uea.shtml.

[52] *Guardian* (16 June 2006) *The Media's MMR shame*, available at:
http://commentisfree.guardian.co.uk/brendan_oneill/2006/06/when_journalism_kills.html.

[53] Wakefield AJ, Murch SH, Anthony A *et al.* (1998) Ileal-lymphoid-nodular hyperplasia, non-specific colitis, and pervasive developmental disorder in children *Lancet* **351**: 637–41.

[54] The journal that published the paper has since stated that the study was flawed and that it should never have published it. In 2004, six years after its publication, ten of the 13 authors of the paper issued a retraction. Further studies, in particular a Cochrane systematic review published in 2005, have found insufficient evidence for the claimed link between the MMR vaccine and either autism or inflammatory bowel disease. Dunne R (2004) Inside the world of medical journals *BBC News Online* 23 February, available at: http://news.bbc.co.uk/1/hi/health/3513791.stm; Murch SH, Anthony A, Casson DH *et al.* (2004) Retraction of an interpretation *Lancet* **363**: 750; Cochrane Library (2005) *The Cochrane Library publishes the most thorough survey of MMR vaccination data which strongly supports its use*, available at: http://www.cochrane.org/press/MMR_final.pdf.

[55] Hargreaves I, Lewis J and Speers T (2003) *Towards a Better Map: Science, the public and the media* (London: Economic and Social Research Council).

[56] For example Dr Arpad Pusztai's views on the dangers of genetically modified foods (discussed in Nuffield Council on Bioethics (1999) *Genetically Modified Crops: The ethical and social issues* (London: NCOB), Appendix 1) and the Hooper theory on AIDS (see WHO (2000) *Statement on the Hypothesis that an Experimental Polio Vaccine was Origin of HIV*, available at: http://www.who.int/inf-pr-2000/en/state2000-04.html).

business.[57] More generally, governments are under pressure from industries that emphasise the value they bring to a country in terms of employment opportunities and tax revenues. This may discourage politicians from taking action to protect health if it comes at an economic cost.

3.46 Political interests can also have significant impact on public health matters when politicians are motivated by the need to be seen to be 'doing something'. They may have to choose between an intervention that would be popular straight away but ineffective, and another having less immediate appeal but more likely to be successful in public health terms. For example, discussions about banning 'junk food' appear to have enjoyed some popularity with the electorate. Yet, although important issues are raised by the quality of food available in schools and other places, it is important not to oversimplify a complex problem, diverting attention from other more promising strategies.

Economics

3.47 Economic considerations affect policy making in numerous ways. We have already alluded to possible tradeoffs between employment and health. The economic arguments for supporting different types of intervention vary with different ethical frameworks and assumptions about health behaviour.

3.48 In the UK the healthcare system is financed from general taxation. Any healthcare intervention that affects individual choices and health outcomes will have a potential impact therefore, albeit indirect and financial, on others through its cost to the system. The Wanless Report drew sharp conclusions about the lack of affordability of treatment by the NHS if the population remained reluctant to engage more actively in improving its own health. The report concluded that if the public were 'fully engaged' with improving their own health, the NHS would be spending £154 billion a year by 2022–3.[58] In the worst-case scenario – that of a slow uptake – the figure would be £184 billion. The report argued that improving healthy behaviours will have benefits in reducing the potential burden on the NHS as well as improving health.

3.49 Another potential impact of poor health is on the productivity of the workforce. The implication is that healthy populations will have fewer absences for sickness, a higher proportion of the population able to work and no loss of skills through premature deaths. Conversely, actions that impact adversely on public health can lead to loss in productivity.

3.50 Taxing unhealthy behaviours would be one method of reducing harm to others and ensuring that the 'polluter pays'.[59] The aim of such policy interventions is to ensure economic efficiency and that we make the best use of scarce resources. There are, however, issues of fairness or equality attached to different interventions. The tax burden on individuals will be uneven if the same tax is applied to all, as there is variation in disposable income and in health behaviour. Using a purely economic criterion of fairness, it might be argued that smokers do not impose particular strain on the healthcare system, as they contribute much in taxes (see Box 6.7).

---

[57] For example, the Rt Hon Kenneth Clarke MP has been involved with, and latterly the Deputy Chairman of, British American Tobacco for much of his time in parliament, where he has held positions including Secretary of State for Health and Chancellor of the Exchequer. See British American Tobacco *Who we are*, available at: http://www.bat.com/oneweb/sites/uk__3mnfen.nsf/0/09586a20b7eede4980256bf400019873?OpenDocument. See also Daube M (2005) Why Ken Clarke is unfit to be Tory leader *Br Med J* **331**: 912.

[58] Wanless D (2002) *Securing our Future Health: Taking a long-term view*, available at: http://www.hm-treasury.gov.uk/consultations_and_legislation/wanless/consult_wanless_final.cfm.

[59] According to the 'polluter pays' principle, more generally used in relation to the environment, where environmental damage occurs it is the polluter that pays the costs of the damage.

3.51 We have already recognised that some health-related behaviours may not be regarded as 'free choices' (see paragraphs 1.4, 3.20–3.21) because they are affected, for example, by addiction, or by economic and social environments. This may lead to public support for government interventions that support restrictions of individual choice. Other public health interventions may need to be made at a population level to be successful, for example the design of environments that encourage people to walk rather than take transport. Such policies can have economic consequences in terms of jobs or changes in government revenue patterns. From an economic perspective the question is whether there is an overall gain in benefits from a programme in cost terms compared with not having this intervention. However, in policy terms any costs might be outweighed by the value of individuals being able to make choices.

3.52 Other values might also be considered when examining the potential cost-effectiveness of different policy options, such as quality and quantity of life, public good and altruistic aspects of improving public health and reducing health inequalities.

The policy-making debate

3.53 The policy-making process is an exercise in collective judgement. It requires debate on the evidence about particular risks, and about what these mean in a particular context. Debate is required not merely about ethical principles, but about how those principles should be applied in context and how to resolve possible conflicts between principles. The policies debate can also turn on how one particular issue impacts on other policy – for example, the creation (or reduction) of employment, the diversion of limited resources from other deserving causes, and so on – and the relative importance and urgency of this issue compared with competing issues.

3.54 The example of smoking (see Chapter 6) illustrates some of these challenges. Few people contest that passive smoking can cause harm, and few people object to the principle that, broadly speaking, air in public places should be smoke-free. However, the question of whether this principle is relative or absolute, and the question of how far the state should interfere to enforce it, is a matter for debate. Some people would argue that smoking is acceptable 'between consenting adults' and that the policy maker's role is to ensure that a proportion of pubs, restaurants and workplaces are smoke-free so that non-smokers can 'choose' to avoid contaminated air. Others might contest that the sale of cigarettes should be made illegal and those who 'deal' these addictive and dangerous drugs should be penalised. These two 'framings' of the policy debate on smoking – and the many additional framings in between – each represent a different way of conceptualising the issue and a different combination of values and priorities. In practice, conflicts about substantive differences help to focus attention on the procedural arrangements that are put in place to resolve those conflicts (see paragraph 2.25).

Summary

3.55 We emphasised in this chapter that policy decisions are not made mechanically when a set of evidence is added to a set of ethical principles and economic considerations. We have described several criteria that can ensure that evidence has some degree of robustness (peer review, not using research findings selectively or overstating them, acknowledging openly where there is disagreement). However, we recognise that, in practice, information about evidence and risks is often incomplete, ambiguous and contested, and may not lead by itself to a clear indication of which policy is likely to be the most effective.

3.56 We noted that reducing health inequalities is a crucial part of health policy in the UK, and we considered a range of issues arising from different strategies used for this end (targeting the disadvantaged, targeting at-risk groups and universal approaches). We also noted that some plausible and well-intentioned public health measures may actually do more harm than good, and some may even increase, rather than decrease, inequalities. We suggest therefore, that all approaches require careful design and monitoring to ensure population health can be improved overall, while health inequalities are reduced.

3.57 In presenting the intervention ladder, we offered a tool for thinking about the acceptability and justification of different policy initiatives, focusing on the degree of invasiveness in relation to a particular goal. We also gave examples of a range of liberty-reducing legislative or regulatory measures that have been introduced by the state, for example in the form of health and safety regulation. In the last section we commented on the role of other parties, such as journalists or commercial companies, underlining the notion that public health engages the collective efforts of society (see paragraph 1.6). In the next four chapters we illustrate in more detail how these considerations relate to issues of infectious disease, obesity, smoking and alcohol, and fluoridation of water.

Chapter 4

Case study – Infectious disease

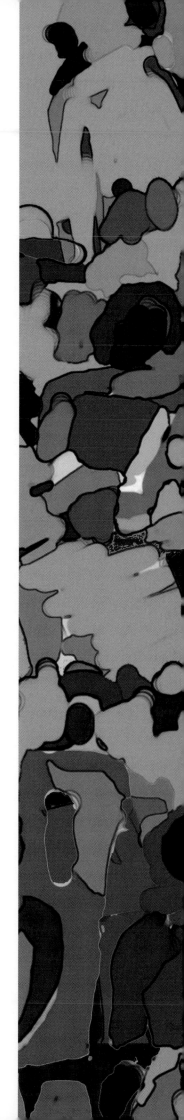

Chapter 4

Case study – infectious disease

Case study – Infectious disease

Introduction

4.1 In this chapter we outline some of the main ethical and policy issues raised by public health measures relating to infectious disease. The chapter is divided into three sections, focusing on: prevention through vaccination (paragraphs 4.7–4.35); surveillance (paragraphs 4.36–4.55); and control strategies (paragraphs 4.56–4.72). Regarding vaccination schemes, we examine the tension between individual choice over receiving or not receiving vaccination, and the potential benefits or risks to the community. We also discuss the policy options of voluntary, quasi-mandatory and incentivised vaccination programmes. We next consider surveillance for identifying infectious disease trends, for researching the nature and epidemiology of a disease and for detecting cases of disease for which control interventions may be needed. The ethical issues raised here include the acceptability of surveillance measures for which people do not give individual consent. In the final section we consider whether approaches for the control of infectious diseases that infringe personal liberty, such as quarantine and isolation, can be justified. As in other chapters, our main focus is on the situation in the UK and in the context of the developed world,[1] but in the sections on surveillance and control we also consider the global context of infectious disease, especially with regard to preparedness for a pandemic (paragraphs 4.47–4.55, 4.66–4.68).

Background

Effects and 'costs' of infectious diseases

4.2 Infectious diseases are a leading cause of illness and death worldwide. Globally, infections cause over a fifth of all deaths and a quarter of all illnesses, disproportionately affecting poorer communities and resource-poor countries.[2] It is estimated that worldwide each year around 5.5 million people die from malaria, tuberculosis (TB) and human immunodeficiency virus (HIV)-related infections, 1.8 million die from diarrhoeal disease and more than a million children die from other diseases that are preventable through vaccines.[3] The vast majority of these deaths are in the developing world, and similarly it has been suggested that in the case of an influenza pandemic up to 96% of deaths could occur in developing countries (see paragraphs 4.65–4.66).[4]

4.3 In Europe and other Western countries, death rates from infectious diseases have reduced over the past century. This trend results from factors such as improvements in living conditions, antimicrobial treatments and the introduction of vaccination programmes. However, in the UK infectious diseases still account for over 10% of deaths and around one

---

[1] We note that in 2007 the Department of Health for England held a consultation relating to a review of parts of the Public Health (Control of Disease) Act 1984, which included proposals relating to several of the topics discussed in this chapter, including disease notification, detention of individuals with serious infections, and vaccination, and more generally to principles that should be applied in considering issues relating to infectious disease control. Department of Health (2007) *Review of Parts 2, 5 and 6 of the Public Health (Control of Disease) Act 1984: A consultation*, available at: http://www.dh.gov.uk/en/Consultations/Closedconsultations/DH_073452.

[2] Foresight (2006) *Infectious Diseases: Preparing for the future. Executive summary* (London: Office of Science and Innovation).

[3] Estimates for 2002 by the World Health Organization, see World Health Organization (2004) *World Health Report 2004* (Geneva, Switzerland: WHO), Statistical Annex; available at: http://www.who.int/whr/2004/en/.

[4] Murray CJ, Lopez AD, Chin B, Feehan D and Hill KH (2006) Estimation of potential global pandemic influenza mortality on the basis of vital registry data from the 1918-20 pandemic: a quantitative analysis *Lancet* **368**: 2211–8; Uscher-Pines L, Duggan PS, Garoon JP, Karron RA and Faden R (2007) Planning for an influenza pandemic – Social justice and disadvantaged groups *Hastings Cent Rep* **37**: 32–9.

in three consultations in primary care.[5] There are also marked inequalities in morbidity due to common infectious diseases. For example, within the UK, hospitalisation rates for respiratory infections in children under five are twice as high in the economically most deprived fifth of the population as they are in the least deprived fifth of the population.[6]

4.4 While prevention and control of many infectious diseases has improved in recent decades, they continue to pose major challenges to public health, both in the UK and internationally. These stem from, for example, the emergence of new infections in humans such as HIV and SARS (severe acute respiratory syndrome),[7] the emergence of old disease problems with new complexities[8] and the continued periodic occurrence of worldwide epidemics of influenza resulting from new strains of the virus.[9] Since AIDS (acquired immune deficiency syndrome) was first described in 1981, and the causative virus HIV was subsequently identified, over 25 million people have died of HIV/AIDS, and in 2006 it was estimated that around 40 million were infected with the virus.[10] Although the outbreak of SARS in 2002/3 was controlled, it caused 774 documented deaths and was estimated to have cost over $12 billion in the affected Asian countries alone (see also Box 4.6).[11] Other potential costs of infectious diseases include reductions in the capacity of the health service to deal with other conditions and restrictions or changes affecting the lives of individuals and their businesses where an outbreak occurs. Higher levels of international travel and trade increase the risk of infectious agents spreading rapidly around the world, causing epidemics and pandemics (worldwide epidemics); meanwhile, changing behavioural, environmental, economic and migration patterns create new ecological niches for the multiplication and spread of infectious agents.[12]

Causes of infectious diseases

4.5 Infectious diseases in humans are caused by a wide range of disease agents including viruses, bacteria, fungi and protozoa (single-celled organisms including amoebae). They vary widely in their ability to be transmitted in human populations, and different infections are transmitted by different means. The means of spread include:

■ airborne and aerosol, e.g. measles, influenza, TB;

■ food/water, e.g. typhoid, cholera, hepatitis A;

■ close contact, e.g. scabies, impetigo, MRSA (methicillin-resistant *Staphylococcus aureus*);

■ sexual intercourse, e.g. gonorrhoea, syphilis, chlamydia, HIV;

■ blood, e.g. hepatitis B and C, HIV;

■ insect vectors, e.g. malaria, dengue, plague; and

■ from animal to man (zoonoses), e.g. rabies, avian influenza.

---

[5] Health Protection Agency (2005) *Health Protection in the 21st Century – Understanding the Burden of Disease; Preparing for the future, Part 4 Infectious diseases*, available at: http://www.hpa.org.uk/publications/2005/burden_disease/.

[6] Health Protection Agency (2005) *Health Protection in the 21st Century – Understanding the Burden of Disease; Preparing for the future, Part 12 Health inequalities*, available at: http://www.hpa.org.uk/publications/2005/burden_disease/.

[7] Indeed, new infectious diseases are emerging at the "historically unprecedented" rate of one per year. WHO (2007) *The World Health Report 2007: A safer future* (Geneva: Switzerland).

[8] Such as TB associated with HIV infection, malaria resistant to previously curative drugs, bacteria resistant to antibiotics, and the resurgence of sexually transmitted infections due to changes in sexual behaviour.

[9] Influenza pandemics typically recur two or three times per century. Department of Health (2007) *Pandemic Influenza: A national framework for responding to an influenza pandemic – Draft for comment* (London: Department of Health).

[10] Joint United Nations Programme on HIV/AIDS (UNAIDS) and World Health Organization (2006) *2006 AIDS Epidemic Update*, available at: http://www.who.int/hiv/mediacentre/2006_EpiUpdate_en.pdf.

[11] World Health Organization (2003) *Severe Acute Respiratory Syndrome (SARS)*, available at: www.wpro.who.int/sars/docs/RC54-08.pdf.

[12] WHO (2007) *The World Health Report 2007: A safer future* (Geneva: Switzerland).

4.6   The range of prevention and control strategies that may be used is wide, depending in part on the nature of the infectious agent and its mode of spread. It includes, for example, advice about safer sex, regulations on food hygiene, advice about hand-washing, and precautions taken in hospitals to prevent infections spreading between individuals, as well as vaccines. We focus first on vaccinations, which raise several particular ethical issues.

Prevention of infectious diseases through vaccination

4.7   The World Health Organization (WHO) estimates that vaccination programmes averted over two million deaths worldwide in 2002.[13] The incidences of diseases such as tetanus, measles, hepatitis B and polio have been greatly reduced by vaccination programmes in the UK and worldwide, and smallpox has been eradicated.[14]

4.8   In the UK, vaccination rates differ between socio-economic groups, with children from lower socio-economic groups being less likely to receive the full suite of recommended vaccinations. Of children born between September 2000 and January 2002 in the UK, 3.3% were only partly immunised by the age of nine months.[15] This percentage was higher among those living in areas that were deprived, or that had a high proportion of inhabitants from ethnic minorities. However, the proportion of children who received no vaccinations at all (overall rate being 1.1%) was higher among those whose mothers were educated to degree level, were older or were of Black Caribbean ethnicity. The often-observed tendency is for affluent groups to be the quickest to take up practices that are protective of child health.[16] However, if doubts are cast, such as when public confidence in the combined measles, mumps and rubella (MMR) vaccine declined (see paragraphs 4.33–4.35 and Box 4.3), they may also be the first to refuse vaccination.[17]

Why vaccinate?

4.9   Vaccinations involve treating a healthy person with a substance that is derived from (or similar to) a particular infectious disease agent. The purpose is to induce a response by the body that leads to enhanced immunity, and consequent protection, when exposed to the infectious agent in the future.

4.10   Vaccines can be used in controlling an outbreak of infectious disease, either in the case of a pandemic or in the case of a localised outbreak, and we consider their use in this context later in the chapter (see paragraphs 4.63–4.68). More often, however, vaccines are used as a routine public health measure to prevent infectious diseases. Routine vaccination strategies can be designed with three different (but not necessarily exclusive) aims:

■ *Population-wide vaccination to protect individuals*: Such vaccines are usually given during childhood. In the UK, childhood vaccination programmes exist for a number of diseases, including: diphtheria, tetanus, whooping cough, polio, some types of meningitis (*Haemophilus influenzae* type b (HiB) and meningitis C), measles, mumps and rubella.

[13] World Health Organization (2005) *Fact sheet No. 288: Immunization against diseases of public health importance*, available at: www.who.int/mediacentre/factsheets/fs288/en/index.html.

[14] *Ibid*.

[15] Samad L, Tate AR, Dezateux C, Peckham C, Butler N and Bedford H (2006) Differences in risk factors for partial and no immunisation in the first year of life: prospective cohort study *Br Med J* **332**: 1312–3.

[16] Middleton E and Baker D (2003) Comparison of social distribution of immunisation with measles, mumps, and rubella vaccine, England, 1991–2001 *Br Med J* **326**: 854.

[17] *Ibid*. The uptake of the MMR vaccination (introduced in 1988) was initially and consistently higher in more affluent areas. From 1997 to 2001 coverage declined in all areas but more so in more affluent areas, leading to an overall reduction in coverage but also a reduction in social inequality.

■ *Selective vaccination to protect individuals who are vulnerable or at-risk*: Examples include: annual influenza vaccines for health professionals, elderly and disabled people; and vaccinations advised for people travelling to regions where specific infectious diseases are common.

■ *Population-wide vaccination to achieve/maintain 'population immunity'*: Some of the vaccinations given to protect individuals, including measles, polio and mumps, contribute to what might be called 'population immunity', also commonly known as 'herd immunity'. For some diseases that are transmitted from person to person, a 'herd effect' occurs when a sufficiently high proportion of the population is vaccinated for there to be a high likelihood that if a case of disease is introduced, all the people that the infectious person comes into contact with are already immune, and thus there is no onward transmission. As a consequence, the small proportion who are unvaccinated[18] are at a much reduced risk of disease, because the chance of outbreaks of disease is much reduced. The level of vaccination cover required for sufficient population immunity to virtually eliminate the risk of significant disease outbreaks varies from around 80% to over 90%, depending on how infectious the disease is, the effectiveness of the vaccine, and various other factors.[19] For diseases in which population immunity can be achieved, very high vaccination levels around the world, combined with outbreak control, may eventually bring about the global eradication of the infection. Smallpox has been eradicated in this way, and there is currently a global eradication programme in progress for polio.

4.11 Vaccination can therefore have an important role in protecting individuals from infection, and in reducing the transmission of infections in the population through population immunity and eradication. Furthermore, vaccination can have an effect on reducing health inequalities. This may be achieved through the targeting of vaccinations at those who are particularly susceptible to ill health, as in the case of influenza vaccines, or through the protection offered by population immunity as it will clearly extend to the most vulnerable (paragraph 3.22).

4.12 Population immunity can confer a substantial collective benefit. At the same time, achieving it requires the organised efforts of society in establishing vaccination schemes, and the collective action and cooperation by the population in taking part to achieve high levels of vaccination coverage. We next consider what kinds of vaccination policy might be used to achieve the high population coverage required for population immunity, and what ethical issues might be raised.

Benefits and risks of vaccination

Risks

4.13 Several consultation respondents expressed concerns about the safety and potential harms of vaccination and argued that on this basis they should not be used at all (see Box 4.1). While it is not our role to review the evidence for the safety of vaccines, we note that extensive reviews of vaccination programmes and rigorous regulatory processes generally

---

[18] In vaccination programmes directed at children there may be various reasons why some children have not been or cannot be vaccinated. This might be, for example, because they cannot receive the vaccine for medical reasons, because they have not yet reached the age at which vaccination would be recommended, because they lack access to health services or because their parents have refused the vaccine. It is important to note also that few vaccines give total protection to all those vaccinated, so some people who have been vaccinated may not be immune from the disease, and would therefore depend on population immunity for protection from the disease.

[19] Malone KM and Hinman AR (2003) Vaccination mandates: The public health imperative and individual rights, in *Law in Public Health Practice*, Goodman RA, Rothstein MA, Hoffman RE et al. (Editors) (New York: Oxford University Press), pp.262–84.

ensure that vaccine safety is at a very high level.[20] No vaccine can be said to be without risk, and for each vaccine an assessment will always be needed of the associated risks and benefits. Such assessments will be characterised by some degree of uncertainty (see paragraphs 3.10–3.11), and there will also be individual variation in response to vaccines, including the possibility of some rare unpredictable reactions. In the view of the Working Party it would be wrong, however, to suggest that the risks and/or variability in response to vaccination were a basis for undermining categorically the case for their use. To do so would be an abuse of the precautionary approach, paying insufficient attention to the criterion of 'proportionality' (paragraphs 3.15–3.19). We also note that in recognition of the potential risks that individuals bear in contributing to population immunity, a Vaccine Damage Payment Scheme exists in the UK.[21]

Box 4.1: Concerns about vaccination expressed by respondents to the consultation

Although the vast weight of scientific evidence supports vaccination, and generally most children receive the interventions, there are some people that criticise them, as illustrated by the following views expressed by respondents to the consultation[22]:

"I believe that vaccinations are harmful and dangerous. I believe that we are compromising our children's health with numerous vaccinations they receive nowadays. There has not been enough research done to show us that vaccinations are safe, effective and do not cause any long-term health problems." *Mrs Marijke Roberts*

"The chances are that the vaccinations cause more health problems than they solve, ... the disease the vaccination is trying to prevent is, in the huge majority of cases, treatable with no side effects." *C Buckley and S Nolan*

"Many of the diseases for which people are vaccinated were already coming under control through improved sanitation, healthcare, and measures such as quarantine. [...] Apart from all the uncertainty surrounding the MMR vaccine there is also a suggested link between other vaccines and various degenerative illnesses. [...] Some vaccines are not producing the herd immunity they are supposed to." *Mrs Esther Hollands*

Weighing up benefits and risks

4.14 Benefits and risks of vaccinations need to be considered from two different perspectives: first, in relation to oneself or, more often, one's children, on behalf of whom one may make decisions; and secondly, in relation to other people.[23]

4.15 From the first perspective, most people accept vaccines in situations in which the incidence of a vaccine-preventable disease is high, the disease is potentially serious and the risks from the vaccine are proportionately low. The situation is different where incidence is relatively low, as there may be both statistical and perceptual changes in the assessments of risks and benefits. Statistically, where there is fairly high vaccine coverage, the risks of disease for those who are unvaccinated may decrease (owing to population immunity) while the risks of vaccination remain. For example, in the USA, as a result of high levels of vaccination for

---

[20] Relevant bodies in the UK that are concerned with such assessments include the following. The Joint Committee on Vaccination and Immunisation (JCVI) is an independent advisory committee whose role is "To advise the Secretaries of State for Health, Scotland, Wales and Northern Ireland on matters relating to communicable diseases, preventable and potentially preventable through immunisation" (see: http://www.advisorybodies.doh.gov.uk/jcvi/). The Medicines and Healthcare products Regulatory Authority (MHRA) is the Government agency that is responsible for ensuring that medicines and medical devices work, and are acceptably safe, and it continually monitors both the safety and quality of the medicines, including vaccines, available on the UK market (see: http://www.mhra.gov.uk). To aid it in this role various expert advisory groups and relevant committees operate, some of which relate specifically to vaccines, including the Committee on Safety of Medicines and the Biologicals and Vaccines Expert Advisory Group of the Commission on Human Medicines (see: http://www.mhra.gov.uk/home/idcplg?IdcService=SS_GET_PAGE&nodeId=908).

[21] Under this scheme, individuals who have been severely mentally or physically disabled as a result of vaccination, or their families, can claim a one-off payment, currently £100,000. This payment is not intended to be considered as compensation but a payment to ease the financial burdens on the disabled person and their family. For further information see: Department of Health (2006) *Immunisation Against Infectious Disease: The Green Book* (London: The Stationery Office), available at: http://www.dh.gov.uk/en/Policyandguidance/Healthandsocialcaretopics/Greenbook/DH_4097254.

[22] Please note that these views should not be taken to be representative of all respondents.

[23] Bauch CT, Galvani AP and Earn DJD (2003) Group interest versus self-interest in smallpox vaccination policy *Proc Natl Acad Sci USA* **100**: 10564–7.

measles, the risk of exposure to the disease-causing virus is very low, while the vaccine used causes fever or rash in around 5% of cases and very occasionally causes more severe reactions.[24] Although healthcare professionals consider the risks of such trade-offs carefully, low incidence of a disease may also affect people's perceptions of it.[25] They may view the risks of contracting a vaccine-preventable disease not to be serious,[26] since they are less familiar with its symptoms or severity as a result of its low prevalence (owing to a high level of vaccination coverage), and may be more likely to refuse vaccination.[27]

4.16 We noted above that population immunity has two main benefits: first that of protecting individuals within the population, including those who are vulnerable;[28] and secondly that of reducing health inequalities. Population immunity also, however, raises particular issues about the distribution of costs and benefits across individuals and society. Where population immunity exists, the additional benefit to the individual from being vaccinated is very small because if they were not to be vaccinated it is likely that they would be protected from the disease as a result of those around them who had been. The main benefit from their being vaccinated is at the community level through the maintenance of population immunity, which includes the protection of those who, for various reasons, have not been vaccinated themselves.[29]

4.17 The population immunity scenario also raises the 'free-rider' issue. Free-riders are individuals who take more than their fair share of the benefits, or do not bear their fair share of the costs, of a resource or institution that is contributed to by many.[30] Where population immunity exists and provides protection for those who refuse vaccination, it could be suggested that individuals who are not vaccinated are free-riders, as they do not share their fair burden, while nevertheless benefiting from population immunity. However, we find this suggestion unhelpful for understanding the complexities raised by vaccines. Although it is true that people pursuing such self-serving strategies would receive a personal benefit, not all who object to vaccinations or refuse them are motivated in this way. There are a range of other reasons for their objections: for example, people may not be convinced of the need for the vaccine, or may be concerned about its effects on themselves or their children.

4.18 Finally on population immunity, we consider a scenario that arises in a few cases where an infection causes serious disease in only some sectors of the population: for example those that seriously affect females rather than males or vice versa. In such scenarios, if there was a vaccine strategy aiming to achieve population immunity, this could mean that some individuals may receive a vaccine that protected against a disease that would not cause them serious harm, for the sake of achieving population immunity to protect others who could be more seriously harmed by it. An interesting example is the triple vaccine MMR, which confers protection against mumps, measles and rubella (see also paragraphs 4.33–4.35). MMR is

---

[24] Severe reactions including aseptic meningitis, encephalitis, and encephalopathy occur in less than one case per million vaccinated. Centers for Disease Control and Prevention, *Prevention of specific diseases: Measles*, available at: http://www2.ncid.cdc.gov/travel/yb/utils/ybGet.asp?section=dis&obj=measles.htm.

[25] Bauch CT, Galvani AP and Earn DJD (2003) Group interest versus self-interest in smallpox vaccination policy *Proc Natl Acad Sci USA* **100**: 10564–7.

[26] Alternatively, it could be suggested that the risks from a threat that is 'natural' such as the infection itself, are perceived differently from the risks associated with a more 'unnatural' procedure such as vaccination.

[27] For example, very few people in developed countries now know of people who have experienced polio, whereas it used to be widespread, and the implications of this serious condition were well known.

[28] In addition, where global eradication of disease is achieved through population immunity, this has benefits for individuals outside the immediate population and for future generations.

[29] Bauch CT, Galvani AP and Earn DJD (2003) Group interest versus self-interest in smallpox vaccination policy *Proc Natl Acad Sci USA* **100**: 10564–7. See also footnote 18.

[30] Cornes R and Sandler T (1996) *The Theory of Externalities, Public Goods and Club Goods*, 2nd Edition (Cambridge: Cambridge University Press).

given to both boys and girls, even though mumps is generally most serious for males[31] and rubella is serious only for women during pregnancy.[32] The rubella vaccine was previously given selectively only to girls, but this strategy was changed as pregnant women continued to contract the infection. Similarly, there has been some debate about whether males should be expected to receive a vaccination for a virus that causes cervical cancer in women,[33] with some suggesting that they should, in order to reduce overall virus prevalence and transmission to women.[34]

4.19 The paragraphs above illustrate that there is a wide range of different risks and benefits, affecting a variety of people, that need to be considered when deciding whether or not to introduce or change a particular vaccination programme. This may give rise to competing interpretations about whether or not a vaccination presents an acceptable balance of risks and benefits. So although a healthcare professional may be keen to enrol a person in a programme, taking the view that the risks are acceptable and that the benefits to the person concerned and/or others are substantial, the individual may be undecided, or not persuaded, for whatever reason. The fact that some healthcare professionals receive payments for meeting vaccination targets may further complicate such situations.[35] Also, the interests of companies involved in the (expensive and potentially risky) business of developing and producing vaccines may need to be considered. Some are critical of the extent to which these industries influence debate and policies on vaccines, and are sceptical as to whether these interventions are genuinely offered on the basis of medical need only.[36] One consultation respondent who took this viewpoint commented that:

> "those who support vaccination most strongly are the drug companies, who stand to profit the most". *Mrs Esther Hollands*

Alternative approaches to vaccination: voluntary, quasi-mandatory and incentivised schemes

4.20 Where vaccination programmes are introduced, there is a range of approaches for ensuring uptake. These vary from simply providing information and encouragement to take up the vaccine, to influencing or reducing choices more directly. In the UK, vaccinations are voluntary; however, other countries have different approaches, and we consider these next.[37] The main argument for policies that go beyond voluntary participation is based on the ethical considerations of stewardship, especially in relation to reducing health inequalities, and of reducing the risks of harm to others (see paragraphs 2.41–2.44). The latter is particularly relevant as there will always be people who have not been vaccinated because

---

[31] Mumps can, however, sometimes cause swelling of the ovaries in women. Health Protection Agency, *Mumps – General Information*, available at: http://www.hpa.org.uk/infections/topics_az/mumps/gen_info.htm.

[32] Health Protection Agency, *Rubella – General Information*, available at: http://www.hpa.org.uk/infections/topics_az/rubella/gen_info.htm.

[33] This virus does, however, cause infection in males and could also be linked with penile cancer, so there may be some benefits to the males themselves.

[34] The Lancet (2006) Should HPV vaccines be mandatory for all adolescents? *Lancet* 368: 1212; Elbasha EH, Dasbach EJ and Insinga RP (2007) Model for assessing human papillomavirus vaccination strategies *Emerg Infect Dis* 13: 28–41.

[35] In the UK, GPs are eligible for two bonus payments when over 70% and over 90% of children registered at their practice are immunised against certain diseases.

[36] For example, there is some controversy about initiatives by the pharmaceutical company Merck. The company was criticised in 2007 for its campaign in the USA to persuade state legislators to add its vaccine against the virus that can cause cervical cancer to their mandatory vaccine programmes. In February 2007, an announcement was made that Merck was ceasing its lobbying activities, after criticism that it was more interested in profits than health concerns and that this was fuelling objections to the vaccine, making the campaign "counterproductive". Merck intended nevertheless to continue to provide education about the vaccine to health officials and legislators, and to lobby for more financing of vaccines in general. Pollack A and Saul S (2007) Merck to halt lobbying for vaccine for girls, *New York Times* 21 February, available at: http://www.nytimes.com/2007/02/21/business/21merck.html?ex=1177473600&en=9ad641d15c1e7da1&ei=5070.

[37] We do not deal separately with incentives for healthcare professionals who meet certain vaccination targets.

of their vulnerable status (see paragraph 4.30) or because they have not been reached for logistical or other reasons, and these people would suffer from the loss of population immunity. Furthermore, such strategies may have the advantage of ensuring that children are not missed out from a childhood vaccination programme, for example if they were immigrants or if their parents might not otherwise have known of or considered vaccination for their child. It could also be suggested that such strategies are more easily justified where the disease that would be prevented is severe or where the eradication of a serious disease is in reach.

4.21 While we are not aware of any countries that go as far as to force individuals to be vaccinated, there are several approaches that may be used to influence their behaviour. We consider three main types: quasi-mandatory programmes, in which individuals are required to be vaccinated unless they qualify for an exemption and where there are penalties for those who do not comply; incentivised programmes, in which vaccinations are optional but individuals who comply receive some reward, usually financial; and approaches focusing on voluntariness, in which vaccinations are optional and complying or not complying involves no penalties or incentives. In all cases, education and information campaigns are generally used to promote the benefits of vaccination and improve uptake. Incentivised and quasi-mandatory programmes can be viewed as more directive than purely voluntary policies, although they may vary in their directiveness according to, for example, the size of the incentive or penalty, or the ease of securing an exemption. In Box 4.2 and Appendix 3 we outline different vaccination policies used in different countries and indicate some of the vaccine coverage rates achieved in these countries.

Box 4.2: Vaccination policies

Under quasi-mandatory vaccination policies, parents are required to have their child vaccinated, unless they qualify for an exemption. The penalties for those who do not comply vary: in Belgium, Italy and Poland parents can be fined and/or sent to prison;[38] in France, Spain and the USA children cannot enrol for school unless they have received certain vaccinations.[39] Countries that operate quasi-mandatory vaccination policies often do so for only some vaccines, and have voluntary policies for others.

In Canada, vaccinations are not quasi-mandatory, but some states require proof of vaccination status for a child to enrol for school, such that the child must either have been vaccinated or have documentation to indicate that their parents have actively refused vaccination. Throughout Canada unvaccinated children can be excluded from school during outbreaks of vaccine-preventable disease.

Most countries provide vaccines free of charge, or the costs may be covered through health insurance schemes. In addition, some countries with voluntary schemes give parents incentives for vaccinating their children, or give health professionals incentives relating to their vaccine coverage rates. The incentives for parents are typically financial, and vary in size. In some cases there are 'lottery-style' incentives, whereby parents who comply with the vaccination schedule are eligible for a prize.[40]

An overview of some of the policies applied in different countries and the vaccination uptake rates can be found in Appendix 3.

Comparing and assessing vaccination strategies

4.22 Assessing the effect of alternative strategies on vaccination coverage is not easy because of the interaction of many factors that affect the vaccination uptake rate, including cultural, historical, political and social factors that influence attitudes towards healthcare, as well as educational background and the accessibility of health services. Nevertheless, comparisons

---

[38] Moran NE, Shickle D, Munthe C et al. (2006) Are compulsory immunisations and incentives to immunise effective ways to achieve herd immunity in Europe? in *Ethics and Infectious Disease*, Selgelid MJ, Battin MP and Smith CB (Editors) (Malden, MA: Blackwell Publishing), pp.215–31.

[39] *Ibid.*; Wellborn AA (2005) *Mandatory Vaccinations: Precedent and current laws*, available at: www.fas.org/sgp/crs/RS21414.pdf.

[40] Moran NE, Shickle D, Munthe C et al. (2006) Are compulsory immunisations and incentives to immunise effective ways to achieve herd immunity in Europe? in *Ethics and Infectious Disease*, Selgelid MJ, Battin MP and Smith CB (Editors) (Malden, MA: Blackwell Publishing), pp.215–31; Achat H, McIntyre P and Burgess M (1999) Health care incentives in immunisation *Aust N Z J Public Health* **23**: 285–8.

between countries or areas within countries, and evaluations of new policies can provide some insight into the implications of different strategies.

4.23 In France the coverage rates for quasi-mandatory vaccinations such as diphtheria, tetanus and polio (83–98%) are generally higher than for those that are voluntary, such as hepatitis B and measles (26–84%).[41] Similar trends are observed for some other countries.[42] However, this is not necessarily to suggest that quasi-mandatory vaccination schemes are the most effective.[43] Some of the highest levels of coverage in Europe, across all vaccines, are seen in Sweden, where vaccinations are voluntary.[44] Even where quasi-mandatory vaccination policies are effective in increasing vaccination rates, they can have some negative effects on vaccination uptake patterns. First, there may be lower uptake of any other vaccinations for which a quasi-mandatory approach is not adopted, as noted above for France. Secondly, where vaccination is required for school admission it has been suggested that parents might only get their children immunised just before starting school rather than at the recommended age for vaccination; this would mean that they may be susceptible at ages when their risk of contracting and spreading the disease is highest.[45] Further questions may be asked over whether quasi-mandatory policies are just, as the punishments for refusal to vaccinate, such as fines or refusal of access to education may disproportionately affect those on lower incomes.[46]

4.24 Regarding providing incentives for parents, an international review and other studies of their use in immunisation have found that they have a positive influence on immunisation uptake, although cost-effectiveness varies.[47] Incentives of modest value can be effective, which is particularly relevant in ethical terms, as higher-value incentives may lead people to take risks they might not wish to take had no incentive been provided.

4.25 Those favouring an entirely voluntary approach will generally do so by focusing on the values of individual autonomy and consent, and they may emphasise the possible harms involved in vaccination. The case of vaccination illustrates important limitations of purely voluntary approaches in the context of public health, because the consequences of decisions about

CHAPTER 4 CASE STUDY – INFECTIOUS DISEASE

---

[41] Antona D, Bussière E, Guignon N, Badeyan G and Lévy-Bruhl D (2003) Vaccine coverage of pre-school age children in France in 2000 *Euro Surveill* **8**: 139–44; available at: http://www.eurosurveillance.org/em/v08n06/0806-224.asp.

[42] *Ibid.*

[43] The coverage rates can also be affected by how strictly the quasi-mandatory policies are applied; for example, not all countries actively enforce the penalties for non-compliance, particularly when the level for population immunity is already reached. Moran NE, Shickle D, Munthe C *et al.* (2006) Are compulsory immunisations and incentives to immunise effective ways to achieve herd immunity in Europe? in *Ethics and Infectious Disease*, Selgelid MJ, Battin MP and Smith CB (Editors) (Malden, MA: Blackwell Publishing), pp.215–31.

[44] According to WHO, 99% coverage was recorded in 2005 for diphtheria, tetanus, polio, pertussis and HiB, see WHO, *Sweden Reported Immunization Coverage*, available at: http://www.who.int/vaccines/globalsummary/immunization/timeseries/tscoveragebycountry.cfm?country=Sweden; Swedish Institute for Infectious Disease Control, *The Swedish Vaccination Program*, available at: http://www.smittskyddsinstitutet.se/in-english/activities/the-swedish-vaccination-program/.

[45] Moran NE, Shickle D, Munthe C *et al.* (2006) Are compulsory immunisations and incentives to immunise effective ways to achieve herd immunity in Europe? in *Ethics and Infectious Disease*, Selgelid MJ, Battin MP and Smith CB (Editors) (Malden, MA: Blackwell Publishing), pp.215–31.

[46] *Ibid.*

[47] Achat H, McIntyre P and Burgess M (1999) Health care incentives in immunisation *Aust N Z J Public Health* **23**: 285–8. In 1998 Australia implemented several broad vaccination incentives for parents, and two subsequent studies investigating the effect of these strategies found that vaccination coverage increased significantly in the populations studied. However, one incentive was the payment of child care benefit only where the child was up-to-date with vaccinations, and it was reported in one study in 2004 that only 31% of the parents who were receiving this benefit could have afforded child care without it. Bond L, Davie G, Carlin JB, Lester R and Nolan T (2002) Increases in vaccination coverage for children in child care, 1997 to 2000: an evaluation of the impact of government incentives and initiatives *Aust N Z J Public Health* **26**: 58–64; Lawrence GL, MacIntyre CR, Hull BP and McIntyre PB (2004) Effectiveness of the linkage of child care and maternity payments to childhood immunization *Vaccine* **22**: 2345–50.

vaccinations affect not only the people who are considering whether to receive a vaccination, but also others. Quasi-mandatory approaches tend therefore to shift the emphasis away from protecting the interests of the individual, and towards providing benefits to others.[48]

4.26 **In general, public health policies should use the least intrusive means to achieve the required public health benefit. Directive vaccination approaches that go further than simply providing information and encouragement to take up the vaccine may, however, be justified on the basis of minimising risks of harm to others, or protecting the health of children and other vulnerable people. A case-by-case assessment will always be required. When assessing whether more directive policies are acceptable, the following factors should be taken into account: the risks associated with the vaccination and with the disease itself, and the seriousness of the threat of the disease to the population. In the case of incentivised policies, the size of the incentive involved should be appropriate so that it would not unduly compromise the voluntariness of consent.**

4.27 **We identified two circumstances in which quasi-mandatory vaccination measures are more likely to be justified. First, for highly contagious and serious diseases, for example with characteristics similar to smallpox. Secondly, for disease eradication if the disease is serious and if eradication is within reach.**

4.28 A more difficult case is raised by a few diseases for which vaccinations could be targeted at the whole population to achieve population immunity, but where the disease would not have been a significant threat to all those vaccinated (paragraph 4.18). In this situation there is no substantial personal benefit to some of the people who might be included in the vaccination programme. Vaccination of males against rubella and a virus that causes cervical cancer or of females against mumps would be examples (see paragraph 4.18). These disease prevention strategies may not be successful if all involved take purely self-interested approaches.

4.29 **On the basis of the value of community and stewardship considerations, it is in principle ethically justified to encourage individuals to take part in vaccination programmes when there is no, or only a small, personal benefit, but significant benefits for others. However, consent is essential, and there should be careful assessments of the benefits to be gained for the population and the possible harm that may result for the people who receive the vaccination.**

Children as special cases

4.30 Special consideration of the role of consent (paragraphs 2.22–2.26) is required in the case of children, who are usually, and legally, unable to consent for themselves. Children are one of the more vulnerable groups in society, and the decision about whether to vaccinate a child may have significant implications for their prospect of leading a healthy life. A small number of children are unable to receive vaccinations for medical reasons, but for most the parents will decide whether they should be vaccinated. To decide such matters, it is reasonable to expect that parents should focus on best interest considerations. Where they fail to do so,

---

[48] We note that there may be other cases where quasi-mandatory vaccinations may be acceptable, where the aim is not to achieve population immunity. For example, the harm principle and the value of the community, as well as pragmatic considerations, could be invoked to support vaccination of all healthcare workers against specific serious diseases as a condition of their employment, as there might be a risk that they could otherwise infect their patients. In addition it could be argued that their professional role in the case of an epidemic is of such central importance that they need to be protected in order to protect others.

the stewardship-guided state may intervene in exceptional cases to ensure that the welfare of children is protected (paragraph 2.44). We therefore agree with the following response to our consultation:

> "Ordinarily, ... parents are deemed to be the best judges of their [children's] interests and ... make decisions [on] vaccination [etc.]. [...] Where parents make choices that seem ... seriously at odds with the child's interests, legally and ethically such choices can be overridden. The courts have shown themselves willing to intervene to consent or refuse treatment on behalf of a child, even in the face of concerted parental opposition. Such cases have usually involved potential serious harm, and in relation to vaccination in the face of parental refusal, a risk of serious harm would have to be demonstrated." *British Medical Association*

4.31 The best-interests standard can be difficult to apply in some scenarios raised by vaccinations. In particular, in the case of vaccinating against a disease for which population immunity exists, the additional benefit to the child from being vaccinated is very small since they would otherwise be protected by population immunity. As such it could be considered that it is rational, or possibly in an individual's best interests, not to receive the vaccine (see paragraphs 4.14–4.19).[49] Nonetheless, there is a benefit to the community in contributing to the maintenance of population immunity. We therefore take the view that best interests considerations should take into account not only the health needs of the individual, but also the wider context of the decision, and that it is appropriate to appeal to parents to vaccinate their children on the basis of the value of community (paragraph 2.34).[50]

4.32 We concluded above (paragraph 4.26) that when assessing whether more directive vaccination policies are acceptable, the following factors should be taken into account: the risks associated with the vaccination and with the disease itself, and the seriousness of the threat of the disease to the population. In addition, there needs to be consideration of whether directive measures would be more effective than voluntary ones. The evidence on this for routine childhood vaccinations is complex and limited. Therefore, **at present, there is not sufficient justification in the UK for moving beyond the current voluntary system and implementing incentivised or quasi-mandatory policies for routine childhood vaccinations.**

Vaccinations in the media

4.33 As we noted above, achieving population immunity through vaccination depends to a significant degree on the cooperation of very many individuals. Any situation that brings about a lack of cooperation by some of these individuals to the extent that population immunity is jeopardised has the potential to have a highly damaging effect on population health. This is a potential consequence where evidence or risk relating to vaccination is portrayed poorly or inaccurately by media reporting (see paragraphs 3.3–3.14, 3.44). A salient example is that of the MMR vaccine, and we outline the background to the controversy in Box 4.3.

---

[49] Bauch CT, Galvani AP and Earn DJD (2003) Group interest versus self-interest in smallpox vaccination policy *Proc Natl Acad Sci USA* **100**: 10564–7.

[50] *Ibid.*

> **Box 4.3: MMR and the media**
>
> A childhood vaccination scheme for measles has been in operation in the UK since 1968, initially with the single measles vaccine, and since 1988 with the combined MMR vaccine.[51] In the 1950s the number of cases of measles reported in England and Wales regularly reached 500,000, but by the 1990s this number had fallen considerably, with fewer than 200 cases each year between 1996 and 2000.[52]
>
> In 1998 a paper suggesting a link between the MMR vaccine, and autism and bowel disease was published in *The Lancet*.[53] The study was weak and considerable other evidence did not support its findings,[54] but it was widely reported in the media, causing misperceptions of the strength of the evidence.[55] The journal has since stated that the study was flawed, that the lead author had a serious conflict of interest, and that as such it should never have published the paper.[56] In addition, ten of the 13 authors of the paper issued a retraction relating to the paper in 2004.[57] Further poor media coverage casting doubts over the safety of the MMR vaccine has, however, continued.[58]
>
> Public confidence in the vaccine declined after the publication of the 1998 paper, and the vaccine coverage decreased below the minimum population immunity level of 90% across the UK.[59] A low of 80% vaccine coverage was reached in 2003–4 in England and Wales, although uptake has now begun to increase in all areas. A number of large measles outbreaks have occurred since the vaccination rate began to fall,[60] and during 2006 the number of cases in England and Wales reached its highest level for 20 years, and the first death caused by measles for 14 years was reported.[61]

4.34 The MMR example illustrates how media reports can influence public perceptions, potentially hindering public health measures and affecting population health. The Council noted the importance of accurately reporting evidence in one of its previous Reports, on the example of genetic research.[62] In the context of public health we consider this to be particularly important given the potential for adverse consequences on population health. As in our previous Report, **we consider that researchers, journalists and others who report**

---

[51] Asaria P and MacMahon E (2006) Measles in the United Kingdom: can we eradicate it by 2010? *Br Med J* 333: 890–5.

[52] Health Protection Agency, *Annual Measles Notifications and Vaccine Coverage 1950–2000*, available at: http://www.hpa.org.uk/infections/topics_az/measles/vaccine_coverage.htm; Health Protection Agency, *Confirmed cases of Measles, Mumps & Rubella 1996–2006*, available at: http://www.hpa.org.uk/infections/topics_az/measles/data_mmr_confirmed.htm.

[53] Wakefield AJ, Murch SH, Anthony A *et al.* (1998) Ileal-lymphoid-nodular hyperplasia, non-specific colitis, and pervasive developmental disorder in children *Lancet* 351: 637–41.

[54] Further studies, in particular a Cochrane systematic review published in 2005, have found insufficient evidence for the claimed link between the MMR vaccine and either autism or inflammatory bowel disease. Demicheli V, Jefferson T, Rivetti A and Price D (2005) Vaccines for measles, mumps and rubella in children *Cochrane Database of Systematic Reviews* Issue 4, Art. No.: CD004407, DOI: 10.1002/14651858.CD004407.pub2.

[55] Hargreaves I, Lewis J and Speers T (2003) *Towards a Better Map: Science, the public and the media* (London: Economic & Social Research Council). For further information about the safety of the MMR vaccine and its review, see Medicines and Healthcare products Regulatory Authority, *MMR Vaccine*, available at: http://www.mhra.gov.uk/home/idcplg?IdcService=SS_GET_PAGE&nodeId=237.

[56] Dunne R (2004) Inside the world of medical journals *BBC News Online* 23 February, available at: http://news.bbc.co.uk/1/hi/health/3513791.stm.

[57] Murch SH, Anthony A, Casson DH *et al.* (2004) Retraction of an interpretation *Lancet* 363: 750.

[58] On 8 July 2007 *The Observer* ran a front-page story on the issue entitled "New health fears over big surge in autism", with the subheading "Questions over triple jab for children". This piece received considerable criticism elsewhere, see Goldacre B (2007) The MMR story that wasn't *The Guardian* 18 July, available at: http://www.guardian.co.uk/comment/story/0,,2128807,00.html; Ahuja A (2007) Autism: The truth *The Times* 12 July, available at: http://www.timesonline.co.uk/tol/life_and_style/health/article2060575.ece; Bad Science Blog, available at: http://www.badscience.net/?p=464. We note also that in February 2007 the BBC OneLife website carried an article on autism suggesting that "many people are convinced [a link between MMR and autism] exists" (copy available from the Nuffield Council on Bioethics), although by August 2007 a search for similar articles on autism revealed none that reported such a link as favourably.

[59] The Information Centre, NHS (2006) *NHS Immunisation Statistics (England) 2005–6*, available at: http://www.ic.nhs.uk/webfiles/publications/immstats2005to2006/ImmunisationStatistics280906_PDF.pdf; Scottish Executive (2003) *Latest Immunisation Statistics*, available at: http://www.scotland.gov.uk/News/Releases/2003/06/3625; National Statistics (2005) *NHS Immunisation Statistics (Wales) 2004–5*, available at: http://newydd.cymru.gov.uk/legacy_en/keypubstatisticsforwales/content/publication/health/2005/sdr109-2005/sdr109-2005.pdf; Department of Health, Social Services and Public Safety (Northern Ireland) (2006) *Community Statistics: 1st April 2005 – 31st March 2006*, available at: http://www.dhsspsni.gov.uk/community_stats_06.pdf.

[60] Jansen VAA, Stollenwerk N, Jensen HJ, Ramsay ME, Edmunds WJ and Rhodes CJ (2003) Measles outbreaks in a population with declining vaccine uptake *Vaccine* 301: 804.

[61] Health Protection Agency (2006) *Health Protection Matters*, Issue 5, available at: http://www.hpa.org.uk/publications/HPM/summer_2006.pdf.

[62] Nuffield Council on Bioethics (2002) *Genetics and Human Behaviour: The ethical context* (London: Nuffield Council on Bioethics), paragraphs 11.12–11.14.

research have a duty to communicate findings in a responsible manner. Those who report research should take account of the *Guidelines on Science and Health Communication* published by the Social Issues Research Centre, the Royal Society and the Royal Institution of Great Britain.[63] In particular we emphasise that the source and the status of scientific evidence alluded to should be identified (for example, whether it is preliminary findings or a conference presentation, and whether it has been peer reviewed).

4.35 We also encourage initiatives that provide independent information that is accessible to the public on the accuracy and reliability of medical stories reported in the media. An example of such an initiative is the National Library for Health's 'Hitting the Headlines' resource,[64] which provides summaries relating to media reports within two days of their publication.

Surveillance

4.36 We examine the ethical issues raised by two distinct types of infectious disease surveillance. First, we consider population surveillance methods to detect important risks and trends in infectious diseases, and to inform the planning of public health interventions or further investigations. Secondly, we discuss schemes aiming to detect individual cases of diseases that might require control measures to be implemented, in particular through notifiable disease strategies.

Broad surveillance for research and monitoring trends

4.37 Surveillance involving the systematic collection, analysis and interpretation of data about incidence and prevalence of infectious diseases, and factors that may contribute to them, forms an integral part of the protection of population health. Data used in this context are generally collected in anonymised form, although the degree of anonymisation can vary. Such data can provide important insights into basic epidemiological questions and trends, and identification of emerging strains and novel infectious agents. Surveillance information is also important in identifying groups who are at risk of certain infections, and for devising strategies for preventing and controlling outbreaks. For example the Health Protection Agency uses data on the incidence of influenza and the uptake of influenza vaccines to guide policies on protecting the UK population from this infection.[65]

Collection and use of surveillance data and consent

4.38 There are various benefits to this type of infectious disease surveillance, but there are also objections to the collection and use of surveillance data, in particular regarding consent.[66] We have noted that obtaining consent is crucial in legitimising interventions that involve some risk to the patient or research participant. There is no question that this requirement is important where there are potentially serious health risks to the individual, for example, in the case of clinical medicine or research involving a new medicine. However, it is far less clear whether people should necessarily have the same authority and control over, for example, biological samples or medical data, particularly where these are anonymised, because it is more difficult to identify relevant harms.[67] Overall the Working Party is not persuaded that there are significant harms involved where the data are suitably anonymised.

---

[63] Social Issues Research Centre, the Royal Society and the Royal Institution of Great Britain (2001) *Guidelines on Science and Health Communication*, available at: http://www.sirc.org/publik/revised_guidelines.pdf.

[64] See: http://www.library.nhs.uk/hth/ and http://www.library.nhs.uk/rss/newsAndRssArchive.aspx?storyCategory=0.

[65] Health Protection Agency *Seasonal influenza*, available at: http://www.hpa.org.uk/infections/topics_az/influenza/seasonal/default.htm.

[66] For further discussion of issues raised in this section see: Verity C and Nicoll A (2002) Consent, confidentiality, and the threat to public health surveillance *Br Med J* **324**: 1210–3.

[67] We note that indeed the Human Tissue Act (2004) excludes public health monitoring from the purposes for which consent to tissue storage and use is required.

4.39 The collection of anonymised surveillance data on trends in infectious disease ranks low on the intervention ladder. Without sufficient data, it may not be possible to assess and predict trends and risks in infectious diseases. **It is acceptable to collect and use anonymised data for assessing and predicting trends in infectious disease without consent, as long as any invasion of privacy is reduced as far as possible.**

4.40 In some circumstances it may be necessary to collect surveillance data in a non-anonymised way, but provided adequate systems are in place to ensure confidentiality of the collected data, it may be justifiable to collect such data without consent. We are aware of several examples of surveillance policies in which consent requirements have had, or could have had, serious negative consequences for the surveillance in question. Some of these are discussed in Box 4.4.[68]

Box 4.4: Consent and population health surveillance

Here we describe two policies that illustrate how consent requirements for population health surveillance schemes can be overly onerous, with implications for the research and surveillance being conducted:

1) Research and surveillance using newborn blood spots

At present in the UK, four 'blood spots' are routinely taken from newborn babies on a blood spot card, which is used for screening for certain diseases, including phenylketonuria and sickle cell disorders. In addition, these blood spot cards can subsequently be stored and used, after being unlinked and anonymised, for research. Because these blood spot cards are collected from nearly all newborn children,[69] they are very useful for surveillance, for example on HIV prevalence,[70] and other research purposes. Parents are given the choice over whether or not their baby has blood spots taken and screened,[71] but there has been debate over whether their consent should also be required for the storage of the blood spot cards and research using these. In 2003, the consent process was changed in Scotland to require a parental signature for each of several elements of the programme, including taking and screening blood spots, storing residual specimens, and research on these specimens.[72] Following this change more parents were found to refuse blood spot screening altogether, which became a cause of concern.[73] In 2005, the UK Newborn Screening Programme Centre published new guidelines on this matter, stating that "Residual newborn blood spots may also be used for research where the samples have been anonymised and the research project has ethical approval, as outlined in the Human Tissue Act and in MRC Guidance, without individual informed consent."[74] It should be noted though, that the parental information leaflets on blood spot screening do state that the blood spots may be used for public health monitoring and research.[75]

2) Research using human tissue, e.g. tonsils

The National Anonymous Tonsil Archive (NATA) began collecting and archiving tonsil tissue from individuals undergoing routine tonsillectomy in 2003, except where individuals opted out, and hopes to collect 100,000 tonsils.[76] The tonsils collected would otherwise have been destroyed routinely after removal. One use of the archive is to study the prevalence of the prion protein that is believed to cause variant Creutzfeldt-Jakob disease (vCJD). In 2004 an early version of the Human Tissue Bill was drafted that required the consent of patients for the storage and use of these leftover tissues, which would have severely affected the NATA and other similar projects.[77] A number of groups including the British Medical Association (BMA) and the Royal College of Pathologists lobbied for changes on this. They suggest that such requirements would be costly in terms of money and human resources for the administration and infrastructure needed, and hence jeopardise the future of this form of surveillance. The Bill was subsequently amended to allow such storage and use without consent, although with safeguards, including the requirements that that the research is approved by a Research Ethics Committee, and that the samples are anonymised.[78]

---

[68] For further examples of surveillance systems that could be jeopardised if it became necessary to either obtain explicit patient consent or totally anonymise data, see additional online materials from: Verity C and Nicoll A (2002) Consent, confidentiality, and the threat to public health surveillance *Br Med J* **324**: 1210–3.

[69] It has been reported that over 99% of newborn babies are screened; UK Newborn Screening Programme Centre, *Why we need a newborn screening programme*, available at: http://www.newbornscreening-bloodspot.org.uk/.

[70] Health Protection Scotland, *Unlinked Anonymous HIV Testing of Dried Blood Samples from Newborn Infants (The Guthrie study)*, available at: http://www.hps.scot.nhs.uk/bbvsti/ssdetail.aspx?id=52.

[71] UK Newborn Screening Programme Centre (2005) *Newborn Blood Spot Screening in the UK – Policies and standards*, available at: http://www.ich.ucl.ac.uk/newborn/download/policies_standards.pdf.

[72] UK Newborn Screening Programme (2004) *Proposed Standards and Policies for Newborn Blood Spot Screening – An integrated consultation*, available at: http://www.ich.ucl.ac.uk/newborn/download/proposed_standards_consultation.pdf.

[73] *Ibid.*

[74] UK Newborn Screening Programme Centre (2005) *Newborn Blood Spot Screening in the UK – Policies and standards*, available at: http://www.ich.ucl.ac.uk/newborn/download/policies_standards.pdf.

[75] Available to download at: http://www.ich.ucl.ac.uk/newborn/resources/delivery.htm#parents.

[76] Health Protection Agency (17 January 2007) *The National Anonymous Tonsil Archive (NATA)*, available at: http://www.hpa.org.uk/infections/topics_az/cjd/tonsil_archive.htm.

[77] Dyer C (2004) Human Tissue Bill is modified because of research needs *Br Med J* **328**: 1518.

[78] This ensures that there is no information that would allow the identification of the person from whom the tissue was taken.

Surveillance to detect cases of disease that require intervention

4.41 Medical practitioners have a statutory obligation to report cases of certain infectious diseases to local authorities (see Box 4.5). The list of diseases that are 'notifiable' in this way varies from country to country, illustrating, in part, the international diversity in the cultural, ethical and regulatory frameworks that governs the control of infectious diseases.

Box 4.5: Notifiable diseases in the UK and elsewhere

UK policy

In the UK the statutory requirement for notification of infectious diseases was first established in London in 1891, when cholera, diphtheria, smallpox and typhoid had to be reported by the head of the family or the landlord to the local authority. Nowadays, doctors in the UK have a statutory duty under public health legislation[79] to notify the relevant officer of the local authority of suspected cases of around 30 infectious diseases, including, for example, measles, mumps, rabies and smallpox.[80] In addition, childminders, day care centres and schools that cater for children under eight years old are required to notify Ofsted (Office for Standards in Education, Children's Services and Skills) of any cases of notifiable diseases and of food poisoning affecting two or more children.[81] Two main purposes of the notifiable disease system are for the rapid detection of outbreaks and epidemics and for the implementation of measures to control such outbreaks by local public health officials. Some of the information relating to each notification is passed on, in an anonymised form, to the Health Protection Agency for England and Wales and the Information Services Division (ISD) in Scotland for evaluation at a national level.[82]

Policy in other countries

Notifiable disease schemes exist in other countries and internationally. The diseases included in each country are usually revised periodically, but, for example, at present in New Zealand there around 50 such diseases and in the USA around 60, with some variations between states.[83]

WHO policy

Under the revised *International Health Regulations* of 2005, a few diseases considered to have a "serious public health impact" (smallpox, poliomyelitis caused by wild-type poliovirus, human influenza caused by a new subtype, and SARS) must additionally be reported to WHO. So too must any other cases of infectious diseases deemed to constitute, under WHO definitions, a "public health emergency of international concern".[84]

4.42 After a notification, the relevant authorities may take action to investigate the outbreak and implement measures to prevent the spread of the disease. For example, under UK legislation, in some circumstances an individual with an infection could be detained at a treatment centre,[85] or, more commonly, excluded from the work place if the infection represents a threat to the community (for example if they work in food production).[86] Where medical professionals pass on details of cases of notifiable diseases for the purposes of control, it is not required that the individual agrees to them doing so and the data passed on necessarily include information that identifies the individual. Some might take the view that consent and privacy considerations make this unacceptable. However, we noted previously the different roots of the concept of

---

[79] In England and Wales: the Public Health (Control of Disease) Act 1984 and the Public Health (Infectious Diseases) Regulations 1988; in Scotland: the Public Health (Notification of Infectious Diseases) (Scotland) Regulations (1988).

[80] The list of notifiable diseases is different in Scotland (see Schedule 1 of the Public Health (Notification of Infectious Diseases) (Scotland) Regulations (1988), available at: http://www.opsi.gov.uk/SI/si1988/Uksi_19881550_en_2.htm) and England and Wales (see: http://www.hpa.org.uk/infections/topics_az/noids/noidlist.htm).

[81] Health Protection Agency, *Day Care and Child Minding (National Standards)*, available at: http://www.hpa.org.uk/infections/topics_az/noids/day_care.htm.

[82] The information collected nationally is the age and sex of the individual, the disease, the local authority and the year and week of notification. Health Protection Agency, *General Information – Notifications of Infectious Diseases (NOIDS)*, available at: http://www.hpa.org.uk/infections/topics_az/noids/gen_info.htm; ISD Scotland, *Infectious Diseases*, available at: http://www.isdscotland.org/isd/1522.htm.

[83] Centers for Disease Control (2006) Summary of notifiable diseases – United States, 2004 *Morb Mortal Wkly Rep* **53**: 1–79, available at: http://www.cdc.gov/MMWR/preview/mmwrhtml/mm5353a1.htm; Ministry of Health (New Zealand) (2005) *Notifiable Diseases*, available at: http://www.moh.govt.nz/moh.nsf/wpg_index/About-notifiable+diseases.

[84] World Health Assembly (2005) *International Health Regulations (2005)*, available at: http://www.who.int/csr/ihr/IHRWHA58_3-en.pdf.

[85] For example an individual with multi-drug-resistant tuberculosis who refuses to take precautions to prevent transmission to others. Public Health Laboratory Service (2002) Hospital acquired multi drug resistant tuberculosis *Commun Dis Rep CDR Wkly* [serial online] **12** (42), available at: http://www.hpa.org.uk/cdr/archives/2002/cdr4202.pdf.

[86] For example, in the case of typhoid or another serious gastrointestinal infection. In such circumstances the person may receive compensation for their loss of earnings.

consent in the context of clinical medicine and public health (paragraphs 2.22–2.26), and the role of proportionality (paragraph 3.18). Both of these are relevant where a public health intervention has significant potential benefits for the population and no substantial risks to the individual.[87]

4.43 Infectious disease monitoring strategies involving the collection of information including identifying data for the purpose of implementing control measures for individuals, as for some notifiable diseases, rank higher on the intervention ladder than surveillance based on anonymised data (see paragraphs 4.37–4.39). The aim of such measures is generally to prevent harm to others from the spread of disease, which means that they can be justified under the classical harm principle. **The avoidance of significant harm to others who are at risk from a serious communicable disease may outweigh the consideration of personal privacy or confidentiality, and on this basis it can be ethically justified to collect non-anonymised data about individuals for the purposes of implementing control measures. However, any overriding of privacy or confidentiality must be to the minimum extent possible to achieve the desired aim.**

HIV and AIDS as notifiable diseases

4.44 Particular controversy surrounds the question of whether HIV and/or AIDS should be included as notifiable diseases. In the UK they are not, although there is a voluntary national reporting system, as well as other surveillance systems, but elsewhere, including the USA and Australia, these are included as notifiable diseases.[88] In some places, including New York State, the HIV notification legislation requires that infected individuals name their sexual partners and these people are notified by health professionals of their risk of having the infection, although no details will be given about the individual who named them.[89] This 'partner notification' law is controversial, but has been proposed as a means of limiting the spread of communicable disease.[90]

4.45 The question of whether to include HIV/AIDS as notifiable diseases in the UK[91] has raised concerns about human rights, discrimination,[92] stigma and penalties from insurance companies.[93] Another concern was that mandatory notification might 'drive the disease underground', as it was feared that potentially infected people might avoid contact with healthcare professionals. Whether these negative consequences would have occurred in practice has been the subject of debate, but we use this example to note that the case of HIV/AIDS illustrates the importance of taking into account the particular context of the disease in question.

4.46 First, a main argument for making HIV/AIDS notifiable diseases would be the classical harm principle, i.e. that this would enable others to be protected from the infection. However, this approach might be of limited utility, as information about people's HIV status cannot easily

---

[87] Verity C and Nicoll A (2002) Consent, confidentiality, and the threat to public health surveillance *Br Med J* **324**: 1210–3.

[88] CDC (USA) (2006) *Nationally Notifiable Infectious Diseases*, available at: http://www.cdc.gov/epo/dphsi/phs/infdis2006.htm; Australian Government Department of Health and Ageing, *Nationally Notifiable Diseases*, available at: http://www.health.gov.au/internet/wcms/publishing.nsf/Content/cda_surveil-nndss-dislist.htm#dislist.

[89] New York State Department of Health, *HIV/AIDS Laws and Regulation: What you need to know about the law*, available at: http://www.health.state.ny.us/diseases/aids/regulations/notification/hivpartner/qanda.htm.

[90] We note that in 2006 the Department of Health for England held a consultation "Confidentiality and Disclosure of Patient Information: HIV and Sexually Transmitted Infection (STIs)", which relates to some of the issues discussed here. See http://www.dh.gov.uk/prod_consum_dh/groups/dh_digitalassets/@dh/@en/documents/digitalasset/dh_4137711.pdf.

[91] Similar issues arise in the debate about proposals for the routine screening of immigrants for infectious diseases such as tuberculosis.

[92] We note that the existence and enforcement of anti-discrimination laws and protection of privacy varies greatly among countries, and that this influences policy on HIV surveillance.

[93] Berridge V (1996) *AIDS in the UK: The making of a policy, 1981–1994* (Oxford: Oxford University Press).

be used to protect others.[94] Secondly, it may be that the surveillance objectives of notifiable disease programmes could be realised without the full regime entailed by such schemes. HIV is subject to several surveillance and reporting systems[95] that allow the collection of useful data, but these data are either fully or partly anonymised, protecting as far as possible the individual from personal identification.[96] Indeed, because HIV often remains undiagnosed for some time after initial infection, case notification or reporting of cases would not necessarily give a full picture of the prevalence of the disease, whereas one of the surveillance programmes in use in the UK assesses prevalence across the population by testing unlinked anonymised samples from a large number of patients.[97] The information gained is used to plan and evaluate health promotion programmes and services for those affected by HIV/AIDS, and is likely to be better suited to this purpose than a notifiable disease scheme would be. Hence the question of whether or not a disease should be notifiable requires ethical consideration of issues such as the classical harm principle and the role of consent, in combination with evaluation of the empirical context of the disease.

Surveillance in an international context

4.47 Outbreaks of infectious disease can have global implications. We note that in 2007 the Department of Health for England published a report on the international context of health, which included discussion of infectious disease.[98] It describes "the need for an international approach if we are to protect the health of the UK population, reduce global poverty and harness the opportunities of globalization", and suggests a UK Government-wide strategy in this area. In addition in 2007 the Department for International Development published a new health strategy, based on the principle that "improving health is crucial in the fight against global poverty".[99]

4.48 In relation to surveillance, the very nature of infectious diseases and the context of global travel and trade, which may assist in spreading diseases very rapidly, underline the fact that effective surveillance programmes are not simply a national matter.[100] The sharing of surveillance data is increasing through international agencies such as WHO, the European Centre for Disease Prevention and Control, the Centers for Disease Prevention and Control (CDC) in the USA and regional disease surveillance networks and initiatives. It is through these systems that emerging outbreaks such as SARS (see also Box 4.6) and avian influenza may be identified, and the information gained can be used to inform interventions and raise professional and public awareness. The global *International Health Regulations*, revised in 2005, now require member states to notify WHO of any potential international public health emergency.[101]

---

[94] Although, we note that Cuba has a quarantine policy for individuals infected with HIV, see: Hansen H and Groce N (2003) Human immunodeficiency virus and quarantine in Cuba *J Am Med Assoc* **290**: 2875.

[95] These include the HIV and AIDS patient reporting system (HAP), the Survey of Prevalent HIV Infections Diagnosed (SOPHID), the Unlinked Anonymous HIV Surveillance Programme and the National Study of HIV in Pregnancy and Childhood; see Health Protection Agency, *Epidemiology – HIV and AIDS*, available at: http://www.hpa.org.uk/infections/topics_az/hiv_and_sti/hiv/epidemiology/introduction.htm.

[96] See Health Protection Agency, *The Unlinked Anonymous Prevalence Monitoring Programme*, available at: http://www.hpa.org.uk/infections/topics_az/hiv_and_sti/hiv/epidemiology/ua.htm.

[97] Health Protection Agency, *Epidemiology – HIV and AIDS*, available at: http://www.hpa.org.uk/infections/topics_az/hiv_and_sti/hiv/epidemiology/introduction.htm; Health Protection Agency, *The Unlinked Anonymous Prevalence Monitoring Programme*, available at: http://www.hpa.org.uk/infections/topics_az/hiv_and_sti/hiv/epidemiology/ua.htm.

[98] Department of Health (2007) *Health is Global*, available at: http://www.dh.gov.uk/en/Publicationsandstatistics/Publications/PublicationsPolicyAndGuidance/DH_072697.

[99] Department for International Development (2007) *Working Together for Better Health*, available at: http://www.dfid.gov.uk/Pubs/files/health-strategy07.pdf.

[100] USA National Intelligence Council (2000) *The Global Infectious Disease Threat and its Implications for the United States – Factors affecting growth and spread: International trade and commerce*, available at: http://www.dni.gov/nic/PDF_GIF_otherprod/infectiousdisease/infectiousdiseases.pdf.

[101] World Health Assembly (2005) *International Health Regulations (2005)*, available at: http://www.who.int/csr/ihr/IHRWHA58_3-en.pdf.

4.49 The stewardship model we introduced in Chapter 2 is usually applied at the national level in relation to obligations that states have towards those affected by their laws and policies. However, it is also reasonable to apply it at a much higher level. In the case of SARS in 2002/3, China was criticised for delays in reporting cases and an initial lack of cooperation with WHO.[102]

4.50 If a country fails to inform other countries of an outbreak of a serious infectious disease, the disease may spread more rapidly across the world. **Based on an application of the stewardship model** (paragraphs 2.41–2.44) **at the global level, countries have an ethical obligation to reduce the risk of ill health that people might impose on each other across borders. Therefore countries should notify other relevant countries and bodies about outbreaks of serious diseases at the earliest stage, following the relevant procedures laid out by WHO.** However, early detection of outbreaks requires an efficient surveillance system, and different countries at present have different capacities for surveillance, monitoring and reporting of infectious diseases. We note that both WHO and a Foresight report have identified a need for greater investment in surveillance capacity in poorer countries.[103] Guided by an application of the stewardship model (paragraphs 2.41–2.44) to the global context, we endorse this conclusion and recommend that **countries such as the UK should seek to enhance the capacities of developing countries to conduct effective surveillance of infectious diseases. The UK health departments, in liaison with the Department for International Development, should work to take this forward with international partners such as WHO, the European Centre for Disease Prevention and Control (ECDC) and the Centers for Disease Prevention and Control (CDC) in the USA.**

4.51 Gathering and passing on data related to infectious diseases that have pandemic potential is one important part of pandemic preparedness strategies, nationally and globally. The interests of many different parties may be affected by such activities, including: populations and governments of different countries, medical professionals, researchers, pharmaceutical companies and WHO. These interests can, however, come into conflict, and a controversy in early 2007 highlighted the fragility of global pandemic preparedness, when the Indonesian Government decided to suspend the sharing of clinical specimens of human avian influenza viruses with the surveillance system managed by WHO.[104]

4.52 Indonesia has had more cases of avian influenza in humans than any other country in recent years and is considered to be a country in which a pandemic of H5N1 influenza might emerge.[105] Indonesian officials ceased cooperation with the surveillance system managed by WHO over concerns that the country would not have reasonable access to the benefits resulting from its contribution to global pandemic surveillance.[106] In particular, it was suggested that any vaccines developed by pharmaceutical companies using the virus isolates processed and made available through the WHO system were unlikely to be available and affordable in developing countries.

---

[102] Fleck F (2003) How SARS changed the world in less than six months *Bull World Health Org* **81**(8): 625–6. Other examples are those of cholera, plague and yellow fever, which are supposed to be reported by all countries. However, WHO reports that countries are sometimes unwilling to notify it of cases because of the fear of economic and political consequences, such as the loss of tourism and trade, and the imposition of travel restrictions. WHO Department of Communicable Disease Surveillance and Response (2000) *WHO Report on Global Surveillance of Epidemic-prone Infectious Diseases*, available at: http://whqlibdoc.who.int/hq/2000/WHO_CDS_CSR_ISR_2000.1.pdf.

[103] Foresight (2006) *Infectious Diseases: Preparing for the future. Executive Summary* (London: Office of Science and Innovation); World Health Organization (2006) *Strengthening Pandemic-Influenza Preparedness and Response, including Application of the International Health Regulations (2005)*, available at: http://www.who.int/gb/ebwha/pdf_files/WHA59/A59_5-en.pdf.

[104] See WHO, *Global Influenza Surveillance*, available at: http://www.who.int/csr/disease/influenza/influenzanetwork/en/index.html.

[105] European Centre for Disease Prevention and Control (July 2007) *Interim ECDC Scientific and Public Health Briefing: Sharing influenza virus samples – July 2007* (Stockholm: ECDC), briefings available at: http://www.ecdc.eu.int/Health_topics/Seasonal%20Influenza/Guidance.html; World Health Organization (2007) *Areas with confirmed human cases of H5N1 avian influenza since 2003*, available at: http://gamapserver.who.int/mapLibrary/app/searchResults.aspx. As of 25 July 2007, the numbers of cases and deaths from H5N1 avian influenza, were 102 and 81, respectively; Viet Nam was the only other country to have over 50 cases.

[106] The Director-General of WHO subsequently thanked the Indonesian government for having "brought the very important issue to the world's attention, and that is access to pandemic influenza [vaccine] by resource-poor countries" CNN (2007) Interview with Dr Margaret Chan, available at: http://www.cnn.com/2007/WORLD/asiapcf/04/13/talkasia.chan.script/index.html.

Instead, Indonesian officials agreed a deal with a USA-based vaccine producer under which Indonesia would receive assistance with improving its capacity for vaccine production. It was reported in the media that the deal gave the company sole commercial rights for the use of virus isolates, and would therefore have prevented access to the isolates for sequencing, analysis and other purposes by WHO,[107] although the company involved has denied that this was the case.[108] There have also been suggestions that another company offered to purchase samples from Indonesia rather than obtaining the virus through the WHO system.[109] The lack of cooperation by Indonesia became a cause for serious concern because of the risk that it would severely hinder international surveillance and preparedness activities, and WHO made efforts to restore collaboration with this country. After several special meetings and a dedicated WHO Resolution[110] passed at the World Health Assembly in May 2007, cooperation briefly resumed; however, this was short-lived and the situation as of July 2007 was that no Indonesian samples were being sent to WHO Collaborating Centres.[111] The nature and details of the deal between Indonesia and the pharmaceutical company remains to be better defined at the time of writing, and many questions remain over details in the developments that led to Indonesia's initial decision to cease collaboration with WHO.

4.53 This case raises issues of considerable complexity about, among other things, intellectual property, global solidarity, and appropriate mechanisms and criteria for the fair and equitable sharing of vaccines and other benefits. We return later in the chapter to consider the issue of vaccine sharing and allocation in a pandemic (paragraphs 4.66–4.68), but for now we make two general observations about the responsibilities of the pharmaceutical industry and WHO in relation to surveillance.

4.54 Further to our observations on corporate social responsibility (paragraphs 2.47–2.50), the effect of commercial interests and intellectual property rights on public health surveillance measures requires careful consideration. From a purely commercial perspective it might be attractive for pharmaceutical companies to seek exclusive access to virus isolates.[112] However, even where such access is combined with measures aimed at benefit sharing, such as capacity-building initiatives, ethical issues still remain. The primary responsibility of pharmaceutical companies, as of any other larger commercial enterprise, is to their shareholders. It is possible therefore that commercial interests will be put before considerations of producing affordable vaccines for the people in developing areas that are most likely to be affected (especially in the early stages of a pandemic). Furthermore, commercial exclusivity would usually mean that access to virus isolates would be limited. Without access to these isolates, the numerous and important processes in which they would normally be used, such as surveillance for numbers of cases, emerging viruses and patterns of spread, would not be possible. Such developments would be detrimental to the ongoing surveillance work that has global benefits,[113] and

---

[107] *New Scientist* (16 February 2007) Poor countries hold out for vaccine, available at: http://www.newscientist.com/channel/health/mg19325914.600?DCMP=NLC-nletter&nsref=mg19325914.600.

[108] Baxter (7 February 2007) *Press Release: Baxter Continues Collaborations With Global Health Authorities To Advance Pandemic Preparedness*, available at: http://www.baxter.com/about_baxter/news_room/news_releases/2007/02-07-07-indonesia.html.

[109] European Centre for Disease Prevention and Control (April 2007) *Interim ECDC Scientific and Public Health Briefing: Sharing influenza virus samples – April 2007* (Stockholm: ECDC); European Centre for Disease Prevention and Control (July 2007) *Interim ECDC Scientific and Public Health Briefing: Sharing influenza virus samples – July 2007* (Stockholm: ECDC), briefings available at: http://www.ecdc.eu.int/Health_topics/Seasonal%20Influenza/Guidance.html.

[110] World Health Assembly (23 May 2007) *Resolution WHA60.28: Pandemic influenza preparedness: sharing of influenza viruses and access to vaccines and other benefits*, available at: http://www.who.int/gb/ebwha/pdf_files/WHA60/A60_R28-en.pdf.

[111] European Centre for Disease Prevention and Control (July 2007) *Interim ECDC Scientific and Public Health Briefing: Sharing influenza virus samples – July 2007* (Stockholm: ECDC), briefings available at: http://www.ecdc.eu.int/Health_topics/Seasonal%20Influenza/Guidance.html.

[112] While we note that it is unclear whether this occurred in the case of Indonesia (see paragraph 4.52), we address this scenario as one that could nevertheless be pursued in the future.

[113] WHO (2007) *The World Health Report 2007: A safer future* (Geneva: Switzerland).

therefore **we urge pharmaceutical companies not to enter into agreements with countries in a way that would potentially undermine the work of the WHO Global Influenza Surveillance Network.**[114] **WHO is in a unique position to enable centralised and transparent determination that a novel virus has emerged, to evaluate pandemic-related evidence, and to develop response strategies, as acknowledged in the** *International Health Regulations 2005.* **This capacity must be sustained.**

4.55 At the same time, it is important to recognise that cooperation between pharmaceutical companies and the WHO-administered surveillance system could also lead to inequalities in access to vaccines (see paragraphs 4.66–4.68). This would also be undesirable from a more technical public health perspective, as the early provision of vaccines to people in the outbreak area could play an important role in limiting or containing an emerging pandemic.[115] **WHO should not merely facilitate access to virus isolates for commercial companies, leaving the question of availability of vaccines to market forces. It should use its authority to impress on pharmaceutical companies their social responsibilities.** Patents and other forms of intellectual property rights can be useful ways of rewarding research investment and stimulating innovation and progress, but they can also come into conflict with the interests of the wider public, as the Council has reported elsewhere.[116] While we cannot address here all the complexities raised by the sharing of virus isolates for the purpose of monitoring and developing vaccines, virus isolates should not be treated like any ordinary commodity, as adequate access and use is of the greatest importance for public health, both on a national and global level. Therefore, **we urge WHO to explore, in liaison with governments and relevant industries, the notion of viewing virus isolates as a form of 'public good'** (paragraphs 1.8–1.10), **and to take a flexible approach to patenting and intellectual property protection.**

Control of infectious diseases

4.56 The control of different infectious diseases involves an extensive range of interventions. These may depend on the nature of the disease, how easily it is transmitted, the mode of transmission, the infectious period, the incubation period (i.e. the time from infection to the appearance of clinical disease), the population at risk, and the severity of its clinical manifestations. Many infections are relatively mild and often self-limiting, and although they may cause significant minor morbidity and be a major burden to the health services, they are not a major threat to population health. In this section, we focus on methods for the management of epidemics or cases of infectious diseases that pose a serious risk to those infected and which may affect the health of others by onward transmission of the infectious agent.

4.57 Measures implemented to tackle the SARS epidemic of 2002/2003 included isolation, quarantine, surveillance, contact tracing and restrictions or advisory warnings about travel (see Box 4.6). WHO judged that rigorous control schemes were responsible for the interruption of transmission in July 2003. However, measures such as these raise ethical issues, particularly about the acceptability of interventions that limit personal liberty for the sake of reducing the risk of disease to others.[117] Control measures such as isolation have also been used for individual cases of serious disease, such as smallpox and drug-resistant tuberculosis,

---

[114] We note that the terms of reference of the WHO Collaborating Centres and National Influenza Centres (which constitute the WHO Influenza Surveillance Network) are, at the time of writing, being revised under the recent WHA Resolution; World Health Assembly (23 May 2007) *Resolution WHA60.28: Pandemic influenza preparedness: sharing of influenza viruses and access to vaccines and other benefits,* available at: http://www.who.int/gb/ebwha/pdf_files/WHA60/A60_R28-en.pdf.

[115] A so-called rapid containment strategy, discussed further in paragraphs 4.65 and 4.68.

[116] Nuffield Council on Bioethics (2002) *The Ethics of Patenting DNA: A discussion paper* (London: Nuffield Council on Bioethics), available at: http://www.nuffieldbioethics.org/go/ourwork/patentingdna/introduction.

[117] For further discussion see: Gostin LO, Bayer R and Fairchild AL (2003) Ethical and legal challenges posed by severe acute respiratory syndrome *J Am Med Assoc* **290**: 3229–3237.

in order to minimise the risk of transmission to others.[118] Here we discuss, in particular, quarantine and isolation measures, and their ethical justification.

Box 4.6: SARS

In 2002/2003 an epidemic occurred of a new infectious disease, severe acute respiratory syndrome (SARS). The first known cases of SARS occurred in China in November 2002, and in total 8,098 cases were recorded in 26 countries, resulting in 774 known deaths.[119] China was criticised by WHO and countries internationally for delays in reporting cases and an initial lack of cooperation with WHO, which in March 2003 classified the disease as a global health threat.[120] This was one of the major precipitants to changes in the *International Health Regulations*, which were published in 2005.

The disease was highly contagious, there was initial uncertainty over the identity of the disease-causing agent and its epidemiology, such as the time and period of infectivity to others, and there was no definitive diagnostic test or effective vaccine or treatment.[121] These and other factors posed particular challenges in establishing an appropriate public health response.

During the epidemic, some countries implemented policies that severely restricted individual freedoms, as part of quarantine and isolation measures.[122] In Beijing around 30,000 people were quarantined,[123] mostly in their own homes, and two major hospitals were sealed, one of which held 2,000 employees and an unreported number of patients.[124] News reports suggested that in Toronto in Canada over 2,000 people who showed no symptoms of SARS were in quarantine at one point, and 141 health workers who showed no symptoms were in "working quarantine", meaning they worked with infected patients and had to take many precautions including isolating themselves from others in their homes.[125]

Additional measures were also put in place for people travelling between countries. For example, quarantine officers at ports of entry and exit in Canada were given the authority to ask a person suspected of having the disease to undergo a medical examination and to detain that person if necessary for up to 20 days (the maximum incubation period set out for SARS).[126] We note, however, that no such detentions were made for SARS, and the amendments to this regulation were made as a "precautionary measure".

Other consequences for individuals included those resulting from reduced travel, either where restrictions were in place or where individuals had voluntarily opted not to travel, and the postponement of some non-emergency medical care. More broadly there were financial implications due to disruption of travel, tourism, trade and production; it was estimated that the outbreak cost $12.3 billion in the Asian countries affected.[127] Healthcare workers also suffered particularly (most transmission was in hospitals); 73 (51%) of the 144 SARS patients included in one study in Canada were healthcare professionals.[128]

WHO has now published guidance on surveillance and management of a future SARS outbreak.[129] Many of the uncertainties that existed during the first outbreak have been resolved, and experience has been gained from this outbreak in dealing with the infection and other outbreaks involving similar infectious agents.[130]

---

[118] Public Health Laboratory Service (2002) Hospital acquired multi drug resistant tuberculosis *Commun Dis Rep CDR Wkly* [serial online] **12 (42)**, available at: www.hpa.org.uk/cdr/archives/2002/cdr4202.pdf.

[119] World Health Organization (2004) *WHO guidelines for the global surveillance of SARS, Updated recommendations, October 2004*, available at: http://www.who.int/csr/resources/publications/WHO_CDS_CSR_ARO_2004_1.pdf.

[120] *Ibid.*

[121] Zhong N and Zeng G (2006) What we have learnt from SARS epidemics in China *Br Med J* **333**: 389–91; Gerberding JL (2003) Faster ... but fast enough? Responding to the epidemic of severe acute respiratory syndrome *N Engl J Med* **348**: 2030–1.

[122] For further details about the quarantine schemes implemented in China and Taiwan, see: Centers for Disease Control and Prevention (2003) Efficiency of quarantine during an epidemic of severe acute respiratory syndrome – Beijing, China, 2003 *Morb Mortal Wkly Rep* **52**: 1037–40; Centers for Disease Control and Prevention (2003) Use of quarantine to prevent transmission of severe acute respiratory syndrome – Taiwan, 2003 *Morb Mortal Wkly Rep* **52**: 680–3.

[123] Centers for Disease Control and Prevention (2003) Efficiency of quarantine during an epidemic of severe acute respiratory syndrome – Beijing, China, 2003. *Morb Mortal Wkly Rep* **52**: 1037–40.

[124] *New York Times* (26 April 2003) The SARS epidemic: SARS; Beijing broadens SARS quarantine; more cases found, available at: http://query.nytimes.com/gst/fullpage.html?res=9B02E5DF153DF935A15757C0A9659C8B63&sec=health&pagewanted=1.

[125] CNN (27 May 2003) Toronto traces SARS cases to 96-year-old patient, available at: http://www.cnn.com/2003/HEALTH/05/26/sars.wrap/index.html.

[126] Public Health Agency of Canada (2003) *Fact Sheet: Quarantine Act and Regulations – SARS Amendment*, available at: http://www.phac-aspc.gc.ca/sars-sras-gen/fact_sheet.html.

[127] World Health Organization (2003) *Severe Acute Respiratory Syndrome (SARS)*, available at: http://www.wpro.who.int/sars/docs/RC54-08.pdf.

[128] Booth CM, Matukas LM, Tomlinson GA *et al.* (2003) Clinical features and short-term outcomes of 144 patients with SARS in the Greater Toronto area *J Am Med Assoc* **289**: 2801–9.

[129] World Health Organization (2004) *WHO guidelines for the global surveillance of SARS, Updated recommendations, October 2004*, available at: http://www.who.int/csr/resources/publications/WHO_CDS_CSR_ARO_2004_1.pdf.

[130] Zhong N and Zeng G (2006) What we have learnt from SARS epidemics in China *Br Med J* **333**: 389–91; Gerberding JL (2003) Faster ... but fast enough? Responding to the epidemic of severe acute respiratory syndrome *N Engl J Med* **348**: 2030–1.

Issues raised by quarantine and isolation

4.58 'Quarantine' refers to restrictions on the activities of a healthy person or group of people suspected of having been exposed to an infectious disease and who therefore might go on to develop it. 'Isolation' refers to restrictions on the activities of a person who is known to be infected, typically at a treatment centre where they can also receive appropriate medical care for the infection. In both cases the aim is to prevent or limit the transmission of disease. These two measures can operate either on a fairly large scale in the case of epidemics or pandemics, or on a smaller scale for individual cases of a serious disease, such as multi-drug-resistant tuberculosis.[131] An alternative measure that may be used in controlling epidemics or pandemics is that of 'social distancing', which would involve, for example, the closure of schools and workplaces, and avoiding large gatherings such as conferences and public events.[132] Although this measure may disrupt the lives of individuals within the population, it does not restrict liberty to the same extent as quarantine and isolation, and we focus here on these. Several respondents to the consultation expressed views on the acceptability of forcefully restricting the movement of people and when this might be acceptable (see Box 4.7).

Box 4.7: Consultation responses on proportionality and control measures

"Decision makers must balance individual freedom against the common good, fear for personal safety against the duty to treat the sick, and short term economic losses against the wider implications of the potential spread of serious diseases." *Health Protection Agency*

"To enforce someone into quarantine is imprisoning them and this can never be right, no matter what the circumstance. Governments could potentially quarantine people for reasons other than disease control, using disease as the reason, and this is a highly questionable practice." *Vaccination Awareness Network (VAN) UK*

"If an individual has a contagious infection and does not comply with treatment maybe then it would be appropriate to enforce quarantine. While it is an individual's choice to accept or not accept treatment, their choice has to have limits when it impinges on another person's right to health." *Fiona Reynolds*

"Quarantine or isolation is a reasonable and responsible action as long as it is in proportion to the seriousness of the disease." *JABS – Justice, Awareness and Basic Support*

4.59 It has been suggested that quarantine and isolation, and particularly the latter, can be an effective part of the control of a serious disease. (It has been suggested that quarantine may add little benefit where effective isolation strategies are in place, although this is likely to depend on many factors.[133]) Compulsory admission and detention in hospital of individual patients who pose a serious risk to the health of others and have refused to take precautions to prevent spread voluntarily is permitted in the UK under public health legislation,[134] and a few such cases have occurred in recent years.[135] In relation to isolation and quarantine in the case of epidemics or pandemics, at the time of writing, draft pandemic-planning documents

---

[131] Public Health Laboratory Service (2002) Hospital acquired multi drug resistant tuberculosis *Commun Dis Rep CDR Wkly* [serial online] **12** (42), available at: http://www.hpa.org.uk/cdr/archives/2002/cdr4202.pdf.

[132] World Health Organization (2005) *WHO Outbreak Communication: Influenza Pandemic*, available at: http://www.who.int/csr/don/Handbook_influenza_pandemic_dec05.pdf.

[133] These factors include some relating to the disease, such as how infectious the disease is and whether it can be transmitted before symptoms occur, and others relating to the society, such as how well the quarantine programme is adhered to. For further discussion see: Day T, Park A, Madras N, Gumel A and Wu J (2006) When is quarantine a useful control strategy for emerging infectious diseases? *Am J Epidemiol* **163**: 479–85. We note that, for example, an assessment of the efficiency of quarantine in controlling SARS suggests limiting its use to only where individuals had contact with actively ill patients (Centers for Disease Control and Prevention (2003) Efficiency of quarantine during an epidemic of severe acute respiratory syndrome- Beijing, China, 2003 *Morb Mortal Wkly Rep* **52**: 1037–40); Wynia MK (2007) Ethics and public health emergencies: restrictions on liberty *Am J Bioethics* **7**: 1–5.

[134] See Section 37 and 38 of the *Public Health (Control of Disease) Act 1984*, and Joint Tuberculosis Committee of the British Thoracic Society (2000) Control and prevention of tuberculosis in the United Kingdom: Code of Practice 2000 *Thorax* **55**: 887–901.

[135] Public Health Laboratory Service (2002) Hospital acquired multi drug resistant tuberculosis *Commun Dis Rep CDR Wkly* [serial online] **12** (42), available at: http://www.hpa.org.uk/cdr/archives/2002/cdr4202.pdf.

from both the Department of Health for England and the Scottish Executive stated that such measures would be "unsustainable after the first hundred or so cases".[136] Nevertheless, it is conceivable that they might be considered in the future.

4.60 Both quarantine and isolation have costs in terms of individual liberty. Quarantining is potentially the more costly of the two as it restricts the liberty of more individuals. In addition it risks placing some individuals who are not infected at a higher risk of becoming infected if groups of people are quarantined together and the disease is transmitted among them. In view of these issues, on the basis of proportionality considerations (see paragraph 3.18, also Box 4.7), quarantine would require a stronger justification than isolation. In addition we note that there is the potential that these types of measures could be implemented inappropriately or abused, or that people may be suspicious of potential abuses, for example, in countries with totalitarian regimes.

4.61 When isolation and quarantine measures are introduced, it may be that some individuals willingly accept their confinement. People who have been found to carry an infectious disease are likely to have a strong personal interest in receiving treatment, and may accept that this is provided in a context of isolation. However, other individuals may be less willing to be confined in this way, especially for diseases for which there are limited treatment options. They are effectively, in this circumstance, being held against their wishes.

4.62 **Liberty-infringing measures to control disease, such as compulsory quarantine and isolation, rank towards the top of the intervention ladder. The ethical justification for such measures involves weighing the classical harm principle on the one hand, and individual consent and the importance of avoiding intrusive interventions on the other** (paragraphs 2.13–2.15, 2.22–2.26, 2.43). **Where risk of harm to others can be significantly reduced, these considerations can be outweighed** (paragraph 3.18).

Use of vaccines in control of infectious diseases

4.63 Whereas the use and effectiveness of quarantine and isolation in an influenza pandemic may be limited, it has been suggested that vaccination has greater potential. In a pandemic context, vaccines have two principal roles: they may be used, first, in the local containment of the epidemic at an early stage (using existing stocks of pre-pandemic vaccine), in a so-called rapid containment strategy.[137] Secondly, they may be used more widely if the pandemic becomes established, initially by using existing stocks of pre-pandemic vaccine[138] and later using pandemic-specific vaccine, once this has been developed. The rapid containment strategy is most relevant in the countries where the epidemic is more likely to emerge, which are generally developing countries, while the use of pandemic-specific vaccines would be relevant worldwide. In 2007, Margaret Chan, Director-General of WHO, stated that "vaccines are the single most important medical intervention for reducing morbidity and mortality during an influenza pandemic".[139] However, the availability of both types of vaccine is

[136] Department of Health (2007) *Pandemic Influenza: A national framework for responding to an influenza pandemic – Draft for comment* (London: Department of Health); Scottish Executive Health Department (2007) *A National Framework for Responding to an Influenza Pandemic – Draft*, available at: http://www.scotland.gov.uk/Resource/Doc/170231/0047533.pdf. Note that a final version of this framework is due to be published in autumn 2007.

[137] A pre-pandemic vaccine, of a known strain, would not necessarily completely match the strain that emerges as the pandemic strain, but might be cross-reactive and therefore provide at least partial protection. The ECDC considers that this strategy could be feasible if the strain was the same subtype (i.e. H5). European Centre for Disease Prevention and Control (2007) *Technical Report: Expert advisory groups on human H5N1 vaccines – Scientific Questions*, available at: http://www.ecdc.eu.int/pdf/Sci%20Questions%20final.pdf.

[138] This vaccine is likely to provide only partial protection against the pandemic strain; however, the ECDC group's view is that it would be of some value even with protectiveness of as low as 15%. European Centre for Disease Prevention and Control (2007) *Technical Report: Expert advisory groups on human H5N1 vaccines – Public Health and Operational Questions*, available at: http://www.ecdc.eu.int/pdf/PH%20Questions%20final.pdf.

[139] Chan M (13 June 2007) *Address to the Pacific Health Summit: Pandemics – working together for an effective and equitable response*, available at: http://www.who.int/dg/speeches/2007/20070613_seattle/en/.

expected to be limited, and therefore difficulties arise in establishing how the available vaccine should be distributed, both on a national and international level.

4.64 There are many different options for allocation strategies.[140] We do not explore them here, but note that various considerations and principles might be involved, for example: even distribution across different sectors of the population; a 'fair innings' approach, whereby the youngest are given preference; focusing on reducing harms, 'fair chance' or saving-most-lives approaches; or preferential treatment of those most at risk through their occupation (healthcare workers) or those who perform critical duties (key workers).[141]

4.65 In the UK there are some stocks of a vaccine that could be considered for use in the pre-pandemic phase, and it is intended that these should be given to healthcare workers.[142] Once a pandemic emerges, it is anticipated that a further vaccine specific to the pandemic strain would be developed and manufactured,[143] but in the UK's draft pandemic framework there is no specific indication as to how these vaccines would be allocated even though clinical prioritisation is described as "inevitable".[144] We noted in paragraphs 2.27–2.32 the importance of public health programmes being sensitive towards health inequalities between different groups. It has been suggested that in the case of a pandemic some groups that are already disadvantaged are likely to experience a further and disproportionate burden as, for example, they may be assigned a low priority on allocation plans.[145] The implications of allocation strategies for disadvantaged groups therefore require careful consideration.

4.66 The international context of pandemics raises further issues relating to the availability of vaccines at a global level. First, rapid containment strategies, if employed, would require a large-scale vaccination programme in whichever country it was that the pandemic strain emerged. Secondly, the likely global scale of the disease would lead to demand for pandemic vaccines that is likely to far exceed their supply.[146] We noted above the concerns expressed by Indonesia that it would have little access to vaccines in the case of an influenza pandemic

---

[140] We note the work by WHO and others in seeking to establish criteria for allocating resources in situations of scarcity exacerbated by emergency. World Health Organization (2007) *Global Consultation on Addressing Ethical Issues in Pandemic Planning: Summary of Discussions*, available at: http://www.who.int/trade/Ethics_PI_consultation_report_WHO_2006.pdf; The Hastings Center (2006) *Bioethics Backgrounder: Flu Pandemic and the Fair Allocation of Scarce Life-Saving Resources: How can we make the hardest of choices?*, available at: http://www.thehastingscenter.org/pdf/avian_flu_backgrounder.pdf; University of Toronto Joint Center for Bioethics Pandemic Influenza Working Group (2005) *Stand on Guard for Thee. Ethical Considerations in Preparedness Planning for Pandemic Influenza*, available at: http://www.utoronto.ca/jcb/home/documents/pandemic.pdf.

[141] See also: Brock D and Wikler D (2006) Ethical issues in resource allocation and new product development, in *Disease Control Priorities in Developing Countries*, 2nd edition, Jamison DT, Breman JG, Measham AR *et al.* (Editors) (New York: Oxford University Press), pp.259–70.

[142] The UK stockpile includes 3.5 million doses. Department of Health (2007) *Pandemic influenza: A national framework for responding to an influenza pandemic – Draft for comment* (London: Department of Health).

[143] It is estimated that it would take four to six months for manufacturing of such a vaccine to begin, and that therefore they would not be ready in time for the first wave of the pandemic. Department of Health (2007) *Pandemic influenza: a national framework for responding to an influenza pandemic – Draft for comment* (London: Department of Health).

[144] The Department of Health's draft ethical framework for pandemic influenza lists seven general principles to draw on in the case of a pandemic, although these are not specifically discussed in relation to allocation of vaccine or treatment; See Department of Health (2007) *The Ethical Framework for the Response to Pandemic Influenza – Draft for Comment*, available at: http://www.dh.gov.uk/en/Publicationsandstatistics/Publications/PublicationsPolicyAndGuidance/DH_073179; Department of Health (2007) *Pandemic influenza: A national framework for responding to an influenza pandemic – Draft for comment* (London: Department of Health); Scottish Executive Health Department (2007) *A National Framework for Responding to an Influenza Pandemic – Draft*, available at: http://www.scotland.gov.uk/Resource/Doc/170231/0047533.pdf. Note that a final version of this framework is due to be published in autumn 2007.

[145] For example, the "entrenched poor, institutionized populations, and people with mental and physical disabilities." Gostin L (2007) Why should we care about social justice? *Hastings Cent Rep* **37**: 3. See also: Uscher-Pines L, Duggan PS, Garoon JP, Karron RA and Faden R (2007) Planning for an influenza pandemic – Social justice and disadvantaged groups *Hastings Cent Rep* **37**: 32–9.

[146] The WHO estimates suggest that there are likely to be enough pandemic vaccines for perhaps a quarter of the World's population and in addition these would not be available when they are first needed. Chan M (13 June 2007) *Address to the Pacific Health Summit: Pandemics – working together for an effective and equitable response*, available at: http://www.who.int/dg/speeches/2007/20070613_seattle/en/.

(see paragraphs 4.51–4.52), and similar concerns are reported to have been raised by other countries such as Thailand.[147] We also noted above that the burden of an influenza pandemic is expected to fall disproportionately on developing countries, and that therefore the international context of such an outbreak raises particular issues around equity, and these should clearly be considered in relation to vaccine distribution (see paragraph 4.2).

4.67 In response to the situation in Indonesia, in May 2007 the World Health Assembly (WHA) passed a Resolution[148] that intended, among other things, to promote the access of developing countries to pre-pandemic and specific pandemic influenza vaccines. The WHA Resolution calls on WHO's Director-General to:

> "formulate mechanisms and guidelines in close consultation with Member States aimed at ensuring fair and equitable distribution of pandemic influenza vaccines at affordable prices in the event of a pandemic in order to ensure timely availability of such vaccines to Member States in need."

While the aspiration behind this provision is commendable, we note several significant practical challenges to its implementation. First, there are problems over timeliness: manufacture of the pandemic vaccine will only begin a few months after the pandemic strain has been established, during which time the first wave of the infection may already have passed around the world. Secondly, there are problems over fairness and equity, given that the vaccine will become available progressively, not all at once, and that by WHO estimates there are likely to be enough pandemic vaccines for at most only a quarter of the world's population.[149] Thirdly, much of the present potential global pandemic vaccine capacity has already been committed for use in developed countries through contracts with the manufacturers.[150] One suggestion that has been made is that developed countries should make commitments to supply sufficient doses for healthcare and other key workers in developing countries, or alternatively that WHO receive additional resources to establish contracts for production of vaccine for developing countries. However, global solidarity might be seriously tested even in such a relatively straightforward case, given that the supply of vaccines to developing countries[151] would result in less access for people in developed countries.

4.68 We also draw attention to two further WHO initiatives relating to this Resolution. First, there is the establishment of an international stockpile of pre-pandemic vaccines for use by countries in need during a pandemic. At the time of writing, at least one pharmaceutical company had publicly offered to donate vaccines for this stockpile,[152] and we encourage continued cooperation and discussion between vaccine-producing companies, WHO and its member countries so that they are all partners in this endeavour.[153] This initiative is at a fairly

---

[147] *New Scientist* (16 February 2007) Poor countries hold out for vaccine, available at:
http://www.newscientist.com/channel/health/mg19325914.600?DCMP=NLC-nletter&nsref=mg19325914.600.

[148] World Health Assembly (23 May 2007) *Resolution WHA60.28: Pandemic influenza preparedness: sharing of influenza viruses and access to vaccines and other benefits*, available at: http://www.who.int/gb/ebwha/pdf_files/WHA60/A60_R28-en.pdf.

[149] Chan M (13 June 2007) *Address to the Pacific Health Summit: Pandemics – working together for an effective and equitable response*, available at: http://www.who.int/dg/speeches/2007/20070613_seattle/en/.

[150] European Centre for Disease Prevention and Control (July 2007) *Interim ECDC Scientific and Public Health Briefing: Sharing influenza virus samples – July 2007* (Stockholm: ECDC), briefings available at:
http://www.ecdc.eu.int/Health_topics/Seasonal%20Influenza/Guidance.html.

[151] *Ibid.*

[152] GlaxoSmithKline has offered to provide 50 million doses of vaccine. Chan M (13 June 2007) *Address to the Pacific Health Summit: Pandemics – working together for an effective and equitable response*, available at:
http://www.who.int/dg/speeches/2007/20070613_seattle/en/.

[153] We note that there can be potential difficulties in assembling a stockpile from multiple sources, and these should be taken into consideration. European Centre for Disease Prevention and Control (July 2007) *Interim ECDC Scientific and Public Health Briefing: Sharing influenza virus samples – July 2007* (Stockholm: ECDC), briefings available at:
http://www.ecdc.eu.int/Health_topics/Seasonal%20Influenza/Guidance.html.

early stage of development, and further issues to be considered will include policies on the allocation of these vaccines, management of the stockpile and practical arrangements for coordinating the stockpile and for the deployment of the vaccine. Secondly, the Resolution pledged to improve the manufacturing capacity for influenza vaccines in developing countries.[154] While we recognise that endeavours such as these are not without their challenges, we consider them to be important applications of the stewardship model (paragraphs 2.41–2.44, also paragraph 4.50) on a global scale, and encourage further work by WHO, the international community and pharmaceutical companies in this area.[155] Initiatives aimed at strengthening the systems for rapid administration and delivery of vaccines, whether from national production or stockpiles or made available through WHO, are also of crucial importance.

The importance of information in the case of an epidemic or pandemic

4.69 As we have discussed in other contexts, effective communication of risk is often central to the success of the public health response to disease (paragraphs 3.13–3.14). Once there is an outbreak of a harmful infectious disease on a scale that might justify restrictions of movement, the pressure on governments and health protection agencies to be seen to be 'doing something' is substantial. Downplaying the risk of the disease may lead to higher rates of infection. By contrast, a campaign that overstates the risks may lead to panic and lack of trust in healthcare professionals in the longer term.

4.70 The media has an important role to play in this.[156] We note and endorse one of the goals outlined in the UK's 2007 draft influenza pandemic framework: "Active media engagement to ensure that timely and accurate information and technical explanations are available to support informed reporting"[157] (see also paragraphs 4.34–4.35).

4.71 Information is important not only during an outbreak but also in planning for such scenarios. It is appropriate therefore that preparations should be made, and that these should include consultation and engagement with the public and other stakeholders. We note that another of the elements of the draft UK influenza pandemic framework is to encourage "prior public debate to explore the ethical, professional and practical implications of an influenza pandemic, condition public expectations and ensure that decisions are made in an inclusive and transparent way".[158] The Working Party endorses this approach.

---

[154] One aspect of this, which had already been in progress, is the use of grants for developing countries to improve capacity for producing vaccines, and grants to six countries have already been announced. WHO (2006) *Global Pandemic Influenza Action Plan to Increase Vaccine Supply*, available at: http://www.who.int/csr/resources/publications/influenza/CDS_EPR_GIP_2006_1.pdf; *WHO facilitates influenza vaccine technology transfer to developing countries*, available at: http://www.who.int/mediacentre/news/notes/2007/np18/en/index.html.

[155] We note that the Department of Health's draft ethical framework for pandemic flu comments on the need to "help other countries to fight a pandemic if it starts abroad"; Department of Health (2007) *The Ethical Framework for the Response to Pandemic Influenza – Draft for Comment*, available at: http://www.dh.gov.uk/en/Publicationsandstatistics/Publications/PublicationsPolicyAndGuidance/DH_073179. In addition the Department for International Development's 2007 health strategy commits to "strengthen the capacity of partner countries to plan for and manage emerging health challenges that affect poor people"; Department for International Development (2007) *Working Together for Better Health*, available at: http://www.dfid.gov.uk/Pubs/files/health-strategy07.pdf.

[156] See also World Health Organization (2005) *WHO Handbook for Journalists: Influenza pandemic*, available at: http://www.who.int/csr/don/Handbook_influenza_pandemic_dec05.pdf.

[157] Department of Health (2007) *Pandemic influenza: A national framework for responding to an influenza pandemic – Draft for comment* (London: Department of Health); Scottish Executive Health Department (2007) *A National Framework for Responding to an Influenza Pandemic – Draft*, available at: http://www.scotland.gov.uk/Resource/Doc/170231/0047533.pdf.

[158] *Ibid.*

4.72 **Where a potentially serious infectious disease outbreak or incident occurs, the relevant authorities should ensure that they neither downplay the risks, which may lead to higher rates of preventable infections, nor overstate the risks, as this may result in panic or a lack of public trust that could be long-lasting. The UK health departments and health protection agencies,[159] in particular, have a responsibility to ensure the timely provision of adequate and appropriate information about the nature of an infectious disease outbreak or incident, the type of interventions to be implemented and the rationale for their use.**

Summary

4.73 The principal ethical issue raised in relation to the prevention, surveillance and control of infectious diseases is how to reconcile consent and civil liberty concerns with community benefit. In the cases of infectious disease surveillance and control measures, we concluded that where harm to the population could be prevented through implementing measures that restrict civil liberties (isolation and quarantining) and challenge the notion of individual consent, this may be justified, particularly when the risks to the individual are minimal and/or the potential harms to others are substantial. We noted that it would be inappropriate to deny use of anonymised samples for epidemiological research and monitoring of trends in infectious disease, because it is unclear that there are significant harms involved where the data are suitably anonymised and this is the most effective way of ensuring thorough assessment and prediction of the risks of infectious diseases.

4.74 Regarding vaccination policy, we focused on vaccines given across the population both to protect individuals and to achieve or maintain population immunity. Here we concluded that in general, voluntary vaccine programmes should be preferred, but more coercive policies might be acceptable in some circumstances, depending on the risks of the vaccination, the seriousness of the disease, the degree of coerciveness involved, and the benefit to the community of implementing such a policy.

4.75 The international context of infectious disease requires consideration, perhaps more than in other areas of public health considered in this Report, and especially in relation to surveillance and control measures. We commented on the need for well-functioning surveillance systems for infectious diseases, and the central role of WHO in, for example, managing systems for receiving and distributing information and biological material (such as virus isolates), and ensuring transparent criteria for the allocation of vaccines internationally in the case of a pandemic.

CHAPTER 4 CASE STUDY – INFECTIOUS DISEASE

---

[159] By this we refer to the Health Protection Agency, Health Protection Scotland, the National Public Health Service for Wales and the Communicable Disease Surveillance Centre (Northern Ireland).

Chapter 5
Case study – Obesity

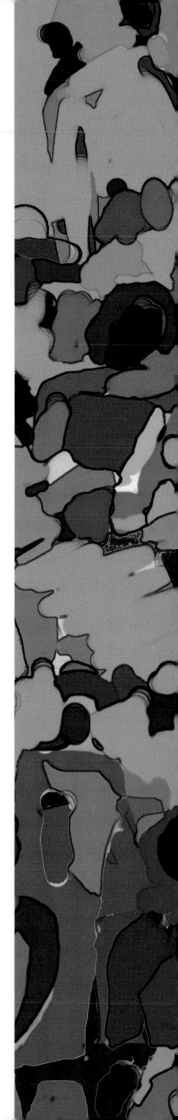

Case study – Obesity

Introduction

5.1 The prevalence of obesity has increased dramatically over the past few decades in the UK and in many other countries, and being overweight or obese is a risk factor for several other health conditions. In this chapter we discuss the public health issues raised by obesity and outline the complex range of factors contributing to the prevalence of obesity.[1] We comment on relevant ethical issues, considering in particular whether people are able to make genuine choices about the types of food they eat and the amount of physical activity they take, and how environmental and other constraints impact upon those choices. The focus of this chapter is on the roles and responsibilities of various agents including: individuals; the government; industries such as those that produce, market and sell food and drinks; and industries involved in the designing of buildings, towns and transport networks. Consideration is also given to protecting vulnerable groups, especially children.

Obesity: impact upon health, prevalence and causes

5.2 There are several definitions of 'obese'. The Royal Society suggests that a person who is obese has an "excess of body fat that imparts a health risk."[2] Although this is a useful conceptual definition, it is of more limited use in practical terms. A widely accepted, although not uncontested,[3] definition is that of the World Health Organization (WHO), based on 'body mass index' (BMI), which is a measure of weight relative to height (see Box 5.1).

Box 5.1: The body mass index (BMI) measurement

BMI = weight (in kilograms) divided by height (in metres) squared

$$= \frac{weight(kg)}{height(m)^2}$$

***WHO definitions for adults**[4]

Underweight	BMI < 18.5
Normal range	BMI = 18.5 to 24.9
Overweight	BMI ≥ 25
Obese	BMI ≥ 30

BMI should only be considered as an approximate guide to overweight and obesity because it may not correspond to the same level of fat in different individuals. For example, differences in distribution of fat around the body, higher or lower than average amounts of muscle, and ethnic differences may mean that people with the same BMI have different levels of fat, and this may affect the associated health risks.

Effects of obesity on health

5.3 There is evidence from epidemiological research that obesity is an important risk factor for a wide range of chronic diseases, including type 2 diabetes, hypertension, coronary heart disease,

---

[1] We note that there is a spectrum between being slightly overweight and being obese. Generally speaking, the more overweight a person is, the higher are the health risks from the range of conditions outlined in this chapter.

[2] Royal Society (2006) *Report of Royal Society Policy Seminar on the Scientific Understanding of Obesity* (London: The Royal Society).

[3] We acknowledge that there are difficulties with the BMI measurement (see Box 5.1), but because it is in such wide current use, we adopt it as the current, if imperfect, operational scale. We note that other measures, including those of central adiposity, may in future prove more valuable in predicting health risks associated with obesity.

[4] World Health Organization, *BMI Classification*, available at: http://www.who.int/bmi/index.jsp?introPage=intro_3.html.

stroke, osteoarthritis, some cancers, respiratory dysfunction, liver dysfunction, gall-bladder diseases and metabolic syndrome.[5] As with any epidemiological correlation, separating the effects on health of obesity from the associated effects of other factors such as lack of physical exercise and poor nutrition is not straightforward.[6] Nevertheless, globally, being either overweight or obese has been estimated to be the seventh most significant risk factor for mortality and the eighth most significant risk factor for disease.[7] As an example, it has been estimated that 30,000 deaths a year in England are attributable to obesity and that deaths linked to obesity shorten life by an average of nine years.[8]

Prevalence of obesity

5.4 Obesity is increasingly common in developed countries (see Box 5.2).[9] The prevalence of obesity in children under eleven years old in England increased from 9.9% in 1995 to 13.7% in 2003.[10] Generally, prevalence in England has trebled since the 1980s,[11] to 23% of both men and women in 2004.[12] Similar trends have occurred in Scotland and Northern Ireland, where the proportion of adults who were obese in 2003 was 24% in both countries.[13] The prevalence in Wales is lower, at 18%.[14] According to research commissioned by the Department of Health for England it is predicted that, if current trends continue unchanged, in 2010 the proportion of adults in England who are obese would reach approximately 30%.[15] Although there are some exceptions, there are general patterns of obesity across wealth and social groups in developed and developing countries: in developed countries, obesity is more prevalent among people in lower socio-economic groups, whereas in developing countries it is more common in higher socio-economic groups (see also Boxes 5.5 and 5.6).

Understanding the causes of obesity

5.5 Although it may seem at first that individuals are exclusively responsible for their own food intake and exercise levels, and consequently their weight, closer analysis reveals that this is too simplistic, as a complex mix of factors contribute to weight gain. Understanding the causes of

[5] See, for example, National Audit Office (2001) *Tackling Obesity in England* (London: The Stationery Office); Hu G, Tuomilehto J, Silventoinen K *et al.* (2005) The effects of physical activity and body mass index on cardiovascular, cancer and all-cause mortality among 47,212 middle-aged Finnish men and women *Int J Obes* **29**: 894–902; Calle EE, Thun MJ, Petrelli JM, Rodriguez C and Heath CW (1999) Body-mass index and mortality in a prospective cohort of US adults *N Engl J Med* **341**: 1097–105.

[6] Hu G, Tuomilehto J, Silventoinen K, Barengo N and Jousilahti P (2004) Joint effects of physical activity, body mass index, waist circumference and waist-to-hip ratio with the risk of cardiovascular disease among middle-aged Finnish men and women *Eur Heart J* **25**: 2212–9.

[7] The risk factors for mortality are (in order, starting with the highest risk and listing those higher than overweight and obesity): high blood pressure, smoking, high cholesterol, child underweight for age, unsafe sex, low fruit and vegetable intake. The risk factors for disease burden are (in order, starting with the highest risk and listing those higher than overweight and obesity): child underweight for age, high blood pressure, unsafe sex, smoking, alcohol use, high cholesterol, unsafe water, sanitation and hygiene. See Lopez AD, Mathers CD, Ezzati M, Jamison DT and Murray CJL (2006) Global and regional burden of disease and risk factors, 2001: systematic analysis of population health data *Lancet* **367**: 1747–57.

[8] National Audit Office (2001) *Tackling Obesity in England* (London: The Stationery Office), p.1.

[9] *Ibid.*

[10] Figures are only available for children from 1995. Department of Health, *Obesity*, available at: http://www.dh.gov.uk/en/Policyandguidance/Healthandsocialcaretopics/Obesity/index.htm.

[11] *Ibid.*

[12] NHS (2005) *Health Survey for England 2004: The Health of Minority Ethnic Groups – headline tables*, available at: http://www.ic.nhs.uk/webfiles/publications/hlthsvyeng2004ethnic/HealthSurveyForEngland161205_PDF%20.pdf.

[13] Sprosten K and Shelton N (Editors) (2005) *The Scottish Health Survey 2003 Volume 2: Adults* (Scottish Executive); Department of Health, Social Services and Public Safety (2007) *Northern Ireland Health and Social Wellbeing Survey 2005/06 Topline Results*, available at: http://www.dhsspsni.gov.uk/hwb_topline_bulletin.pdf.

[14] Health of Wales Information Service (2006) *Welsh Health Survey 2004/05*, available at: http://www.wales.nhs.uk/newsitem.cfm?contentid=5137.

[15] Zaninotto P, Wardle H, Stamatakis E, Mindell J and Head J (2006) *Forecasting Obesity to 2010*, available at: http://www.dh.gov.uk/en/Publicationsandstatistics/Publications/PublicationsStatistics/DH_4138630.

Box 5.2: The prevalence of obesity in the UK and internationally

The UK currently has the highest prevalence of obesity within Europe (23%), with France having the lowest (7%). The USA has the highest prevalence of obesity of any country in the developed world (39%), although some Polynesian islands such as Samoa have an even higher prevalence (48%).

Projections from WHO indicate that globally in 2005 approximately 1.6 billion adults (age 15+) were overweight and at least 400 million were obese. WHO predicts that by 2015 approximately 2.3 billion adults will be overweight and more than 700 million will be obese. Current figures indicate that, globally, at least 20 million children under the age of five are overweight.[16]

Prevalence of obesity in the adult populations of selected countries (2005)*

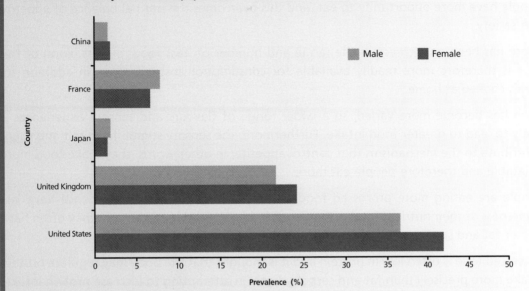

*Source: World Health Organization *Global InfoBase Online*, available at: http://www.who.int/infobase/comparestart.aspx. Reproduced with permission. Prevalences are age-standardised estimates by country for ages 15+ years.

obesity is important for policy and practice aimed at preventing or alleviating excess weight gain, and for examining the ethical issues involved. Understanding the extent to which individuals are able to make genuine choices is also important for discussion of the rights and responsibilities of individuals, industries and the state.

5.6 When more energy is consumed than expended, the excess energy is laid down as fat, and if this process continues over a period of time, the result is an increase in BMI. Although this describes simply the process at the individual level, it is important for public health policy to identify the interventions that might be most effective in preventing or treating obesity at the population level. Yet the underlying factors that contribute to the increase in obesity at the population level are not well understood. Is the root of the problem people eating too much, not using up enough energy or a complex mixture of both? Below, we explore some of the changes relating to food and activity that have occurred in recent years. Additionally, what is the influence of genetics? The speed with which the prevalence of obesity has increased is often thought to show that heritable factors are not relevant. However, studies have indicated that genetic makeup could contribute significantly to the differences in BMI between different individuals.[17] Changing societal and environmental factors, such as availability of food and changes in diet (see below), may have different effects on different individuals depending on their genetic make up.

---

[16] See Box 5.1 for definitions used by WHO. World Health Organization (2006) *Factsheet: Obesity and overweight*, available at: http://www.who.int/mediacentre/factsheets/fs311/en/index.html.

[17] Farooqi IS and O'Rahilly S (2007) Genetic factors in human obesity *Obes Rev* **8** (Suppl. 1): 37–40.

5.7 On the intake side of the energy equation (how much energy is consumed compared with how much is expended), there are several (not mutually exclusive) hypotheses to explain what might have changed in the past few decades:[18]

■ The energy density of food has increased, and this 'short-circuits' normal satiety mechanisms.

■ Food, especially food high in fat and sugar, has become cheaper and more available, so people have more opportunity to eat, and this overcomes the normal balance of appetite and satiety.

■ There has been an increase in the range and number of 'fast food' outlets. Food of this type is therefore more readily available for consumption instead of, or in addition to, meals cooked at home.

■ Food has become more varied, so a wider range of flavours and sensory experiences is likely to lead to greater food intake. Furthermore, the sensory stimuli from salt and sugar contribute to the mechanisms that control appetite; in other words, they make food more palatable and therefore people eat more.

■ People are eating more processed food and are eating out more, and hence have less awareness of their nutrient intake. Processed food and food in restaurants may often have higher fat and sugar content than that prepared in the home.

■ Processed food is often low in protein and it is thought that the body may regulate protein intake more precisely than fat and carbohydrate. In attempting to increase protein intake, excess carbohydrate and fat is taken in as a side effect. Protein is recognised to induce a greater sense of satiety than fat or carbohydrate, and therefore a diet low in protein may lead to a person consuming more in order to achieve satiety.

■ Portion sizes have increased.[19]

■ Home life has changed, and there is some evidence that working parents are less likely to cook more traditional, balanced meals. One reason for this is that many people, especially women, are under greater time constraints than they used to be. Additionally, there has been a loss of cooking skills.[20]

■ Energy-dense foods are heavily advertised and marketed, especially to children.

5.8 On the expenditure side of the equation there are similarly several factors that contribute to what have increasingly been called 'obesogenic' environments that are less conducive to energy expenditure:

■ Patterns and modes of transport have changed, for example, from foot or bicycle to car or other forms of motorised transport. Many planning decisions have resulted in increased use of private vehicles and increased distances from homes to schools, shops, leisure facilities and workplaces, making it difficult to walk or cycle. At the same time, underinvestment in public transport and cycle lanes has discouraged walking or cycling.

■ Manual labour has largely been replaced by sedentary jobs and by mechanisation.

---

[18] For a discussion of some other possible contributing factors to the increase in obesity, see Keith SW, Redden DT, Katzmarzyk PT et al. (2006) Putative contributors to the secular increase in obesity: exploring the roads less travelled *Int J Obes* **30**: 1585–94.

[19] Prentice AM (2001) Overeating: the health risks *Obes Res* **9**: 234S–8S.

[20] One study in the USA has indicated that a child is more likely to be overweight if his/her mother worked more hours per week over the child's life. This trend appeared to particularly affect mothers with higher socio-economic status whose work intensity is particularly disadvantageous for their children's overweight status. Anderson PM, Butcher KF and Levine PB (2003) Maternal employment and overweight children *J Health Econ* **22**: 477–504.

■ Parental concerns about the safety of children have led to reductions in outdoor play and walking or cycling to school.

■ Public and private buildings often include more lifts, moving walkways and escalators.

■ Labour-saving devices in the home have reduced energy expenditure. Central heating encourages people to be less active in the home and may mean that people expend less energy keeping warm.[21]

■ Television, computers and other forms of sedentary entertainment have largely replaced active play among children and teenagers.

5.9 As we have described, obesity is likely to result from a complex mix of causes and the available evidence does not reveal their relative importance at a population level.[22] Likewise, evidence for the efficacy and cost effectiveness of interventions to prevent or treat obesity is very incomplete. There are a limited number of pharmaceutical treatments available to assist people to lose weight. However, these often have side effects and effectiveness is varied. Developing improved pharmaceutical treatments for obesity is an active area of research. Additionally, certain surgical procedures have successfully helped some people to lose weight, although again these often involve considerable risks to the individual concerned.

5.10 Incomplete evidence for the effectiveness of policy options should not be used by industry and government as an excuse for inaction (see paragraphs 3.37–3.38, also paragraph 3.17). We present below a discussion of the responsibilities of various parties and make recommendations for policy that would be desirable under our ethical framework (see Chapters 2 and 3).

The challenge of reducing obesity

5.11 Because of the many factors involved, there is no single 'magic bullet' to reduce obesity, and effective strategies are likely to incorporate many small changes implemented over a long time period by many different agencies. For example, the National Institute for Health and Clinical Excellence (NICE), in a series of recommendations about how to prevent, identify, assess and manage overweight and obesity, targeted the NHS, local authorities and partners, early years settings, schools, workplaces, self-help, commercial and community settings.[23] Given that the prevalence of obesity is expected to rise in the next few years, to bring about any large reduction in mean BMI might require very coercive measures that are unlikely to be politically acceptable. Thus, there is a risk that strategies that could potentially achieve a small decrease in obesity (or even a decrease in the rate of increase of obesity), and therefore benefit some people, might not be implemented by governments. An additional difficulty is that changes are likely to take many years to produce results because food and physical activity habits are deeply ingrained in social and individual patterns of behaviour.[24] People's behaviours may, at least in part, be dependent on the built environment and other factors

---

[21] Keith SW, Redden DT, Katzmarzyk PT *et al.* (2006) Putative contributors to the secular increase in obesity: exploring the roads less travelled *Int J Obes* 30: 1585–94.

[22] Even the basic question of whether energy intake has gone up or expenditure gone down in recent decades is unresolved. At face value, the National Diet and Nutrition Survey indicates that energy intake for men has gone down over the past 15 years, although analysis of under-reporting shows that obese people under-report consumption by over 30% and lean people under-report by about 20%. This could arise for a variety of reasons, for instance because people fail to report snacks (e.g. biscuits and cakes) eaten between meals as part of their daily intake. See Office for National Statistics, Medical Research Council Human Nutrition Research and Food Standards Agency (2004) *The National Diet and Nutrition Survey: Adults aged 19 to 64 years Volume 5: Summary Report*, available at: http://www.food.gov.uk/multimedia/pdfs/ndns5full.pdf.

[23] National Institute for Health and Clinical Excellence (2006) *Obesity: The prevention, identification, assessment and management of overweight and obesity in adults and children*, available at: http://www.nice.org.uk/guidance/CG43#summary.

[24] Although we note that the contemporary rise in obesity has been remarkably rapid. It appears that changes in habits or diet that increase obesity are easier to bring about than those aimed at reducing obesity.

that are only likely to be changed slowly. For individuals, it also takes time to actively reduce obesity. For the government, policies with potential long-term benefits are difficult to reconcile with short-term priorities, but they should not be ignored.

5.12 The notion of individual choice, responsibility and autonomy is especially difficult to apply in relation to obesity. There are barriers for people wishing to achieve behaviour change, as we discuss in paragraphs 3.35–3.36. People's personal behaviour 'choices' are to a substantial degree shaped by their environment, which in turn is heavily influenced by local authorities and national government, industry and others (see paragraphs 1.4, 3.20–3.21). Therefore, policies based on education, information and individual choice alone are not likely to succeed either in reducing inequalities or in reducing prevalence of obesity in the population as a whole. With regard to implementing policies that aim to target interventions to treat or prevent obesity deliberately at specific groups, policy makers would need to be sensitive to the risk of stigmatisation, or of excluding those whose health is at risk, but who lie outside the target groups (see paragraphs 3.29–3.34). For these reasons, the strategies we recommend below are based on the roles and responsibilities in relation to food and the environment that we think various different parties should take based on our ethical framework (see Chapters 2 and 3). They include measures that are aimed both at helping people to make healthier choices and at changing the factors in our environment that contribute to obesity at the population level.

Roles of different parties in reducing obesity

5.13 Many parties could take some responsibility for responding to the problem of obesity, including central and local government, institutions such as schools and employers, charities and the voluntary sector, the corporate sector, and families and individual citizens. Several respondents to the consultation expressed strong views on whether such agents should intervene on the issue of food selection, for example, as illustrated by the following:

"Choosing food is one of the most personal choices. Attempting to justify political intervention into this area of personal choice is wrong. A person's lifestyle is their own, and in a truly free society, individuals should be free to choose what experts may think of as a wrong choice. It is not the place of government or indeed health officials to pronounce on lifestyle choices." *Anon*

"Why would anyone think that attempts to influence people's eating habits were *particularly* intrusive? If we confine ourselves to the promotion of healthy eating, and (potentially) to legislation aimed at food manufacturers to design and market their products responsibly, I don't think there are any special sensitivities connected with food to be taken into account." *Dr Peter Lucas*

5.14 We highlighted in Chapter 2 the reasons why the Working Party regards making genuine choices as an integral part of living a meaningful and autonomous life (see paragraphs 2.19, 3.20–3.21). However, we have also noted powerful constraints on choice, imposed by the environment in which people (have to) live (see paragraph 1.4). The interactions between individuals and their environment are therefore such that the government acts as a *facilitator* of choices: for example, urban planning policies may encourage or discourage walking or cycling, and regulations imposed on food and drinks industries might influence the availability of foods with different nutritional profiles. However, while government policies establish the 'playing field', responsibilities of the food and drink industries involved in producing, marketing and selling products go further than simply complying with mandatory regulations.

Role of the food and drink industries – corporate social responsibility

5.15 Consumers' choices of food and drink are at least partly driven by the products available and the way they are promoted, priced and distributed. Consultation responses included the following observations on the responsibilities of corporations:

> "We feel that manufacturers who produce foods high in salt, fat, sugar and also those who produce tobacco and alcohol should be fully responsible for any harm caused from the use of their products." *British Association for the Study of Community Dentistry*

> "Food industry should price healthy options more competitively and provide clear labelling." *PR Myles*

5.16 Although the regulation of industry can be necessary, much can be achieved through industry self-regulation. There are several examples where voluntary commitments may lead to healthier choices being offered to consumers. For example, although there has been criticism of the speed of implementation, the Food and Drink Federation has pledged that its members would reduce levels of fat, salt and sugar in their products.[25] Some major UK retailers made a commitment early in 2007 to stop adding trans-fats to their own-brand products to help cut rates of heart disease and obesity.[26] Such initiatives form an important part of corporate social responsibility and are to be encouraged.

5.17 We noted in Chapter 2, however, that it is not always clear whether corporate social responsibility initiatives are driven by governance or marketing aims, as some companies may simply seek to establish themselves as providers of healthier food because they perceive an associated market advantage (see paragraphs 2.47–2.50). It might be considered naïve, therefore, to appeal to corporate social responsibility as, ultimately, companies are concerned primarily with maximising returns. We make three observations in this respect. First, in practice what matters is whether healthier foods are available. If companies are offering this for 'the wrong reasons', namely for purely economic ones, a more healthy option has nevertheless been made available. Secondly, in seeking market advantages through being known as a provider of healthier food, companies might also contribute to a shift in attitudes, and more people may become aware of the importance of a healthy and balanced diet. Lastly, there are concerns that industry will generally be reluctant to adopt corporate social responsibility because this might have negative effect on their returns. Although major returns are made on unhealthy foods, it is not necessarily true that healthier options will always be less economically attractive. Hence, drawing on our discussion, it is reasonable to appeal to industries to explore as creatively as possible the options of improving the nutritional values of foods.

5.18 We focus below on two specific examples: the promotion to children of foods and drinks high in fat, salt and sugar, which raises important ethical issues because children constitute an especially vulnerable group (see Chapter 2); and the labelling and composition of food. We then consider issues about corporate social responsibility as it relates to the food industry more generally. We have identified the implementation of information and education strategies, and the avoidance, where possible, of coercive measures, as being important overarching themes in good public health policy (see Chapters 2 and 3). In policy terms, initiatives in these two areas are of further significance because their influence is designed to be primarily *preventative* rather than *curative*. Although limited at this time, there is some evidence to suggest that initiatives to prevent obesity are effective and may also be cost-effective.[27]

[25] See Food and Drink Federation, *Policy Position on Reformulation*, available at: http://www.fdf.org.uk/keyissues.aspx?issue=558; see also BBC News (2004) *Firms to cut salt in sliced bread*, 1 July, available at: http://news.bbc.co.uk/1/hi/health/3855807.stm.

[26] British Retail Consortium (2007) Press release: BRC Retailers' Action on Fats Cuts through Legislative Impotence, 31 Jan, available at: http://www.brc.org.uk/details04.asp?id=1081&kCat=&kData=1.

[27] Brown T, Kelly S and Summerbell C (2007) Prevention of obesity: a review of interventions *Obes Rev* **8** (Suppl. 1): 127–30; National Institute for Health and Clinical Excellence (2006) *Obesity: The prevention, identification, assessment and management of overweight and obesity in adults and children*, Section 6: Health economics, pp.773–81.

Food advertising to children

5.19 Advertising food and drink products to children raises the fundamental issue of whether it should be acceptable at all for companies to try to influence the diets of vulnerable groups, and whether restrictions on the industry are justified. In 2003, the Food Standards Agency (FSA) published a review of research examining the way foods are promoted to children and the effects that this promotion has on children's preferences and behaviour. The *Review of Research on the Effects of Food Promotion to Children* (more commonly known as the Hastings Review) concluded that food advertising had some effect which, although small, operates both on choice of food category and on brand selection.[28]

5.20 Reviewers commissioned by the Food Advertising Unit[29] disputed the robustness of the evidence used in the Hastings Review and argued that it paid insufficient attention to the extent to which children's diets are influenced by other factors such as the home environment, school and peers.[30] The Food Advertising Unit reports were subsequently rejected by the FSA after further review processes.[31] There followed further publications on the subject[32] and debate in the media.

5.21 In 2007, the communications regulatory authority, Ofcom[33], introduced restrictions on television advertising of food and drink products high in fat, salt[34] and sugar (HFSS), so as to reduce children's exposure to these advertisements.[35] The new measures included a ban on HFSS food and drink advertisements in and around all children's programmes and during programmes that attract a significantly higher than average proportion of viewers under the age of 16 years. Some health campaigners and lobby groups thought that the restrictions were insufficient, and argued for a 9.00 p.m. watershed, before which the advertising of HFSS foods should be prohibited.[36] Conversely, some representatives of the food, advertising and broadcasting industries stated that the restrictions were too stringent.[37] In April 2007 the Committee for

[28] Hastings G, Stead M, McDermott L et al. (2003) *Review of Research on the Effects of Food Promotion to Children* (Food Standards Agency), available at: http://www.food.gov.uk/multimedia/pdfs/foodpromotiontochildren1.pdf.

[29] The Food Advertising Unit was set up under the auspices of the Advertising Association, see http://www.fau.org.uk. The Advertising Association is a trade federation representing the advertising and promotional marketing industries. It is a non-profit-making company, funded by a combination of subscriptions, donations and revenue-raising activities.

[30] Paliwoda S and Crawford I (2003) *An Analysis of the Hastings Review: "The Effects of Food Promotion on Children"*, available at: http://www.fau.org.uk/hastings_review_analysis_dec03.pdf; Young B (2003) *Advertising and Food Choice in Children: A Review of the Literature* (Food Advertising Unit), available at: http://www.fau.org.uk/brian_youngliteraturereview.pdf.

[31] Food Standards Agency (2003) *Outcome of academic seminar to review recent research on food promotion and children*, available at: http://www.food.gov.uk/multimedia/webpage/academicreview; Food Standards Agency, *Outcome of the review exercise on the Paliwoda and Crawford paper: An Analysis of the Hastings Review: "The Effects of Food Promotion on Children"*, available at: http://www.food.gov.uk/multimedia/pdfs/paliwodacritique.pdf.

[32] See World Health Organization (2006) *Marketing of Food and Non-alcoholic Beverages to Children: Report of a WHO Forum and Technical Meeting* (Oslo, Norway, 2–5 May 2006), available at: http://www.who.int/dietphysicalactivity/publications/Oslo%20meeting%20layout%2027%20NOVEMBER.pdf; World Health Organization Europe (2006) *WHO European Ministerial Conference on Counteracting Obesity* (Istanbul, Turkey, 15–17 November 2006), available at: http://www.euro.who.int/Document/E89567.pdf.

[33] The Office of Communications (Ofcom) is the independent regulator and competition authority for the UK communications industries. Its remit includes television, radio, telecommunications and wireless communications services.

[34] Some of the foods included in the restrictions are high in salt, which is an issue for dietary health separate from obesity.

[35] Ofcom (17 November 2006) Press Release: *New restrictions on the television advertising of food and drink products to children*, available at: http://www.ofcom.org.uk/media/news/2006/11/nr_20061117; Ofcom (22 February 2007) Press Release: *Ofcom publishes final Statement on the television advertising of food and drink products to children*, available at: http://www.ofcom.org.uk/media/news/2007/02/nr_20070222. Previously, televised children's food advertisements had been dominated by foods considered to be, or classified as, 'unhealthy', including certain breakfast cereals, confectionery, savoury snacks, soft drinks and food from fast-food outlets. Hastings G, Stead M and McDermott L (2003) *Review of Research on the Effects of Food Promotion to Children* (Food Standards Agency), available at: http://www.food.gov.uk/multimedia/pdfs/foodpromotiontochildren1.pdf.

[36] See BBC News (2006) *Junk Food Ad Crackdown Announced*, 17 November, available at: http://news.bbc.co.uk/1/hi/health/6154600.stm; National Heart Forum (2006) *Initial Response to OFCOM Announcement on Restrictions of Junk Food Advertising to Children*, available at: http://www.heartforum.org.uk/News_Media_pressreleases_PressRelease_OFCOM.aspx.

[37] Food Advertising Unit, The Advertising Association (2006) *FAU Position on Final Ofcom Consultation: Food and drink advertising to children – extension to under 16s*, available at: http://www.fau.org.uk/FAU_response_to_final_Ofcom_consultation__22.12.06_.pdf.

Advertising Practice announced restrictions, but not a ban, on food and drink advertising to children in non-broadcast media, for example print and press adverts, posters and cinema commercials, as a response "to public concern about rising levels of childhood obesity".[38]

5.22 The example of food advertising to children illustrates that the judgement about a proportionate level of action cannot be determined in a formulaic way. Whether to intervene is a complex decision, not least because the evidence base is incomplete. However, evidence shows that children's early diet affects their health later in life, and that obesity in childhood is strongly associated with obesity in adulthood.[39] Additionally, we consider that children are especially vulnerable because they are more susceptible to external influences, including marketing by industry, and they have limited control and ability to make genuine choices.[40] Children need special protection from harm. Parental influence is central, but other parties have an ethical duty to support parents. Many food and drink companies have established principles of corporate social responsibility. These should be reviewed to ensure that they include appropriate provisions for the protection of children.

5.23 Due to the special vulnerability of children it would be desirable not to advertise to children foods high in fat, salt and sugar by any medium, including on the Internet.[41] The stewardship-guided state should aim to protect children from harm and provide an environment in which they can lead healthy lives. An example of the way in which the state might intervene includes regulation of the promotion of unhealthy foods and drinks to children, if industry fails to adequately regulate itself. A study in Australia published in 2006 suggested that this may be a particularly cost-effective way of reducing obesity in children.[42] We note that, in May 2007, the European Commission published a White Paper entitled *A Strategy for Europe on Nutrition, Overweight and Obesity-related Health Issues*[43], which included details of a best practice model for self-regulation of food advertising for children (see Appendix 4). **Following the planned review of the EU Strategy on obesity in 2010, the European Commission should consider whether there are cases in which self-regulation of food advertising for children has proved unsatisfactory and whether more binding regulation across the EU is required.**

Labelling and composition of food

5.24 Our second example of where we think industry should take a more active role than it has done so far is that of food labelling. There is a strong case for clear labelling of food so that people know what they are choosing. Readily understandable food labelling might also exert consumer pressure on manufacturers and shops to produce and stock foods or 'varieties' that are less unhealthy. There is currently no agreement by the food industry in the UK on appropriate, 'at a glance' front-of-pack labelling for the nutritional composition of food sold in shops. Two different strategies were introduced in 2005–6, though the evidence to date is inconclusive about which scheme is likely to be more effective (see Box 5.3). Additionally, there are no agreed standards or any requirements of an equivalent kind for catered food.

5.25 The stewardship model emphasises providing conditions that make it easy for people to lead healthy lives, paying special attention to vulnerable people and reducing causes of ill health

---

[38] Committee for Advertising Practice (2007) *New food rules for non-broadcast ads*, available at: http://www.cap.org.uk/cap/news_events/news/2007/New+food+rules+for+nonbroadcast+ads.htm.

[39] Deckelbaum RJ and Williams CL (2001) Childhood Obesity: The health issue *Obesity Research* 9: S239–43.

[40] American Academy of Pediatrics Committee on Communications (2006) Children, adolescents, and advertising *Pediatrics* 118: 2563–9.

[41] Some food manufacturers have been accused of irresponsible advertising to children on the Internet: see examples of the criticism in press reports, e.g. Wallop H (2007) Junk food makers reach children on internet *Telegraph*, 2 August, available at: http://www.telegraph.co.uk/news/main.jhtml?xml=/news/2007/08/01/njunk101.xml.

[42] Victorian Department of Human Services (2006) *ACE-Obesity Assessing Cost-effectiveness of obesity interventions in children and adolescents* Summary of Results (Victorian Government Department of Human Services), available at: http://www.health.vic.gov.au/healthpromotion/quality/ace_obesity.htm.

[43] Available at: http://ec.europa.eu/health/ph_determinants/life_style/nutrition/documents/nutrition_wp_en.pdf.

> ## Box 5.3: Food labelling initiatives
> Two types of food labelling system have been introduced on the packaging of some processed foods in the UK.
>
> **'Traffic light' labelling**
>
> Backed by the Food Standards Agency (an independent Government agency) the traffic light system uses a label with coloured panels that indicate the levels of fat, saturated fat, sugars and salt in 100 grams of the food (green, amber and red are used for low, medium and high), and showing the amounts of each that are present in a typical portion or serving (the size of which is assessed by the manufacturer). Several supermarkets and manufacturers are already voluntarily using this system of labelling, including Sainsbury's and Waitrose.
>
> **Guideline Daily Amounts (GDAs)**
>
> Several food manufacturers and retailers backed by the Food and Drink Federation (including Tesco and Kellogg's) have introduced a system called Guideline Daily Amounts (GDAs) labelling. The labels show percentages of GDAs of sugar, salt, fat and calories per serving. This system has been criticised for being more difficult to understand than the traffic light system, for example by the National Heart Forum.[44] The companies behind the GDA system claim that their labels are more helpful to consumers than the traffic light system.

through appropriate regulations (paragraph 2.44). In view of this and our observations on corporate social responsibility (paragraphs 2.47–2.50), we consider that **businesses, including the food industry, have an ethical duty to help individuals to make healthier choices. The food and drink industries should therefore review both the composition of products that they manufacture and the way they are marketed and sold. Where the market fails to uphold its responsibility, for instance in failing to provide universal, readily understandable front-of-pack nutrition labelling or in the marketing of food more generally, regulation by the government is ethically justifiable.** Several different models of providing labelling information have been introduced since 2000. It is premature to judge which of these is most effective in enabling consumers to make appropriately informed decisions. We note that the FSA has commissioned a study[45] to investigate if front-of-pack labels contribute to healthier choices being made and, if so, which elements of the various schemes are the most effective. **When the Food Standards Agency (FSA) has reviewed its commissioned study on the effectiveness of labelling schemes, and the findings have been peer reviewed, they should form the basis for adoption by the food industry of the most effective scheme. If, however, the food industry does not accept the scheme, it would be appropriate for the UK Government to pursue legislation (if appropriate, at the European level). As we have noted elsewhere, such information-based schemes could increase health inequalities, and this should be monitored.**

Role of government and public services

5.26 In liberal market economies there is strong pressure for industries to be only lightly regulated. This is often supported by an interpretation of the supply and demand principle that means that industries should be free to produce what people 'want' (because then both the population and the commercial sector are satisfied). However, in our discussions of individual choice, above and in Chapters 2 and 3, we have already noted that the concept is problematic, and that the government has an important facilitatory role through the policies and laws it puts in place. For example, governments can, through trade arrangements, influence the pricing of different types of food commodity.

5.27 The stewardship model developed in Chapter 2 could support an argument for state intervention on several grounds. We focus on four: promoting healthy living through enabling choice and behaviour change initiatives; strategies for reducing inequalities; interventions for protecting vulnerable groups; and interventions for protecting others from harm. We then discuss the role of government in the provision of obesity-related healthcare.

---

[44] National Heart Forum (8 February 2006) *New food industry health labelling seriously flawed*, available at: http://www.heartforum.org.uk/news_media_pressreleases_archive_foodindustryhealthlabelling.aspx.

[45] Food Standards Agency (2007) Press release: *Front of pack labelling research project moves forward*, 9 July, available at: http://www.food.gov.uk/news/pressreleases/2007/jul/frontpackresearchpress.

Promoting healthy living through enabling choice and behaviour change initiatives

5.28 Under the stewardship framework, public health strategies should "aim to ensure that it is easy for people to lead a healthy life" and promote health "by programmes to help people overcome addictions and other unhealthy behaviours" (paragraphs 2.41–2.44). Therefore, government has a role in ensuring that healthy options are available to people, and in encouraging the uptake of health-promoting behaviours.

5.29 Examples of strategies that enable people to make healthier choices include the building of cycle lanes and providing children and adults with the knowledge and information needed to enable them to make well-informed choices about the food they purchase or eat and the amount of physical activity they take. As we discussed above (paragraph 5.8), many people's energy expenditure levels have changed in recent decades in developed countries. There are a range of measures that could be taken by government to enable people to increase their energy expenditure levels where there are currently barriers to them doing so. For example, planning regulations, either imposed by central government or decided by local government, could take into consideration factors such as segregating walking and cycling routes from heavy traffic, or maintaining public parks and children's playgrounds. More restrictive or mandatory measures have also been suggested, for example banning cars from city centres, compulsory physical education in schools and car exclusion zones around schools. Several examples are given in Box 5.4.

Box 5.4: Examples of initiatives for increasing physical activity[46]

■ Walking school 'buses' (in which a group of children, accompanied by an adult, walk to school), or cycle 'trains' (a similar principle but using cycles) are used in several countries.[47]

■ Cities including Bristol have introduced 'home zones', which are residential areas where pedestrians take priority over traffic, and feature trees, benches and play areas.[48]

■ In Drachten, the Netherlands, traffic lights and road signs at junctions were removed and the roads merged with sidewalks, so that motorists, pedestrians, cyclists and even skateboarders all share the space. This is claimed to have led to more walking and cycling.[49]

■ In 2001 at its headquarters in Brentford, west London, pharmaceutical company GlaxoSmithKline implemented a cycling strategy. The company provided secure parking facilities for 300 bikes and showers and lockers resulted in the number of registered cyclists rising from 50 to 400, representing 13% of the staff on site, with an average daily journey of 14 miles.[50]

■ Since 1977 the city of Groningen has had an integrated policy for town and traffic planning aimed at reducing car traffic while enhancing accessibility and the use of public transport and walking and cycling. City planning requires new residential or office buildings to be built close to the existing city, and restricts the car parking space available for these new developments. There are extensive car-free zones in the city centre, while facilities for bicycles have been extended. In 1990 the modal transport-to-work split was 17% walking, 48% bicycle use, 5% public transport and 30% car use.[51]

■ Some schools have encouraged walking and cycling by regulating the motorised 'school run'. North Yorkshire introduced walking zones with a boundary line set up at five minutes' walk from the school gates, measured by the pupils. Within this boundary parents, children and staff are encouraged to walk. In one school the number of cars outside the school gate dropped from 60 to six when the five minute zone was launched.[52]

---

[46] See also National Heart Forum, in partnership with Living Streets and CABE (2007) *Building Health Creating and Enhancing Places for Healthy, Active Lives: What needs to be done?*, available at: http://www.heartforum.org.uk/downloads/BuildingHealth_Main.pdf.

[47] See Friends of the Earth (2000) *The Walking Bus: A safe way for children to walk to school*, available at: http://www.foe.co.uk/resource/factsheets/walking_bus.pdf.

[48] See Glaskin M (2004) Innovation: The end of the white line *The Sunday Times*, 22 August, available at: http://driving.timesonline.co.uk/tol/life_and_style/driving/article472085.ece; Sustrans, Home Zones, available at: http://www.sustrans.org.uk/default.asp?sID=1095412985125.

[49] Glaskin M (2004) Innovation: The end of the white line *The Sunday Times*, 22 August, available at: http://driving.timesonline.co.uk/tol/life_and_style/driving/article472085.ece; *Traffic Solutions*, available at: http://www.smallingerland.nl/index.cfm?sid=175.

[50] Commission for Architecture and the Built Environment (2006) *Physical Activity and the Built Environment*, available at: http://www.cabe.org.uk/AssetLibrary/8954.pdf.

[51] European Academy of the Urban Environment, *Groningen: Integrated town planning and traffic policy*, available at: http://www.eaue.de/winuwd/95.htm.

[52] Teachernet, *Five Minute Walking Zone*, available at: http://www.teachernet.gov.uk/CaseStudies/casestudy.cfm?id=346.

5.30 Although there is considerable enthusiasm for many of these strategies there is little robust evidence about their effectiveness at increasing physical activity or reducing obesity levels. However, they may bring other benefits (such as other health benefits, including improved mental health, reductions in accidents or air pollution or more opportunities for socialisation) and there is little evidence that they create significant harms or curtailments of individual liberties. In general the population accepts some restrictions on individual or corporate freedoms for the public good in terms of traffic and town planning restrictions and of compulsory standards in schools. Many of these restrictions are subject to democratic inputs through parliament, local government and other local bodies such as boards of governors in schools (see also Box 3.3). Drawing on our discussion of consent and procedural justice arrangements, we do not believe there are ethical objections to such strategies. However, the state should ensure that their implementation is monitored for effectiveness and potential harms such as more pedestrian or cycle injuries, stigmatisation of sedentary people, or increases in socio-economic, ethnic or gender inequalities.

5.31 There is a range of strategies, including those that are considered 'social marketing', that can be successfully used by governments to try to promote behaviour change and improve the health of the population (see paragraph 3.36). However, potential problems with policies that aim to do this should be considered when making policy. First, it might be argued that specific campaigns encouraging people to lose weight could both be seen as undue 'nannying'[53] and also result in stigmatising obese and overweight people. Secondly, not all interventions that come under the term 'social marketing' are effective (and cost-effective) ways of changing behaviour.[54] For example, reviews of attempts to encourage people out of cars and into walking and cycling have shown that publicity campaigns have had little effect on health (although some highly targeted interventions have been effective in increasing walking and cycling among motivated groups).[55] Lastly, and perhaps most importantly, policy makers need to consider the potential consequences of policy decisions on health inequalities. Promoting behaviour change can be incompatible with reducing health inequalities; for example the Government's campaign to encourage people to eat five portions of fruit and vegetables per day[56] or encouraging leisure time physical activity through gym membership, may benefit certain groups more than others and thus contribute to an increase in health inequalities (see paragraph 5.34). Such measures may nonetheless be desirable if complemented by alternative policies that seek to benefit those groups that are disadvantaged.

5.32 Overall, we consider that there is more that could be done in the design of urban environments and buildings to reduce the obesogenic nature of the environment and increase the opportunities for people to increase their energy expenditure with ease. **Planning decisions by central and local government should include the objective of encouraging people to be physically active. This may entail some restrictions of people's freedoms, for instance to drive anywhere they wish to, but these restrictions would be justified in terms of public health benefits.**

---

[53] Although, we note that it is widely accepted that the government has a 'nannying' role whenever it structures our choices in some way, for example when deciding whether or not to provide infrastructure (see also paragraph 8.17). For a discussion of how government interventions in public health are variously seen as 'nanny statism' or stewardship, see Jochelson K (2005) *Nanny or Steward? The role of government in public health* (London: The King's Fund).

[54] For example, see McDermott L, Stead M, Gordon R, Angus K and Hastings G (2006) *A Review of the Effectiveness of Social Marketing: Nutrition Interventions* (Institute for Social Marketing), available at: http://www.nsms.org.uk/images/CoreFiles/NSMC-R2_nutritioninterventions.pdf; see Gordon R, McDermott L, Stead M, Angus K and Hastings G (2006) *A Review of the Effectiveness of Social Marketing: Physical Activity Interventions* (Institute for Social Marketing), available at: http://www.nsms.org.uk/images/CoreFiles/NSMC-R1_Physical_Activity.pdf.

[55] Ogilvie D, Egan M, Hamilton V and Petticrew M (2004) Promoting walking and cycling as an alternative to using cars: systematic review *Br Med J* **329**: 763; Ogilvie D, Foster CE, Rothnie H *et al.* (2007) Interventions to promote walking: systematic review *Br Med J* **334**: 1204 and 1173.

[56] NHS, *5 A DAY*, available at: http://www.5aday.nhs.uk/.

5.33 **The training of architects and town planners should include measures for increasing people's physical activity through the design of buildings and public spaces. This can be viewed as analogous to the recent incorporation of the study of energy efficiency and sustainability of buildings. The recommendation is directed to those who design training programmes, including the Architects Registration Board, the Royal Institute of British Architects and the Royal Town Planning Institute. Planning regulations by local planning authorities should set requirements in this area.**

Strategies for reducing inequalities

5.34 In our stewardship model we suggest that public health policies should aim to eliminate or reduce health inequalities (paragraphs 2.41–2.44). In general in developed countries, obesity is more prevalent in lower income and lower socio-economic groups and in certain ethnic minorities (see Boxes 5.5 and 5.6). A prioritarian approach to reducing obesity might be considered on the basis of reducing inequalities in health (paragraph 2.31). An example would be planning decisions that improve access to sports facilities or shops/markets that sell fresh fruit and vegetables, or the distribution of food vouchers to people of lower socio-economic status. However, although such targeted interventions could benefit people who might not gain from population-wide initiatives, care would be required to avoid actual or perceived stigma that may result from singling out particular social groups in this way.

Box 5.5: The socio-economic pattern of obesity

Rates of obesity tend to rise in association with increasing social disadvantage in developed countries, although the pattern is considerably more marked among women than men. For example, in women, rates of overweight and obesity in England show a consistent rise with increasing social disadvantage, from 19% in the 'managerial and professional' group to 29% in the 'routine and semi-routine' group. For men, the differences in the rates of obesity between different groups are less marked.[57]

Rates of formal, leisure-time physical activity are lower in lower socio-economic status groups. Nevertheless, on average, people in these groups engage in more domestic and work-related physical activity, and in childhood they are more physically active in everyday activities such as walking to school and unstructured play, so that total physical activity levels may differ less across social groups.[58]

Box 5.6: Patterns of obesity and levels of physical activity among different minority ethnic groups in the UK

The prevalence of obesity varies between different ethnic groups in the UK, and within ethnic groups there is large variation between the sexes. As we have said, 23% of men and of women in the general population in England are obese. However, men from most minority ethnic groups have markedly lower obesity prevalence rates, with the exception of Black Caribbean (25%) and Irish (27%) men. Women from several minority ethnic groups also have lower obesity prevalence rates than the general population, with the exception of Black Caribbean (32%), Black African (39%) and Pakistani (28%) women. Low prevalence of obesity is found among Bangladeshi men (6%), and Chinese men (6%) and women (8%).[59]

It is reported that many South Asian individuals who have been resident in the UK for a long time seem to adopt a 'British type' diet, with an increase in fat consumption.[60] Levels of physical activity also vary between different minority ethnic groups, particularly among women. For example, in England, participation in a high level of physical activity[61] ranges from approximately one third of Irish and Black Caribbean individuals compared with 37% of men and 25% of women in the general population. Lowest participation rates in physical activity are reported by Bangladeshi and Pakistani women at less than 15%.[62]

[57] Sprosten K and Primatesta P (2004) *Health Survey for England 2003 Volume 2: Risk factors for cardiovascular disease* (National Statistics), Section 6, available at: http://www.dh.gov.uk/assetRoot/04/09/89/11/04098911.pdf.

[58] Sprosten K and Primatesta P (Editors) (2004) *Health Survey for England 2003 Volume 2: Risk factors for cardiovascular disease* (National Statistics), available at: http://www.dh.gov.uk/assetRoot/04/09/89/11/04098911.pdf; Bromley C, Sprosten K and Shelton N (Editors) (2005) *The Scottish Health Survey 2003 Volume 3: Children* (Scottish Executive); Bromley C, Sprosten K and Shelton N (Editors) (2005) *The Scottish Health Survey 2003 Volume 2: Adults* (Scottish Executive); Macintyre S and Mutrie N (2004) Socio-economic differences in cardiovascular disease and physical activity: stereotypes and reality *J R Soc Health* **124**: 66–9.

[59] All figures from NHS (2005) *Health Survey for England 2004: The Health of Minority Ethnic Groups – headline tables*, available at: http://www.ic.nhs.uk/webfiles/publications/hlthsvyeng2004ethnic/HealthSurveyForEngland161205_PDF%20.pdf.

[60] Williams R, Bush H, Lean M, Anderson A and Bradby H (1998) Food choice and culture in a cosmopolitan city: South Asians, Italians and other Glaswegians, in *The Nation's Diet: The social science of food choice* Murcott A (Editor) (London: Longman), pp.267–84.

[61] A 'high' activity level is defined as achieving the government recommendations of participating in activity of moderate to vigorous intensity for at least 30 minutes on five or more days a week on average.

[62] All figures from NHS (2005) *Health Survey for England 2004: The Health of Minority Ethnic Groups – headline tables*, available at: http://www.ic.nhs.uk/webfiles/publications/hlthsvyeng2004ethnic/HealthSurveyForEngland161205_PDF%20.pdf.

Interventions for protecting vulnerable groups

5.35 The increase in the prevalence of obesity among children is a particular concern, invoking from the stewardship model the principle of providing special care for the vulnerable (paragraphs 2.41–2.44). In July 2004, the Government set itself a public service agreement (PSA) target specifically on obesity – "halting the year-on-year rise in obesity among children aged under eleven by 2010 in the context of a broader strategy to tackle obesity in the population as a whole".[63] Much attention has been focused on the role of schools, as education plays a central role in providing individuals with the capacity to choose healthy behaviours. Schools are only part of a bigger picture. It is unreasonable to expect interventions in schools alone to be sufficient to reduce the prevalence of obesity, given the vast array of other influences experienced by children. However, school communities do provide an important means of influencing many of the socio-cultural factors that have a lasting impact on both food choices and exercise habits. They have a prominent role in the community, are a source of support for parents and families, and can produce community change in environments, knowledge and behaviour. For these reasons, it is appropriate for schools to seek to influence positively the food and exercise habits of children. Recognition of this was evident from many responses to the consultation, of which these are examples:

> "…schools should be responsible for promoting healthy eating habits and physical activity in children. School-food providers should provide healthy food choices to children."
> *PR Myles*

> "State schools are a direct agency of the government, and are charged with direct resonsibility for promoting the wellbeing of children. It is appropriate that schools should both disseminate information about healthy eating and exercise, and reinforce these messages through their own provision of foods, and by ensuring that exercise is a fundamental part of the curriculum." *British Medical Association*

5.36 **The stewardship model's emphasis on circumstances that help people to lead healthy lives, especially if they are in vulnerable positions** (paragraphs 2.41–2.44), **leads to an ethical justification for the state to intervene in schools to achieve a more positive culture towards food, cooking and physical activity.** As in many other areas of public health policy, the only way of establishing whether a new policy is likely to lead to improved health is by trialling it. **Because the need being addressed is an important one, it is desirable to explore the potential of promising policies, even if evidence for their effectiveness is incomplete.** In addition, changes in attitudes and culture towards food and physical activity are likely to take a long time. For example, the effectiveness of recent initiatives to introduce healthier meals and free fruit and vegetables in schools needs to be evaluated over many years.[64] Although short-term targets may be useful as milestones for monitoring progress, care is required not to measure success by reference to short-term targets alone. **The UK Government departments responsible for food, health and education should develop long-term strategies for schools with the aim of preventing obesity, and changing food and exercise culture, accompanied by monitoring and follow up.**

---

[63] Department of Health, *Obesity PSA Target*, available at: http://www.dh.gov.uk/en/Policyandguidance/Healthandsocialcaretopics/Obesity/DH_4133951. As this Report went to press, the Government announced a new PSA target to reduce the proportion of overweight and obese children to 2000 levels by 2020, see Department of Health (2007) *Long-term ambition on obesity*, available at: http://www.dh.gov.uk/en/Policyandguidance/Healthandsocialcaretopics/Obesity/DH_079307.

[64] These programmes, introduced over the past few years, have not yet been shown to result in long-term dietary changes or health benefits, although some researchers have observed evidence of increased knowledge of healthy eating, particularly in children from deprived areas. Some commentators hope that there will be longer-term impacts on children who are exposed to the free fruit and vegetables scheme for a longer period of time, and in the context of a whole-school policy designed to promote healthy eating. See Ransley JK, Greenwood DC, Cade JE *et al.* (2007) Does the school fruit and vegetable scheme improve children's diet? A non-randomised controlled trial *J Epidemiol Community Health* **61**: 699–703; Schagen S, Blenkinsop S, Schagen I *et al.* (2005) *Evaluation of the School Fruit and Vegetable Pilot Scheme: Final Report* (London: Big Lottery Fund).

5.37 In 2006, the Department of Health for England concluded that there were no existing comprehensive and reliable data at local level on child obesity to inform local planning and targeting of resources and interventions, and to enable tracking of progress against the PSA target (see paragraph 5.35). As a result, primary care trusts (and also local health authorities elsewhere) have been made responsible for measuring the height and weight of children in maintained schools at age four to five years and age ten to eleven years.[65] Although in its early stages, there is evidence that some children, and possibly in particular those who are overweight or obese, are declining to participate in the weighing and measuring programmes that are being implemented.[66]

5.38 **Data on the prevalence of obesity are a crucial part of understanding trends and the impact of interventions. Weighing and measuring young children is ethically justifiable, provided the data are anonymised and collected in a sensitive way. The collection of the data on obesity in children should be managed in a way that minimises the risks of stigmatisation, for instance by encompassing it within a broader programme of health checks. The UK health departments should give consideration to how this could be best realised in practice.**

Interventions for protecting others against harm

5.39 The classical harm principle (paragraph 2.14) could be invoked to justify severe interventions where children become obese as a direct result of their parents' preferences for food and exercise. The justification would rest on the special vulnerability of children and on the need to reduce the risks of ill health that people, in this case parents, impose upon others (see paragraphs 2.41–2.44). We note that if parents were to severely harm the health of their children, for example by underfeeding them, action would be taken by social services and they could be charged with neglect. There have now been at least a few cases in the UK where issues of neglect were raised in relation to a child who became severely obese.[67] **In general, direct regulation of food provided to children in the home would be disproportionate, as any health benefits achieved would be outweighed by the value of private and family life** (see also paragraph 6.15). **However, where severe obesity is caused by overfeeding by parents or guardians, child protection issues would be raised if the child was at risk of significant harm to health.**[68] High-profile cases of families with severely obese children have led to debate about whether it is appropriate for authorities to intervene in such situations. **The Secretary of State for Children, Schools and Families, with the advice of the Office of the Children's Commissioner, should develop criteria for deciding when interventions, such as removing a child from their home, would be appropriate under the Government's *Every Child Matters* approach.**[69]

Consideration of obesity-related treatments and costs to the NHS

5.40 We have suggested elsewhere that the NHS is an important part of the UK's public health system, and that the provision of a healthcare system such as this fulfils an important part of the stewardship function of the state (paragraph 1.11). Treating obesity and obesity-related

---

[65] Department of Health *Guidance for Measuring Childhood Obesity*, available at: http://www.dh.gov.uk/en/Policyandguidance/Healthandsocialcaretopics/Obesity/DH_4134095; NHS National Services Scotland (2006) *Childhood Obesity – Statistics and Information*, available at: http://www.isdscotland.org/isd/3640.html.

[66] Crowther R, Dinsdale H, Rutter H and Kyffin R (2006) *Analysis of the National Childhood Obesity Database 2005–06* (NHS), available at: http://www.apho.org.uk/apho/publications/childhoodobesity.pdf.

[67] See, for example, BBC News (2007) *Child obesity 'a form of neglect'*, 14 June, available at: http://news.bbc.co.uk/1/hi/health/6749037.stm.

[68] The fact that state intervention in home life is generally considered a last resort in a liberal state may in part explain why the focus of much government action (whether on eating or exercise habits) is often directed towards the school rather than home environment.

[69] *Every Child Matters* is the Government's approach to the well-being of children and young people from birth to age 19.

illnesses accounts for a large and increasing part of NHS expenditure (see Box 5.7). A significant number of respondents to our consultation expressed strong views about the way in which obesity should be considered in the context of limited resources within the NHS:

"It is acceptable for those who allow themselves to become so obese to the point where they are placing such a burden on their skeleton and organs … should contribute more into the system. They are responsible for their own state of health, and others who maintain their health reasonably should not share the costs." *Ms Magda Taylor*

"The ethos of the NHS is that services are based on need and are free at the point of delivery. […] There are many factors, for example obesity, over indulgence in alcohol, dangerous sports, which can result in the need for NHS input. To decide who 'deserves' treatment and who does not is against the ethos of the NHS and would require considerable investment in determining the rights and wrongs of each case." *Anon.*

"We do not believe that it is acceptable to make NHS services dependent on individuals losing weight, for two reasons: first, the degree of control that individuals have (given their individual histories, their socio-economic situation, and their genetics) is not clear and probably much less than is often assumed; and second, in a society where there are so many ways in which individuals are encouraged to become obese (advertising; food industry products) it is then unfair to penalise those affected by these encouragements." *Ethox Centre, Division of Public Health and Primary Care, University of Oxford*

Box 5.7: Economic factors

The rising prevalence of obesity has several economic consequences including: the treatment of obesity itself and its direct consequences; social care costs; and higher levels of sickness and absence from work. It is difficult to make precise or comprehensive estimates of the costs but it has been estimated that they amount to many billions of pounds per year in the UK.[70]

As an example, in the 2004 Wanless report to the Treasury, the direct cost of treating obesity was estimated at £9.4 million in England in 1998, and the cost of treating diseases attributable to obesity was £470 million. It was predicted that if present trends continue, by 2010 the annual cost to the economy would be £3.6 billion.[71]

In terms of total costs to the economy as a result of obesity, the House of Commons Select Committee on Health estimated that this amounted to between £3.3–3.7 billion in England in 2002.[72] Of this, approximately £1 billion was accounted for by the direct costs of treating obesity and its consequences (2.5% of net NHS expenditure in 2001–02). The remainder was attributed to loss of earnings (including 45,000 lost working years due to premature death and nearly 16 million lost working days because of sickness attributable to obesity). These very large contemporaneous costs of obesity are offset by reduced demands on expenditure such as pensions, as a result of shortened lifespans.

5.41 We have noted that the healthcare system in the UK is organised on a principle of community in which people are treated according to need (see paragraphs 1.11, 2.39). For such a system to be sustainable without increasing contributions, all members of the population need, to the greatest extent possible, to minimise relying on its resources. It may therefore be legitimate for the state to consider measures that ensure the sustainability of the NHS. One way of justifying this might be to appeal to a notion of community (paragraph 2.34) which is sensitive to the opportunity costs of expenditure on 'unnecessary' or avoidable treatment. Hence, it might be legitimate to appeal to individuals to change behaviours that have a significant financial cost to the public healthcare system. However, in our view any considerations about making treatment for obese people conditional on behaviour change

---

[70] McCormick B and Stone I (2007) Economic costs of obesity and the case for government intervention *Obes Rev* **8** (Suppl. 1): 161–4.

[71] Wanless D (2004) *Securing Good Health for the Whole Population* (London: HM Treasury), Chapter 4: Case Studies, available at: http://www.hm-treasury.gov.uk/media/B/4/Wanless04_ch4.pdf.

[72] It is expected that these figures are likely to underestimate the true costs to the economy. House of Commons Health Committee (2004) *Obesity*, Annex 1, available at: http://www.publications.parliament.uk/pa/cm200304/cmselect/cmhealth/23/23.pdf.

do not fall within the remit of public health, but rather each case needs to be assessed in its clinical context.

5.42 Obesity has complex causes. It is usually not easy to determine to what extent a person's weight is under their own control, and to what extent it is influenced by factors, such as their environment, that make it difficult to exercise or eat healthily. There is a significant risk of stigmatisation and unfair 'victim-blaming', where already-disadvantaged people are held unduly responsible for their poor health state. Any policies that single out obese people could also substantially undermine the concept of solidarity and the value of community, as people might come to regard each other merely as self-interested competitors for scarce resources. **It would not generally be appropriate for NHS treatment of health problems associated with obesity to be denied to people simply on the basis of their obesity. However, appeals to change behaviour before or subsequent to an intervention could be justified, provided that the change would enhance the effectiveness of the medical intervention, and people were offered help to do this.** On the whole, although the case of obesity raises some valid considerations about making the most efficient use of resources at the point of providing treatment, and although difficult decisions have to be made in allocating necessarily limited resources, in terms of public health policy the focus of efforts should be on *avoiding* the need for treatment in the first place. This is a fairer approach, and seems likely to be more promising in economic terms.

Role of civil society and individuals

5.43 We recognise that institutions of civil society such as charitable and community groups take valuable action through local initiatives to promote healthy eating or exercise, for example through organising or lobbying for sports clubs, cycle tracks or pedestrian areas. Such organisations can be very effective in facilitating governments to implement public health measures. For example, they might commission research, lobby the government and raise public awareness. These activities help to give governments the public mandate and therefore the political will to act.

5.44 Lastly, although this chapter focuses on public health measures that are designed to operate at the population level, we note that it would be wrong to ignore the contribution of people's individual behaviour in strategies seeking to prevent obesity. While the organised efforts of society can seek to generate an environment that promotes, as far as possible, opportunities for exercise and healthy food, these interventions are unlikely to 'engineer away' obesity completely without efforts by people to manage their weight, including taking up the opportunities provided.

Summary

5.45 There are complex causes for the rise of obesity worldwide. Although some of the contributing factors have been identified, their relative importance is unclear. In general terms, obesity is the result of many changes in our environment that make it easier to consume a large amount of calorie-rich food while expending little energy. Obesity is a risk factor for many chronic health conditions, such as diabetes and heart disease.

5.46 We have considered several salient policy issues in this chapter and emphasised throughout that the complex and multi-factorial causes of obesity mean that no single policy option will act as a 'magic bullet' to reduce the rising incidence of obesity. There is a role to be played by many agents, including central government, local government, industries that manufacture, market and sell food and drinks, public transport agencies, architects and building designers, clinicians and medical advisers, catering outlets, media businesses, institutions of civil society, parents and schools, and, last but not least, individuals. We commented on the importance of corporate social responsibility and concluded that where industry fails to satisfy reasonable expectations by a stewardship-guided state, regulation is ethically justifiable within the stewardship model set out in Chapter 2. We noted that it is necessary to consider the potential effects on social inequalities of any policy options under consideration.

Chapter 6

Case study – Alcohol and tobacco

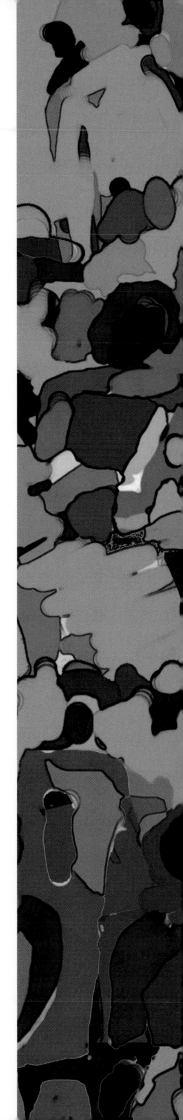

Case study – Alcohol and tobacco

Introduction

6.1 Alcohol and tobacco are enjoyed legally by many people in the UK and elsewhere (for further information on policy internationally see Appendix 6). Alcohol is of considerable social significance and it features as part of many religious and cultural events. Many people take pleasure in drinking moderate amounts of alcohol without any demonstrable harm. At this level it has been shown to have some health benefits, although it is disputed whether these are offset by other harms (see Box 6.1). However, excessive consumption[1] is extremely harmful to individual consumers and is often also linked to public safety problems that impact upon third parties, such as drink-driving. For tobacco, even smoking a small number of cigarettes regularly is harmful to the individual and people around them.

6.2 Public health measures aimed at limiting the harms caused by alcohol and tobacco raise some similar ethical issues. We therefore consider alcohol and tobacco together in this case study, comparing and contrasting similarities and differences where they occur. In particular, both alcohol and tobacco are supported by major manufacturing, advertising and distribution industries, and we consider the role of these industries.

6.3 To be effective and enforceable, public health policies aimed at reducing the consumption of substances that people enjoy usually require a certain threshold of public support. Governments might also decide to take political considerations into account. As expressed by one respondent to our consultation: "If most people smoke, then restricting their activities is not going to win an election; public opinion had to be changed first" (Les Dundon). It is notable that in the UK there were major policy initiatives to try to reduce smoking and passive smoking by the incoming Labour Government in 1998,[2] whereas strategies for alcohol[3] were not forthcoming until much later and they have been much less far-reaching.

> **Box 6.1: Does drinking a moderate amount of alcohol confer health benefits?**
>
> It is widely reported that consuming a small amount of alcohol, particularly red wine, leads to a reduction in risk of coronary heart disease.[4] The amount of alcohol that offers this protection without increasing risk of other health problems is disputed but thought to be low, in the region of one or two alcoholic drinks a few times a week. Some researchers dismiss the theory that alcohol can be protective, and have concluded that coronary protection from light to moderate drinking of alcohol is very limited and unlikely to outweigh the harms caused.[5]

---

[1] In this Report we use 'excessive' alcohol consumption to refer to drinking that leads to alcohol use disorders as defined in the Alcohol Needs Assessment Research Project (ANARP). The report used the World Health Organization categorisation of disorders of alcohol use, which specifies three categories: 'hazardous drinking', people drinking above recognised 'sensible' levels but not yet experiencing harm; 'harmful drinking', people drinking above 'sensible' levels and experiencing harm; and 'alcohol dependence', people drinking above 'sensible' levels and experiencing harm and symptoms of dependence. Department of Health (2005) *Alcohol Needs Assessment Research Project (ANARP): The 2004 national alcohol needs assessment for England* (London: Central Office of Information).

[2] Department of Health (1998) White Paper: *Smoking Kills*, available at: http://www.archive.official-documents.co.uk/document/cm41/4177/contents.htm.

[3] Scottish Executive (2002) *Plan for Action on Alcohol Problems* (Edinburgh: Scottish Executive); Prime Minister's Strategy Unit (2004) *Alcohol Harm Reduction Strategy for England*, available at: http://www.cabinetoffice.gov.uk/strategy/downloads/su/alcohol/pdf/CabOffce%20AlcoholHar.pdf; Department of Health, Home Office, Department for Education and Skills and Department for Culture, Media and Sport (2007) *Safe. Sensible. Social. The next steps in the National Alcohol Strategy* (London: Department of Health Publications).

[4] For example, see Mukamal KJ, Chiuve SE and Rimm EB (2006) Alcohol consumption and risk for coronary heart disease in men with healthy lifestyles *Arch Intern Med* **166**: 2145–50; Britton A and Marmot M (2004) Different measures of alcohol consumption and risk of coronary heart disease and all-cause mortality: 11-year follow-up of the Whitehall II Cohort Study *Addiction* **99**: 109–16.

[5] For example, see Jackson R, Broad J, Connor J and Wells W (2005) Alcohol and ischaemic heart disease: probably no free lunch *Lancet* **366**: 1911–2.

Harms caused by alcohol and tobacco to drinkers and smokers themselves

6.4   Excessive alcohol consumption and the use of tobacco are major contributors to ill health. However, while the association of smoking with disease and premature death is well known, it is less clear that the long-term risks of consuming excessive amounts of alcohol are as well understood across the population, or at least taken as seriously.[6] Analysis for the World Health Organization (WHO) suggests that in developed countries tobacco is the leading single risk factor for mortality while alcohol is third (with blood pressure being the second most significant risk factor).[7] A study published in the *Lancet* in 2007 compared the 'harm scores' for several illegal drugs and also alcohol and tobacco. Alcohol scored more highly than tobacco in this assessment based on judgements of doctors about physical harms, dependence and social harms caused by these substances.[8]

Alcohol

6.5   Alcohol-related harms are usually the result of chronic and dependent drinking, and/or episodic 'binge' drinking.[9] Excessive consumption on a single occasion can also be damaging and even, on very rare occasions, fatal. The health effects of alcohol misuse include high blood pressure, cirrhosis of the liver, pancreatitis, cancer and mental health problems.[10] Increases in consumption correlate with rises in the alcohol-related death rate throughout the 1990s (see Box 6.2 and Figure 6.1). National Statistics has calculated that the annual number of alcohol-related deaths in the UK has more than doubled from 4,144 in 1991 to 8,386 in 2005,[11] although figures from different sources vary. Worldwide, WHO

Figure 6.1: Alcohol-related death rates by sex in the UK, 1991–2005*

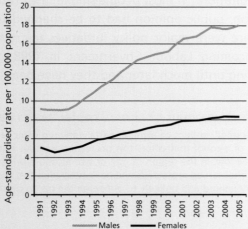

*Source: National Statistics *Alcohol-Related Deaths*, available at:
http://www.statistics.gov.uk/CCI/nugget.asp?ID=1091&Pos=2&ColRank=1&Rank=192, Crown copyright material is reproduced with the permission of the Controller of HMSO under the terms of the Click-Use Licence.

---

[6] Rates of smoking have reduced in recent years (see Box 6.4) whereas alcohol consumption has increased, despite indications of the risks involved. See Association of Public Health Observatories (2007) *Indications of Public Health in the English Regions 8: Alcohol*, available at: http://www.apho.org.uk/apho/publications/Alcohol_Indications.pdf; Rose D (2007) Alcohol abuse undoing gains from curbs on smoking *The Times* 14 August, available at:
http://www.timesonline.co.uk/tol/life_and_style/health/article2253774.ece.

[7] Lopez AD, Mathers CD, Ezzati M, Jamison DT and Murray CJL (2006) Global and regional burden of disease and risk factors, 2001: systematic analysis of population health data *Lancet* **367**: 1747–57; Yach D, Hawkes C, Gould CL and Hofman KL (2004) The global burden of chronic diseases: Overcoming impediments to prevention and control *J Am Med Assoc* **291**: 2616–22.

[8] Nutt D, King LA, Saulsbury W and Blakemore C (2007) Development of a rational scale to assess the harm of drugs of potential misuse *Lancet* **369**: 1047–53.

[9] See Plant M and Plant M (2006) *Binge Britain: Alcohol and the national response* (Oxford: Oxford University Press).

[10] National Statistics (2004) *Health Survey for England 2003 Volume 2 Risk factors for cardiovascular disease*, available at: http://www.dh.gov.uk/en/Publicationsandstatistics/Publications/PublicationsStatistics/DH_4098712.

[11] The definition of alcohol-related deaths used by National Statistics includes those causes regarded as most directly due to alcohol consumption; National Statistics (2006) News Release: *Alcohol-related death rates almost double since 1991*, 7 November, available at: http://www.statistics.gov.uk/pdfdir/aldeaths1106.pdf.

estimates that there are approximately 76.3 million people with diagnosed disorders caused by alcohol, with consumption of alcohol the cause of 3% of all deaths (one third due to unintentional injuries) and 4% of all disability-adjusted life years.[12] In all regions, more males than females were found to suffer from disorders for which alcohol is considered to be causal, and these conditions were found at a higher level in developed countries than developing countries (see also Box 6.3).[13]

6.6 Drinking even small amounts of alcohol is not without risk of harm if combined with other behaviours such as driving or workplace activities, and drinking larger quantities of alcohol is associated with the risk of personal injury. Together with the health risks posed by alcohol directly, alcohol thus has a major impact on the cost and workload of the NHS (see also Box 6.7).[14]

Box 6.2: Prevalence of drinking

■ In 2005, a survey found that 72% of men and 57% of women in Great Britain had had an alcoholic drink on at least one day during the previous week.[15]

■ Levels of alcohol consumption have risen significantly over the past 50 years. During this time, the per capita consumption in the UK has doubled from approximately four litres to over eight litres of pure alcohol per year.[16] Since 1978, when questions about alcohol consumption were first asked as part of the General Household Survey (a population survey), men have reported a slight increase in overall weekly alcohol consumption and women have reported a much more marked increase.[17] There is clear evidence of a relationship between increased overall consumption and an increase in the harm caused.[18]

■ A national survey of Great Britain in 2005 found that exceeding the Government's recommended 'sensible drinking benchmarks' on at least one day in the week prior to the survey was more common among men (35%) than women (20%). These proportions had reduced since 2003.[19] Heavy drinking was also more common among men (19% in 2005) than women (8%).[20]

■ Younger people were more likely than older people both to exceed the daily benchmarks (see graph below) and to drink heavily.[21] Thirty-one per cent of men and 22% of women aged 16 to 24 years had drunk heavily on at least one day during the week prior to the national survey in 2005. Among those aged 65 years and over, these proportions were just 4% and 1%, respectively.[22]

■ An assessment in England in 2004 found that approximately 8.2 million people (38% of men and 16% of women) had an 'alcohol use disorder', meaning that their drinking is judged 'hazardous', 'harmful' or 'dependent' as defined by WHO.[23] The prevalence of alcohol dependence was 3.6% of the population of England, equating to 1.1 million people.[24]

■ Across Great Britain, the proportion of adults exceeding the daily benchmarks is highest in the North East (39%) followed by Scotland and Wales (both 35%). The lowest prevalence is in London and the East of England (both 25%), the South East and the West Midlands (both 27%).[25]

Continued overleaf

---

[12] World Health Organization (2004) *Global Status Report on Alcohol 2004* (Geneva, Switzerland: WHO), p.1.

[13] *Ibid.*, p.52.

[14] Department of Health (2005) *Alcohol Needs Assessment Research Project (ANARP): The 2004 national alcohol needs assessment for England* (London: Central Office of Information), p.2; Royal College of Physicians (2001) *Alcohol – can the NHS afford it?* (London: RCP).

[15] National Statistics *Drinking*, available at: http://www.statistics.gov.uk/cci/nugget_print.asp?ID=1027, data from the General Household Survey 2005 and the National Statistics Omnibus Survey 2006. National Statistics notes that: "Obtaining reliable information about drinking behaviour is difficult. Surveys consistently record lower levels of consumption than would be expected from data on alcohol sales. This is partly because people may under-estimate how much alcohol they consume."

[16] Academy of Medical Sciences (2004) *Calling Time: The nation's drinking as a major health issue* (London: Academy of Medical Sciences), pp.12 and 16.

[17] National Statistics *A summary of changes over time: Drinking*, available at: http://www.statistics.gov.uk/CCI/nugget.asp?ID=829&Pos=3&ColRank=2&Rank=960.

[18] See Academy of Medical Sciences (2004) *Calling Time: The Nation's drinking as a major health issue* (London: AMS), paragraph 2.19.

[19] Government guidelines on sensible drinking are based on daily benchmarks of between three and four units per day for men and two to three units per day for women. National Statistics *Drinking*, available at: http://www.statistics.gov.uk/cci/nugget_print.asp?ID=1027, data from the General Household Survey 2005 and the National Statistics Omnibus Survey 2006.

[20] Heavy drinking is defined as over eight units a day for men and six units a day for women on at least one day during the week prior to the survey.

[21] See footnote 20.

[22] National Statistics *Drinking*, available at: http://www.statistics.gov.uk/cci/nugget_print.asp?ID=1027, data from the General Household Survey 2005 and the National Statistics Omnibus Survey 2006.

[23] For definitions, see footnote 1.

[24] Department of Health (2005) *Alcohol Needs Assessment Research Project (ANARP): The 2004 national alcohol needs assessment for England* (London: Central Office of Information), p.3 and p.6.

[25] 2002–3 figures, National Statistics (2006) *Drinking*, available at: http://www.statistics.gov.uk/CCI/nugget.asp?ID=922&Pos=1&ColRank=2&Rank=128.

Box 6.2 (continued)

Percentage of men and women exceeding daily benchmarks for alcohol consumption by age on at least one day in the week prior to the national survey, Great Britain, 2005*

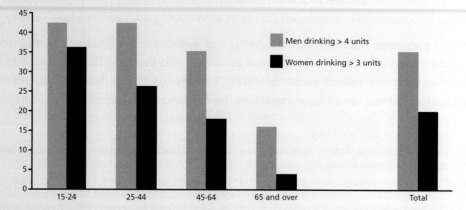

*Source: Goddard E (2006) General Household Survey 2005: Smoking and drinking among adults, 2005 (Office for National Statistics), Crown copyright material is reproduced with the permission of the Controller of HMSO under the terms of the Click-Use Licence.

■ The association of alcohol drinking with socio-economic classifications is complex and varies between the regions and countries of the UK. Although problems caused by alcohol affect people across the socio-economic spectrum, it is recognised that alcohol misuse plays a major role in the experiences of some of the most disadvantaged members of society, especially those who are homeless. The General Household Survey has shown over many years that there is little difference in usual weekly alcohol consumption between those classified as being in non-manual and manual households. Where differences do exist, it has been those in the non-manual categories who tend to have the higher weekly consumption, particularly among women.[26]

■ Minority ethnic groups in this country are more likely to be non-drinkers, particularly Bangladeshis (97% of men and 98% of women) and Pakistanis (89% and 95%), compared with the general population (8% and 14%). However, the drinking habits of Irish people in this country are similar to those of the general population, except that the mean number of days per week when alcohol is consumed is higher.[27]

Box 6.3: Consumption of alcohol – international comparisons

The average amount of alcohol consumed in different countries worldwide ranged from 0 to 19 litres of pure alcohol per adult per year (age 15+) in 2000 or 2001.[28] Countries with no or very little recorded alcohol consumption are mainly Muslim countries, whereas the USA, European countries, Russia, Australia and New Zealand have the highest levels of total alcohol consumption. Several African countries have very high levels, including Uganda, which has the highest recorded alcohol per capita consumption in the world.[29]

Total recorded alcohol per capita (age 15+) consumption per year in selected countries (2000/2001)*

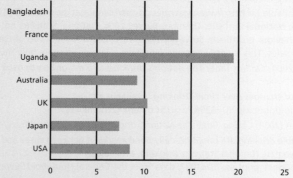

*Source: Figures from World Health Organization (2004) *Global Status Report on Alcohol 2004* (Geneva, Switzerland: WHO), Table 3.

---

[26] Goddard E (2006) *General Household Survey 2005: Smoking and drinking among adults, 2005* (Office for National Statistics), p.50.

[27] Sproston K and Mindell J (Editors) (2006) *Health Survey for England 2004: The health of minority ethnic groups* (Leeds: The Information Centre).

[28] World Health Organization (2004) *Global Status Report on Alcohol 2004* (Geneva, Switzerland: WHO), Table 3.

[29] This is because the calculations included fermented beverages and estimates of locally produced beer.

Smoking

6.7 Smokers suffer considerable ill health and report a lower health-related quality of life than non-smokers at all ages.[30] Smoking causes lung cancer, bronchitis, emphysema, heart disease and cancers in other organs including the mouth, lip, throat, bladder, kidney, stomach, liver and cervix. This ill health translates into more hospital admissions and more sickness absences from work. Smoking was associated with on average 106,000 premature deaths a year in the UK between 1998 and 2002, equating to approximately one in six of all deaths (see also Figure 6.2).[31] Half of all smokers will die prematurely; research has shown that men born in 1900–30 who were lifelong smokers died on average about ten years younger than non-smokers.[32] It has been found that there are gains to stopping smoking at all ages[33] and hence, together with strategies that would reduce uptake, there is considerable potential to reduce the premature loss of life. (See Box 6.4 for data on the prevalence of smoking in various population groups and Figure 6.3 for some international comparisons.)

Box 6.4: Prevalence of smoking

■ There was a dramatic increase and subsequent decline of cigarette smoking in the 20th Century in the UK. In 1974, 45% of people smoked compared with 35% in 1982. Since this time, the rate of decline has slowed. Prevalence has always been higher among men than among women; in 2005, 25% of men and 23% of women were smokers.[34]

■ The proportion of people who smoke declines with age; since the early 1990s, the prevalence of cigarette smoking has been higher among those aged 20–24 years than among those in other age groups.[35]

■ The number of cigarettes smoked per smoker has also declined from 14% of men in 1990 smoking 20 or more cigarettes a day to 10% in 1998 and from 9% to 7% for women in the same period. It has since remained virtually unchanged among both men and women, although there was a suggestion of a slight downturn in the couple of years prior to 2005. Cigarette consumption also varies by age, with those aged 35–59 years smoking the most (men: 16 cigarettes per day; women: 14 per day on average).[36]

■ Smoking has become associated with low socio-economic status and socially disadvantaged groups. One analysis suggests that as well as occupational grouping, socio-economic measures of deprivation such as housing tenure, unemployment and low educational status are independently associated with an increased prevalence of smoking among adults.[37] In the 1970s and 1980s in Britain, the prevalence of cigarette smoking fell more sharply among those in non-manual than in manual occupation groups, so that differences between the groups became proportionately greater. In England in 2005, 29% of those in manual groups and 19% of those in non-manual groups were cigarette smokers.[38] People in manual social classes also have more exposure to other people's cigarette smoke.[39]

■ Scotland generally has a higher smoking prevalence than England. In 2005, 27% of adults in Scotland were smokers, while in Wales 22% of adults were smokers.[40]

■ Smoking prevalence differs between ethnic and cultural groups in the UK. Self-reported cigarette smoking prevalence was 40% among Bangladeshi, 30% among Irish, 29% among Pakistani, 25% among Black Caribbean, 21% among Black African and Chinese, and 20% among Indian men, compared with 24% among men in the general population in England in 2004. For women, prevalence was higher among women in the general population (23%) than in most minority ethnic groups, except Irish (26%) and Black Caribbean women (24%). Ten per cent of Black African, 8% of Chinese, 5% of Indian and Pakistani, and 2% of Bangladeshi women smoked.[41]

---

[30] Kind P, Dolan P, Gudex C and Williams A (1998) Variations in population health status: results from a United Kingdom national questionnaire survey *Br Med J* **316**: 736–41.

[31] Twigg L, Moon G and Walker S (2004) *The Smoking Epidemic in England* (London: Health Development Agency), p.2.

[32] Doll R, Peto R, Boreham J and Sutherland I (2004) Mortality in relation to smoking: 50 years' observations on male British doctors *Br Med J* **328**: 1519–27.

[33] *Ibid.*

[34] Goddard E (2006) *General Household Survey 2005: Smoking and drinking among adults, 2005* (Office for National Statistics), p.4.

[35] *Ibid.*, p.5.

[36] *Ibid.*, p.9.

[37] Jarvis MJ and Wardle J (1999) Social patterning of individual health behaviours: The case of cigarette smoking, in *Social Determinants of Health*, Marmot M and Wilkinson RG (Editors) (Oxford: Oxford University Press).

[38] Goddard E (2006) *General Household Survey 2005: Smoking and drinking among adults, 2005* (Office for National Statistics), p.6.

[39] Whincup PH, Gilg JA, Emberson JR *et al.* (2004) Passive smoking and risk of coronary heart disease and stroke: prospective study with cotinine measurement *Br Med J* **329**: 200–5.

[40] Goddard E (2006) *General Household Survey 2005: Smoking and drinking among adults, 2005* (Office for National Statistics), p.9.

[41] Sproston K and Mindell J (Editors) (2006) *Health Survey for England 2004: The health of minority ethnic groups* (Leeds: The Information Centre).

Figure 6.2: Deaths attributed to smoking ages 35–69 by sex in the UK, 1950–2000*

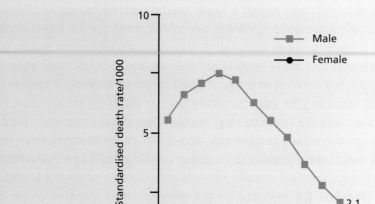

*Source: Peto R, Lopez AD, Boreham J and Thun M (2006) *Mortality from Smoking in Developed Countries 1950–2000: United Kingdom*, 2nd Edition, p.502, available at: http://www.ctsu.ox.ac.uk/~tobacco/C4308.pdf.

Figure 6.3: Proportion of people who smoke: UK, Japan, USA and highest and lowest in EU for teenage and adult populations*

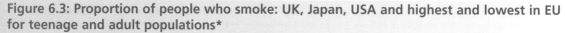
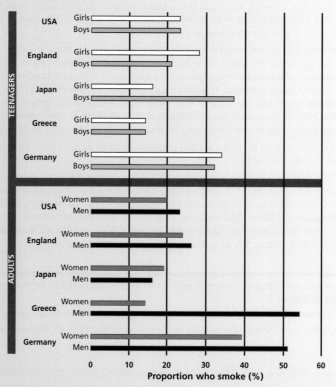

*Figures from: Joossens L (2004) *Effective Tobacco Control Policies in 28 European Countries* (European Network for Smoking Prevention), available at: http://www.ensp.org/files/effectivefinal2.pdf; World Health Organization *The Tobacco Atlas*, available at: http://www.who.int/tobacco/statistics/tobacco_atlas/en/; Osaki Y, Minowa M, Suzuki K and Wada K (2003) Adolescent smoking behavior in Japan, 1996 *Nihon Arukoru Yakubutsu Igakkai Zasshi* **38**: 483–91; Centers for Disease Control and Prevention (2005) Cigarette smoking among adults – United States, 2004 *Morbidity and Mortality Weekly Report* **54**: 1121–4, available at: http://www.cdc.gov/MMWR/preview/mmwrhtml/mm5444a2.htm; Centers for Disease Control and Prevention (2006) Fact Sheet: *Youth and Tobacco Use: Current estimates*, available at: http://www.cdc.gov/tobacco/research_data/youth/Youth_Factsheet.htm.

Note: Figures are only approximately comparable for the different data sets (European countries, Japan and USA) as they may include differences in the way smokers are categorised and in the age of teenagers included. Data from the survey used to obtain figures for European countries are available for the separate countries of the UK only and therefore only data for England are shown in the graph. Figures in this category for the other countries of the UK are similar, although slightly lower than those for England.

Addiction

6.8 Both alcohol and nicotine are addictive substances. Assessment criteria have been developed by WHO (among others) to assist in determining whether someone is dependent on or addicted to psycho-active substances, alcohol or tobacco. A definite diagnosis of dependence should usually be made only if three or more of the following have been present together at some time during the previous year:

■ a strong desire or sense of compulsion to take the substance;

■ difficulties in controlling substance-taking behaviour in terms of its onset, termination or levels of use;

■ a physiological withdrawal state when substance use has ceased or has been reduced, or use of the same (or similar) substance with the intention of relieving withdrawal symptoms;

■ evidence of tolerance (such that more of the substance is needed over time to feel its effect);

■ progressive neglect of alternative pleasures or interests because of the substance, increased amount of time necessary to obtain or drink the substance or to recover from its effects; and/or

■ persistence with substance use despite clear evidence of overtly harmful consequences, such as harm to the liver.[42]

6.9 With regard to tobacco, a report by the Royal College of Physicians concluded that "nicotine obtained from cigarettes meets all the standard criteria used to define a drug of dependence or addiction" and "nicotine is highly addictive, to a degree similar or in some respects exceeding addiction to 'hard' drugs such as heroin or cocaine".[43] The definitions of addiction in the previous paragraph do not imply that people cannot change their behaviour, but that there are physical, psychological and social barriers that restrict their ability to change behaviour and may hinder permanent changes (see paragraphs 3.35–3.36). For many, psycho-social or pharmacological aids may be needed to help behaviour change as information about harms to themselves or others is not sufficient. An important difference between cigarettes and alcohol is that most (but not all) smokers are addicted to nicotine, although a lower, but not insignificant, proportion of drinkers are addicted to alcohol.

Harms to other people associated with alcohol and tobacco

6.10 The consumption of both alcohol and tobacco has an impact not only on the individual consumer but also on other people. Alcohol is associated with major health impacts and public order offences towards others, particularly through drink-driving, other accidents and violence (see Box 6.5). There has been more social recognition of the harms of alcohol in the UK in recent years but this has not been matched by modified behaviour. Wider availability and lower cost have been associated with an increase in consumption[44] and, as a result, harm caused. The exact level of this wider burden is difficult to measure.

6.11 Alcohol use generally increases risk-taking and violent behaviour. Excessive drinkers, as well as being more likely to initiate violence, are also more likely to become victims. There are several

---

[42] World Health Organization *Dependence Syndrome*, available at:
http://www.who.int/substance_abuse/terminology/definition1/en/index.html.

[43] Tobacco Advisory Group of the Royal College of Physicians (2000) *Nicotine Addiction in Britain* (London: Royal College of Physicians).

[44] Academy of Medical Sciences (2004) *Calling Time: The nation's drinking as a major health issue* (London: Academy of Medical Sciences), p.9.

direct impacts associated with drinking alcohol in terms of accidents on the road, at work and in the home, fires (often a joint risk with smoking), domestic violence, and public order and violent offences. It is notable that, of all the case studies reviewed in this Report, drinking alcohol causes the highest level of harm to others and yet new legislation to reduce the harm caused by excessive alcohol consumption has not been introduced in the same way as we have seen for smoking (see paragraph 6.13). Because of the level of harm to others caused by people who have consumed large amounts of alcohol, and in keeping with the classical harm principle (see paragraph 2.14), governments should act to reduce this harm. In some areas, this principle is clearly recognised. For example, coercive measures, such as prohibiting driving or operating machinery with a blood-alcohol level over prescribed limits, are publicly accepted and it is appropriate for the proper authorities to implement surveillance mechanisms to enforce these rules.

Box 6.5: Harm to others associated with alcohol

The UK Government estimated in 2004 that alcohol misuse was involved in the following harms that affect other people:[45]

■ 1.2 million violent incidents (approximately half of all violent crimes);

■ 360,000 incidents of domestic violence (around a third);

■ 530 deaths from drink-driving; and

■ at peak times, up to 70% of all admissions to accident and emergency departments.

6.12 As regards harms caused to others by smoking, evidence has accumulated of the harm caused by environmental tobacco smoke ('passive smoking'). This is associated with lung cancer and heart disease, reduced lung function especially in people with asthma, and irritation of the eye, nose and throat. Passive smoking has been conservatively estimated to account for 12,200 deaths in the UK in 2003 from four conditions that can be caused by smoking or passive smoking.[46]

6.13 In 2006/7, it became illegal to smoke in enclosed public places in all four countries of the UK[47] (this measure has also been taken in other countries, see Box 6.6). **As with alcohol, the harm to others caused by tobacco smoking justifies the implementation of coercive measures. The introduction in the UK of legislation to prohibit smoking in enclosed public places is therefore justified.**

Box 6.6: Bans on smoking in enclosed public places

Several regions and countries have introduced legislation to prohibit smoking in public places. In 2004, the first national comprehensive legislation to ban smoking in workplaces was enacted in Ireland, including restaurants, pubs and bars. It was very soon reported that compliance was "excellent"[48], and medical writers have called the ban "a runaway success".[49] Cigarette sales fell by 8% in the first year of the ban.[50] There is evidence that respiratory symptoms in bar staff who do not smoke have declined.[51] Data collected over time are needed to demonstrate any long-term effect on public health. So far, surveys have revealed that the ban in Ireland is popular, including among smokers.[52] Since 2004, countries that have implemented legislation on smoking in workplaces include Australia, South Africa, Norway, New Zealand, Uganda, Italy, Sweden and Scotland. Certain states in the USA and Canada have had bans on smoking in enclosed public places for several years.

---

[45] Prime Minister's Strategy Unit (2004) *Alcohol Harm Reduction Strategy for England*.

[46] The four conditions were lung cancer, ischaemic heart disease, stroke and chronic obstructive pulmonary disease; Royal College of Physicians (2005) *Going Smoke-free: The medical case for clean air in the home, at work and in public places*, available at: http://www.rcplondon.ac.uk/pubs/contents/fe4ab715-2689-4a4a-b8c7-53e80386c893.pdf.

[47] Smokefree *Smokefree regulations*, available at: http://www.smokefreeengland.co.uk/thefacts/the-regulations.html.

[48] McNicholas WT (2004) Controlling passive smoking through legislation in Ireland: An attack on civil liberty or good public health policy? *Eur Respir J* **24**: 337–8.

[49] Howell F (2005) Smoke-free bars in Ireland: a runaway success *Tobacco Control* **14**: 73–4.

[50] Editorial (2005) Ireland's smoking ban is an admirable achievement *Lancet* **365**: 1282.

[51] Allwright S, Paul G, Greiner B *et al.* (2005) Legislation for smoke-free workplaces and health of bar workers in Ireland: Before and after study *Br Med J* **331**: 1117–20.

[52] Howell F (2005) Smoke-free bars in Ireland: A runaway success *Tobacco Control* **14**: 73–4; Fong GT, Hyland A, Borland R *et al.* (2006) Reductions in tobacco smoke pollution and increases in support for smoke-free public places following the implementation of comprehensive smoke-free workplace legislation in the Republic of Ireland: Findings from the ITC Ireland/UK Survey *Tobacco Control* **15** (Suppl. 3): 51–8.

6.14 Many non-smokers have experienced some exposure to environmental tobacco smoke. In 2003, 500 of the estimated 12,200 deaths from environmental tobacco smoke occurred because of exposure in the workplace.[53] However, even before the smoking bans in public places, most exposure occurred within the home.[54] For example, in Scotland, 61% of boys and 64% of girls aged 8–15 years reported being exposed to environmental tobacco smoke in their own or other people's homes.[55] These figures raise the question of whether the passive smoking legislation should be widened to extend to the home, i.e. whether measures are required to protect the most vulnerable, not only in public places, but also in private spheres. Children exposed to smoke at home have a higher risk of a range of health problems and exacerbation of other illness. These problems include pneumonia and bronchitis, asthma, respiratory symptoms and ear disease.[56] It is established that smoking by pregnant women is harmful to their babies as it increases the risk of low birthweight and miscarriage. It is also likely that pregnant women's exposure to environmental tobacco smoke could impact upon the fetus, and that parental smoking is a major cause of sudden infant death syndrome.[57] We note that some local authorities do not allow people who smoke to adopt children aged under five years old.[58]

6.15 **In principle, the general ethical and scientific arguments that apply to banning smoking in enclosed public spaces also apply to banning smoking in homes (and other places) where children are exposed to environmental tobacco smoke. However, this would be extremely difficult to enforce without compromising privacy. We recommend that the Department for Children, Schools and Families should communicate to local authority children's services that there may be exceptional cases where children, for example, those with a serious respiratory condition, would be at risk of such a substantial level of harm from passive smoking that intervention to prevent such harm may be ethically acceptable. This would usually need to be decided in the courts.**

Entitlement to treatment and costs to the NHS

6.16 Alcohol- and tobacco-related illnesses lead to financial cost to the public healthcare system (see Box 6.7) and questions arise about whether this should affect people's access to treatment. We considered a similar situation in the case of obesity and concluded that treatment should generally not be denied because of reasons including the value of the community and risks of stigmatising or penalising people (see paragraph 5.42). We also found, however, that personal behaviour might need to be considered when assessing the potential effectiveness of a treatment for a patient.

6.17 We note that current Department of Health guidelines on liver transplantation require patients to have abstained from alcohol for six months, and people who are considered likely to continue to consume excessive amounts of alcohol are not offered a transplant.[59] We agree that, as in this example, **it might be justified for doctors to appeal to patients to change their behaviour in relation to alcohol and tobacco before or subsequent to an intervention provided by the NHS, provided that the change would enhance the effectiveness of the intervention, and people were offered help to do this. For example, alcohol treatment programmes might be offered in advance of performing a liver transplant as the cessation of excessive drinking would be likely**

[53] Royal College of Physicians (2005) *Going Smoke-free: The medical case for clean air in the home, at work and in public places*, available at: http://www.rcplondon.ac.uk/pubs/contents/fe4ab715-2689-4a4a-b8c7-53e80386c893.pdf.

[54] *Ibid.*

[55] Bromley C, Sprosten K and Shelton N (Editors) (2005) *The Scottish Health Survey 2003, Volume 3: Children* (Edinburgh: Scottish Executive), p.22.

[56] Royal College of Physicians (2005) *Going Smoke-free: The medical case for clean air in the home, at work and in public places*, available at: http://www.rcplondon.ac.uk/pubs/contents/fe4ab715-2689-4a4a-b8c7-53e80386c893.pdf.

[57] *Ibid.*

[58] See BBC News (2007) *Criticism of Smoker Adoption Ban*, available at: http://news.bbc.co.uk/1/hi/england/hampshire/6730697.stm.

[59] Although, people who are successful in avoiding alcohol for this time period often no longer need a transplant. Department of Health (2005) *National Liver Transplant Standards*, available at: http://www.dh.gov.uk/assetRoot/04/11/78/55/04117855.pdf.

Box 6.7: Economic costs and revenue from taxation of alcohol and tobacco

Economic costs of alcohol consumption

Costs that arise from alcohol consumption include healthcare expenditure, prevention measures, work days lost due to ill health and the ill-effects of excessive alcohol consumption, and treatment and prevention services. Estimates of the cost to the NHS of alcohol misuse vary, ranging between 2% and 12% of the total NHS expenditure on hospitals (£3 billion per year).[60] In 2004, the Government calculated that the cost of alcohol-related harms in England was £20 billion per annum.[61]

Estimates of the cost of alcohol-related harms in England per year by the Prime Minister's Strategy Unit*

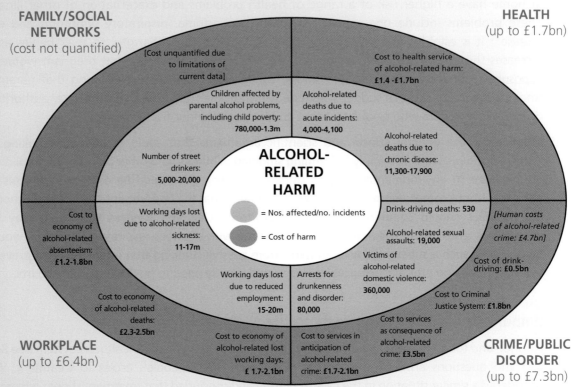

*Source: Prime Minister's Strategy Unit (2004) Alcohol Harm Reduction Strategy for England, available at: http://www.cabinetoffice.gov.uk/strategy/downloads/su/alcohol/pdf/CabOffce%20AlcoholHar.pdf, Crown Copyright, reproduced with permission.

Economic costs of smoking

Smoking is estimated to cost the NHS £1.7 billion per year.[62] A full estimate of the total costs of smoking in the UK has not been calculated. It has, however, been estimated that annual savings of £3.9 billion to the UK economy would result from making workplaces completely smoke-free.[63] Further savings should arise in expenditure on healthcare from reducing childhood exposure to smoke and smoking during pregnancy.

Revenue from alcohol and tobacco

The alcohol and tobacco industries bring economic benefits to governments through taxation and employment. In the UK and many other countries, both alcohol and tobacco are subject to additional taxation over and above value added tax (VAT). The duty on alcohol and tobacco amounted to £8 billion and £7.6 billion respectively in 2006–7 (not including VAT) (each approximately 1.8% of total revenue).[64]

[60] Strategy Unit, Cabinet Office (2003) Alcohol Misuse: How much does it cost?, p.15, available at: http://sia.dfc.unifi.it/costi%20uk.pdf; Royal College of Physicians (2001) Alcohol – can the NHS afford it? (London: RCP).

[61] Prime Minister's Strategy Unit (2004) Alcohol Harm Reduction Strategy for England, available at: http://www.cabinetoffice.gov.uk/strategy/downloads/su/alcohol/pdf/CabOffce%20AlcoholHar.pdf.

[62] Department of Health (1998) White Paper: Smoking Kills, available at: http://www.archive.official-documents.co.uk/document/cm41/4177/contents.htm.

[63] Royal College of Physicians (2005) Going Smoke-free: The medical case for clean air in the home, at work and in public places, p.142, available at: http://www.rcplondon.ac.uk/pubs/contents/fe4ab715-2689-4a4a-b8c7-53e80386c893.pdf.

[64] HM Revenue & Customs (2007) 2006–07 Accounts (London: The Stationery Office), available at: http://www.hmrc.gov.uk/about/hmrc-06-07-acc.pdf.

to increase its clinical effectiveness, or could even make the transplant unnecessary. Generally, as in the case of obesity, we take the view that decisions about healthcare provision for people who smoke and/or drink alcohol excessively raise some valid considerations about the most efficient use of resources. In terms of public health policy, the focus of efforts should be on avoiding the need for treatment for alcohol- and tobacco-related conditions in the first place. This is a fairer approach, and also seems likely to be more effective in economic terms. **The UK health departments should further liaise with employers about how best to offer assistance with behaviour change programmes, such as smoking cessation, which could benefit the employer as well as employees** (see Box 6.7).

Obligations of the alcohol and tobacco industries

6.18 There are differing views on what responsibility industry should take for health problems caused by its products. Some examples from our consultation are:

"If companies are legally entitled to sell their products and the buyers are aware of the dangers to their health that may result, the companies cannot be expected to take responsibility for the illnesses they may cause." *National Council of Women of Great Britain*

"The companies must ... take responsibility for selling hazardous known toxins to the public ... and ... compensation to the damaged people themselves, as well as to their health 'care' should be made available." *Mrs Penny S Pullen*

6.19 For a variety of reasons, businesses have given increasing attention to corporate social responsibility (see paragraphs 2.47–2.50). The Working Party considers that when industry fails to behave responsibly, it is appropriate for government to impose more stringent regulations on the alcohol and tobacco industries to achieve a more effective reduction of the harms caused by their products (see paragraph 2.50). We explore some examples in the paragraphs that follow.

Advertising

6.20 Marketing is acknowledged to be powerful in manipulating people's preferences between alcoholic and non-alcoholic drinks and of which type of drink to choose. For example, cider sales in the UK grew by 23% in 2006 following a widespread advertising campaign costing millions of pounds.[65] The advertising of alcohol is regulated and this could be further extended. For example, one respondent to our consultation proposed that:

"Manufacturers of products known to cause harm ... should not be able to advertise in a way that promotes the idea that their product improves the experience of life. ... they should not be able to sell in ways that take advantage of vulnerable people, including people with poor mental health or people under the influence of alcohol... should not be allowed to advertise unless those advertisements clearly set out the risks." *Anon*

6.21 Companies are allowed to advertise alcoholic drinks much more freely in the UK than in some other countries such as France.[66] By contrast, advertising of tobacco products is almost entirely prohibited in the UK.[67] With certain exceptions (such as that of tobacco), the advertising industry in the UK is generally governed under self-regulation by codes of practice that "are designed to protect consumers and create a level playing field for advertisers".[68] The codes are the responsibility of the Committee of Advertising Practice (CAP)

---

[65] Atkinson S (2007) Cider firms look to build on boom, available at: http://news.bbc.co.uk/1/hi/business/6522855.stm.

[66] See Institute of Alcohol Studies (2005) Fact Sheet *Alcohol and Advertising*, available at: http://www.ias.org.uk/resources/factsheets/advertising.pdf.

[67] Action on Smoking and Health (2006) *Tobacco Advertising and Promotion*, available at: http://www.ash.org.uk/html/factsheets/html/fact19.html.

[68] Committee of Advertising Practice, see http://www.cap.org.uk/cap/.

and are independently administered by the Advertising Standards Authority (ASA). Sanctions available to the ASA against advertisers whose material is in breach of the codes range from a warning to referral to the Office of Fair Trading with the possibility of legal proceedings. For broadcast media (television and radio), the regulator Ofcom can impose fines and withdraw broadcasting licences from those who run advertisements that breach the codes.[69]

6.22 As an example, the *Non-Broadcast Code*[70] advises companies that promote alcoholic drinks that:

■ Marketing communications should not be associated with people under 18 or reflect their culture. They should not feature or portray real or fictitious characters who are likely to appeal particularly to people under 18 in a way that might encourage them to drink.

■ Marketing communications should not suggest that any alcoholic drink has therapeutic qualities (for example, stimulant or sedative qualities) or can change moods or enhance confidence, mental or physical capabilities or performance, popularity or sporting achievements. They should not link alcoholic drinks to illicit drugs.

■ Marketing communications must neither link alcohol with seduction, sexual activity or sexual success nor imply that alcohol can enhance attractiveness, masculinity or femininity.

However, observation of advertisements of alcoholic drinks suggests that not all companies adhere to the ideal proposed in these guidelines.

The tobacco industry: harm reduction

6.23 In one of our fact-finding meetings it was reported to us that the tobacco industry has been aware of the harmful effects of tobacco and pursued a 'harm reduction strategy' since the 1970s (see Appendix 1). It was suggested that this strategy has included the development of regulations for the protection of vulnerable people, making it more difficult for people to take up smoking and easier for those who wanted to cease. We note that all major tobacco companies have corporate social responsibility policies, and although we see a contradiction in marketing very harmful and addictive products and seeking to play a role in reducing harms at the same time, it is clear that that the industry does have a role to play in harm reduction (see paragraph 6.27).

6.24 The tobacco industry has recently been developing a form of smokeless tobacco called 'snus', apparently as a method of harm reduction and also as a response to the increasingly widespread bans on smoking in enclosed public places.[71] Snus, which is placed underneath the lip, has been legally available in Sweden and some other countries for many years although it is banned in all other Member States of the European Union (Sweden has an exemption). It is addictive in the same way as cigarettes and has been found to increase the risk of some diseases but eliminates the risk of harm to third parties. The industry argues that there is epidemiological evidence that this form of tobacco presents considerably lower health risks than cigarette smoking[72] and certain medical bodies and anti-smoking bodies agree.[73] Major tobacco companies have recently lobbied the European Union to change the legislation prohibiting it.[74]

---

[69] Information obtained from the websites of these organisations.

[70] Advertising Standards Authority (2003) *The British Code of Advertising, Sales Promotion and Direct Marketing*, available at: http://www.asa.org.uk/NR/rdonlyres/A44808F1-1573-482A-A0E5-D8045943DA57/0/The_CAP_Code_Ed11_20060901.pdf.

[71] See, for example, British American Tobacco *Selling Snus*, available at: http://www.bat.com/OneWeb/sites/uk__3mnfen.nsf/vwPagesWebLive/DO725M6L?opendocument&SID=&DTC=&TMP=1.

[72] British American Tobacco *Regulation and Bans*, available at: http://www.bat.com/OneWeb/sites/uk__3mnfen.nsf/vwPagesWebLive/DO725MZF?opendocument&SID=&DTC=&TMP=1.

[73] See, for example, Royal College of Physicians *RCP Response to 'Choosing Health': Tobacco*, available at: http://www.rcplondon.ac.uk/college/statements/response_choosehealth_tobacco.asp; Action on Smoking and Health (2004) *Will Europe Lift the Ban on Oral Snuff?*, available at: http://www.ash.org.uk/.

[74] See, for example British American Tobacco *Regulation and Bans*, available at: http://www.bat.com/OneWeb/sites/uk__3mnfen.nsf/vwPagesWebLive/DO725MZF?opendocument&SID=&DTC=&TMP=1; Rose D (2007) Cigarette firms push for tobacco 'teabags' *The Times* 14 May, available at: http://www.timesonline.co.uk/tol/life_and_style/health/article1785028.ece.

6.25 Based on our considerations of the stewardship model, the Working Party is not persuaded that snus should be permitted. Although there may be evidence of lower overall health risks compared with cigarette smoking, there is still evidence of harm and addiction.[75] **In view of the health risks and the possibility that consumers may be led to believe they are using a relatively harmless product, we are not persuaded that permitting snus or conducting further research on the health risks is a helpful approach. Allowing snus might also carry the risk of increasing health inequalities in the UK as members of certain ethnic groups who already have a culture of chewing stimulants, such as betel nut, might more easily take up snus.**

The tobacco industry: international aspects

6.26 While, generally, we focus in this Report on the situation in the UK, in the case of tobacco it is relevant to consider the international context. Tobacco companies operate in many different countries, and increasingly in developing countries, many of which do not have in place stringent regulations on tobacco advertising and promotion. If tobacco companies are sincere in their harm reduction efforts, they are in a unique position to apply best practice that affords the higher level of protection available in some countries to people in countries with less developed regulations. Without this commitment, tobacco companies would be operating 'double standards' in terms of their corporate social responsibility and harm reduction strategies. Parties to the *WHO Framework Convention on Tobacco Control 2003*[76] were "seriously concerned about the increase in the worldwide consumption and production of cigarettes and other tobacco products, particularly in developing countries, as well as about the burden this places on families, on the poor, and on national health systems". The UK has ratified this Convention and it came into force in 2005.

6.27 **It is ethically inconsistent for tobacco and alcohol companies advertising and selling their products in developed countries to claim corporate social responsibility, and yet apply different standards for protecting consumers in different countries, depending on local laws. Acting ethically exceeds simply complying with relevant laws and regulations. Policies on selling and advertising tobacco and alcohol that afford the greatest protection to consumers should be adopted worldwide. The members of the UK Tobacco Manufacturers' Association and other companies that produce or market tobacco products should implement a voluntary code of practice that universalises best practice in terms of consumer protection. One example would be worldwide adherence to standards in advertising that have been developed and agreed by the industry in the EU, and particularly the UK.**

Role of government

6.28 The use of alcohol and tobacco has implications for nearly every government department in the UK. In some cases departments may support the alcohol and tobacco industries despite concerns about population health.[77] This may also be found in devolved administrations and regional and local government, for example where job losses might be caused in that area if sales of these products reduced.

---

[75] For a review article, see Gray N (2005) Mixed feelings on snus *Lancet* **366**: 966–7.

[76] A framework convention is a binding international legal instrument that establishes broad commitments and a general system of governance for an issue area. The *WHO Framework Convention on Tobacco Control* addresses: elimination of illicit trade in tobacco products; banning tobacco sales to and by minors; agricultural diversification and the promotion of alternative livelihoods; and advertising, promotion and sponsorship. For further information see World Health Organization *Frequently asked questions on the WHO FCTC and the context in which it was negotiated*, available at: http://www.who.int/tobacco/framework/faq/en/index.html.

[77] Baggott R (2000) *Public Health: Policy and politics* (Basingstoke: Palgrave Macmillan), pp.196–220.

6.29 In 2004 the Government published its *Alcohol Harm Reduction Strategy for England* followed in 2007 by *Safe, Sensible, Social: The next steps in the National Alcohol Strategy*.[78] A comparison of the Government's Strategy with the findings of the evidence-based study *Alcohol: No ordinary commodity*[79] (sponsored by WHO) finds that there is little consensus. The latter emphasised the effectiveness of increasing taxes, restricting hours and days of sale and the density of outlets that sell alcohol, and possibly of banning advertising, whereas it found little evidence in support of the effectiveness of education about alcohol in schools, and evidence for a lack of effectiveness concerning public service messages and warning labels. The Government's original Strategy, however, concentrated on education and communication, reviewing the advertising of alcohol, enforcement of legal restrictions on selling to under-18s, and voluntary measures for the alcohol industry about labelling and manufacturing. The second part of the Strategy included further measures on guidance and public information campaigns and measures to try to promote a 'sensible drinking' culture. A review of the evidence and a consultation on the relationship between alcohol price, promotion and harm was also announced and the Government pledged to consider the need for regulatory change in the future. We draw attention to the fact that alcoholic drinks in the UK are now less expensive relative to disposable income than they were in the 1970s.[80]

6.30 The areas where *No ordinary commodity* and the UK Government's strategies are in agreement include support for at-risk drinkers and treatment of people with alcohol problems and implementing rules about serving intoxicated people. The evidence presented in *No ordinary commodity* on the effectiveness of restricting the availability of alcohol stands in contrast to the Government's policy since November 2005 of allowing extended opening hours for pubs and bars.[81] The evidence for the effectiveness of some of the interventions aiming to reduce the overall consumption of alcohol is strong.[82] Thus, the Government's failure to take up the most effective strategies cannot be due to lack of evidence.

6.31 **The stewardship model provides justification for the UK Government to introduce measures that are more coercive than those which currently feature in the National Alcohol Strategy (2004 and 2007). We recommend that evidence-based measures judged effective in the WHO-sponsored analysis *Alcohol: No ordinary commodity* are implemented by the UK Government. These include coercive strategies to manage alcohol consumption, specifically in the areas of price, marketing and availability. For example, taxes on alcoholic beverages might be increased, which has been shown to be an effective strategy for reducing consumption. We also recommend that the Home Office, the UK health departments and the Department of Culture, Media and Sport analyse the effect of extended opening hours of licensed premises on levels of consumption, as well as on anti-social behaviour.**

[78] Prime Minister's Strategy Unit (2004) *Alcohol Harm Reduction Strategy for England*, available at: http://www.cabinetoffice.gov.uk/strategy/downloads/su/alcohol/pdf/CabOffce%20AlcoholHar.pdf; Department of Health, Home Office, Department for Education and Skills and Department for Culture, Media and Sport (2007) *Safe. Sensible. Social. The next steps in the National Alcohol Strategy* (London: Department of Health Publications). The original Strategy stated that the Government had consulted with the devolved administrations in Scotland, Northern Ireland and Wales in producing its analysis and would continue to do so as the strategy was implemented. All three devolved administrations produced their own strategies. The follow-up document was also prepared in discussion with the devolved administrations, and reflects programmes developed by each administration.

[79] Babor T, Caetano R, Casswell S *et al.* (2003) *Alcohol: No ordinary commodity – Research and public policy* (Oxford: Oxford University Press).

[80] Academy of Medical Sciences (2004) *Calling Time: The nation's drinking as a major health issue* (London: Academy of Medical Sciences).

[81] See Department for Culture, Media and Sport *Licensing Act 2003 Explained*, available at: http://www.culture.gov.uk/what_we_do/Alcohol_entertainment/licensing_act_2003_explained/.

[82] Academy of Medical Sciences (2004) *Calling Time: The nation's drinking as a major health issue* (London: Academy of Medical Sciences).[78]

Protecting the vulnerable

6.32 Under our stewardship model, public health measures should pay special attention to the health of children (paragraphs 2.41–2.44). As both drinking alcohol and smoking are associated with dependence and harms, there has frequently been concern expressed about any use by children and adolescents (see Box 6.8 for details about consumption in this age group). A considerable number of respondents to our consultation called for vigorous action; for example: "[T]he State should do everything in its power to prevent children and teenagers from becoming addicted to smoking" (Dr V. Larcher). Young people often lack judgement about risk and are vulnerable to the influence of others. Additionally, if people start drinking alcohol and smoking as children and adolescents and continue into adulthood, they will have been exposed to these health harms over a longer period of time than if they had started as adults. Health and other harms (such as any effect on education) caused by misuse of these substances can be very serious for developing children and adolescents.

Box 6.8: Drinking and smoking among children

A national survey conducted in England in 2005 on smoking and drinking among schoolchildren aged 11–15 years suggests the numbers drinking and smoking between 1982 and 2005 had changed little or fallen, but the amount of alcohol consumed has shown a significant increase in recent years, particularly among girls, as illustrated in the figure below.[83] The survey found that 22% of boys and 23% of girls had drunk alcohol in the week prior to the survey. A quarter of all pupils who had drunk in the last week had consumed 14 or more units. The proportion of pupils who had drunk alcohol in the last week increased with age from 3% of 11 year olds to 46% of 15 year olds. The average alcohol consumption of pupils who had drunk alcohol had increased from 5.3 units per week in 1990 to 10.5 in 2005. The prevalence of regular smoking is higher among girls (10%) than boys (7%). Again, regular smoking increased with age, from 1% of 11 year olds to 20% of 15-year-olds (with regular smokers smoking an average of 42 cigarettes). Those who had recently smoked were also more likely to have consumed alcohol.

Mean alcohol consumption of children aged 11–15 who drank in the week prior to the survey, by sex, in England, 1990–2004*

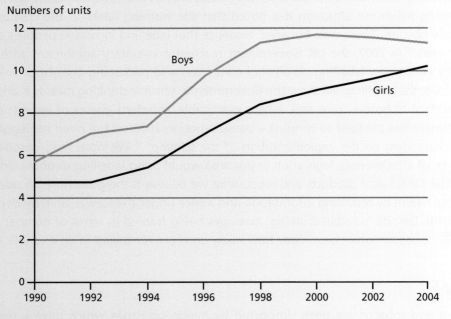

*Source: National Statistics *Drinking*, available at:
http://www.statistics.gov.uk/CCI/nugget.asp?ID=1328&Pos=4&ColRank=2&Rank=800, Crown copyright material is reproduced with the permission of the Controller of HMSO under the terms of the Click-Use Licence.

---

[83] Fuller E (Editor) (2006) *Drug Use, Smoking and Drinking among Young People in England in 2005* (The Information Centre for Health and Social Care).

6.33 **Producers, advertisers and vendors of alcohol and tobacco need to recognise more fully the vulnerability of children and young people, and take clearer responsibility for preventing harms to health. This would include refraining from understating risks, and from exploiting the apparent desirability of drinking alcohol and smoking, particularly in ways that appeal to children and young people. Furthermore, it would appear that whatever the legal position, these products are widely available to underage children, and existing law and policy need to be implemented more stringently. We welcome the raising of the minimum age for the purchase of tobacco from 16 to 18 years that has taken place throughout the UK as part of a strategy to protect vulnerable people. Although thought needs to be given to the way in which this measure can be implemented most effectively, it is an appropriate initiative in the context of the stewardship model, as the market has largely failed to self-regulate in this area.**

Enabling people to live more healthily and make choices (provision of information)

6.34 It is widely recognised that the decrease since the 1970s both in the number of people who smoke and in the amount smoked are, at least in part, the result of an increase in people's knowledge about the dangers of smoking. However, in the case of alcohol, many heavy drinkers still underestimate the risks caused by their drinking and are reluctant or unable to associate their drinking with health risks or their poor health (see paragraph 6.4). Messages about the risks involved with smoking are easier to present, i.e. any amount of smoking is unhealthy and carries risk. Although no less significant, it is harder to present a straightforward picture of the risks associated with drinking alcohol, particularly as the health risks of light or moderate drinking are disputed (see Box 6.1).

6.35 We note that messages and warning notes have been used for several years on tobacco products although the evidence for their effectiveness is still limited. In the WHO-sponsored publication, *Alcohol: No ordinary commodity*, a review of the evidence about warning labels on containers of alcoholic drinks in the USA concludes that labels are not effective in producing a direct change in drinking behaviour although it is noted that the warning labels in the USA are small and relatively obscure. There was, however, evidence that labelling increased people's awareness of health risks.[84] In 2007, the UK Government reached a voluntary agreement with the alcohol industry about new labelling on alcohol containers and packaging bought or sold in the UK. From 2008, the labelling will show the Government's 'sensible drinking message' and the alcohol unit content of bottles, cans and, where practicable, standard glasses of wine and spirits. The Government has pledged to conduct a consultation in 2008 on the need for legislation in this area "depending on the implementation of the scheme".[85] We note that, despite the lack of evidence of effectiveness, legislation in this area would bring labelling alcoholic drinks into line with that for tobacco products and meet what we believe is the government's responsibility to promote health by providing information and advice under the stewardship model (paragraphs 2.41–2.44). Despite 'sensible drinking' messages being framed in terms of number of units (see Box 6.2), it has not often been clear how many units are contained in an alcoholic drink.

Summary

6.36 Alcohol and tobacco are both supported by major industries which have a role to play in reducing the harms caused by their products, both in the UK and around the world. The Working Party concludes that the Government has been justified in trying to reduce the

---

[84] Babor T, Caetano R, Casswell S *et al.* (2003) *Alcohol: No ordinary commodity – Research and public policy* (Oxford: Oxford University Press), pp.192–3.

[85] Department of Health, Home Office, Department for Education and Skills and Department for Culture, Media and Sport (2007) *Safe. Sensible. Social. The next steps in the National Alcohol Strategy* (London: Department of Health Publications).

harms caused to third parties by the introduction of bans on smoking in enclosed public places. However, given the level of harm caused, it would also be justified in taking further action to reduce the harms caused both to people who drink alcohol excessively and smoke tobacco themselves, and also to third parties affected by others' drinking and smoking. This is particularly true for alcohol; per capita consumption is rising and yet there have been few governmental measures to address the resulting consequences for health and public order.

6.37 Socio-economic groups with fewer resources are disproportionately affected by the harms caused by alcohol and tobacco. Therefore any public health policies in this area should aim to reduce health inequalities. Another special case is that of children, who are less able to judge risk to health, are vulnerable to the harms caused by alcohol and tobacco, and may become addicted to these substances at a young age. Promoters of alcohol and tobacco have a role to play in reducing the exposure of young people to harmful products.

6.38 There are a number of measures under the stewardship model that could be introduced and, based on the evidence presented above, could potentially reduce the harms caused by alcohol and tobacco. The Working Party reiterates the theme that if industries do not themselves make sufficient progress towards reducing harm when there is clear evidence that this is possible and desirable for public health, government should take regulatory measures aimed at reducing harm to health.

Chapter 7

Case study –
Fluoridation of water

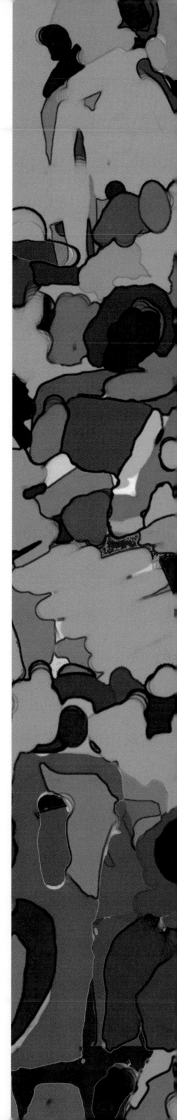

Case study – Fluoridation of water

Introduction

7.1 Water fluoridation is an example of an intervention that directly affects whole populations, in this case for the purpose of improving dental health. Because of the relative difficulty of 'opting out', the measure raises ethical and policy issues: what is the justification for overriding the preferences of those people who wish to receive water that has not been fluoridated? Is the intervention justifiable even if it is not possible (or feasible) to obtain individual consent? In this chapter we begin by providing some background information on dental health, the technical principles behind water fluoridation, and alternative fluoride-based dental health measures. We then consider how different ethical principles outlined in Chapter 2 could potentially be used in support of, or against, water fluoridation, and how the principles should be weighed against one another. The case of fluoridation also raises particular issues about the nature and strength of evidence required in arguments about the acceptability of an intervention, and about ways in which evidence is, and should be, communicated. We therefore, finally, consider the role of evidence and information in policy, and the way different parties in this debate use and communicate evidence.

7.2 Although we focus here on fluoridation, we note that some similar ethical issues are raised about policies on the fortification of foods. Several such programmes are in place in the UK as means of improving the health of a population or sub-population, for example adding vitamins and

> ### Box 7.1: Fortification of flour with folic acid
>
> Folate, a B vitamin, is essential to everyone's health.[1] Insufficient levels during early pregnancy of folate or its synthetic substitute, folic acid, can lead to neural-tube defects in the newborn.[2] For some time, folic acid supplements have been recommended before and during pregnancy. However, research has found that only 55% of women planning a pregnancy increased their folate intake as recommended.[3] Furthermore, because around 50% of pregnancies are unplanned, many women may not start taking folic acid sufficiently early. The recommended folate intake for women of child-bearing age is 600 micrograms (µg) per day, but the National Diet and Nutrition Survey indicates that 34% of women of child-bearing age have intakes of less than 200 µg per day, and this is particularly common in lower socio-economic groups.[4]
>
> Because of this situation, consideration has been given in the UK to fortification of food with folic acid. In 2007 the Board of the Food Standards Agency recommended the mandatory fortification of either bread or flour.[5] This followed a report by the Scientific Advisory Committee on Nutrition (SACN), which recommended fortifying flour with folic acid to a level that they estimated would result in 77–162 fewer pregnancies with neural-tube defects in the UK each year.[6] They also estimated that this level of fortification would reduce the proportion of people across the population consuming less than the recommended amount of folate from 23% to 5%. Flour is already fortified with folic acid in the USA, Canada and Chile.[7]
>
> There have been concerns that folic acid fortification may 'mask' vitamin B12 deficiencies in the elderly. However, SACN has suggested that this effect is not seen with doses of 1 mg/day or less, and that there are no reports of these effects in countries with mandatory folate fortification.[8] The Committee also found insufficient evidence for several other adverse effects that it considered.
>
> Although comparisons between folic acid fortification and water fluoridation are interesting, it should be noted, first, that folic acid fortification is not known to be associated with harms (see paragraphs 7.31–7.32); and secondly, that wholemeal flour/bread would be excluded from the policy, enabling individuals to opt not to receive the fortified foods.

---

[1] Food Standards Agency, *Folic Acid*, available at: http://www.eatwell.gov.uk/healthydiet/nutritionessentials/vitaminsandminerals/folicacid/.

[2] *Ibid.*

[3] Scientific Advisory Committee on Nutrition (2006) *Folate and Disease Prevention*, available at: http://www.sacn.gov.uk/pdfs/folate_and_disease_prevention_report.pdf.

[4] *Ibid.*

[5] Food Standards Agency (2007) Press release: *Board recommends mandatory fortification*, available at: http://www.food.gov.uk/news/newsarchive/2007/may/folatefort. At the time this Report went to press, the Food Standards Agency was in the process of considering whether it should be bread or flour that was fortified and presenting its recommendations to UK Health Ministers.

[6] Scientific Advisory Committee on Nutrition (2006) *Folate and Disease Prevention*, available at: http://www.sacn.gov.uk/pdfs/folate_and_disease_prevention_report.pdf. It is estimated that in 2003 there were 630–850 pregnancies with neural-tube defects in England and Wales, and at least 49 in Scotland and 11 in Northern Ireland. Of these pregnancies, varying proportions (generally at least 50%) were terminated in different UK countries, except in Northern Ireland, where none were terminated.

[7] Scientific Advisory Committee on Nutrition (2006) *Folate and Disease Prevention*, available at: http://www.sacn.gov.uk/pdfs/folate_and_disease_prevention_report.pdf.

[8] *Ibid.*

minerals to margarines and breakfast cereals, while a policy of fortifying flour with folic acid is, at the time of writing, under consideration (see Box 7.1).

Dental health in the UK

7.3 Children's dental health in the UK has been improving over recent decades (see Figure 7.1a). In 2003 the UK Children's Dental Health Survey reported lower levels of obvious dental decay (also called dental caries) than had previously been recorded in the permanent teeth of 8-, 12- and 15-year-olds'.[9] The proportions of children affected by decay in each age group were 14%, 34% and 49%, respectively, compared with 38%, 83% and 91% in 1983.[10] In 2003 the mean numbers of teeth with obvious decay in these age groups were 0.2, 0.8 and 1.6, respectively, compared with 0.8, 3.1 and 5.9 in 1983. These figures are, however, UK averages, and dental health varies considerably across different social groups and areas of the UK (see Figure 7.1). Surveys by the British Association for the Study of Community Dentistry of 5-, 11-, and 14-year-old children in England, Wales and Scotland have all shown wide variation in caries prevalence in different areas (see Figure 7.1b).[11]

Figure 7.1: Children's dental health in the UK*

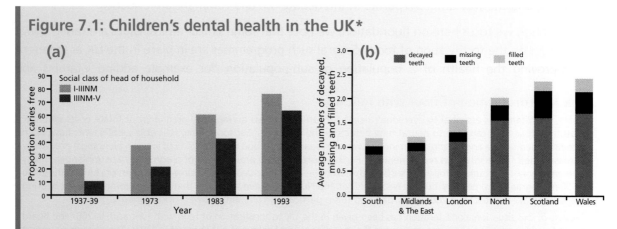

(a) Oral health of children aged 5 in England, 1937–1993. Data: National Children's Dental Health Surveys, 1973 to 1993. Data for other UK countries for 1983 and 1993 indicate that similar trends over time and with socio-economic group were evident in these areas also. The 2003 survey used a different classification system, but indicated further improvements in dental health although socio-economic inequalities persisted.

(b) Occurrence of dental caries, measured as average numbers of decayed, missing and filled teeth, of children aged 5 in Great Britain. Data: The dental caries experience of 5-year-old children in England and Wales (2003/4) and in Scotland (2002/3); surveys co-ordinated by the British Association for the Study of Community Dentistry.

*Figures reproduced under the terms of the Click-Use Licence, from: Department of Health (2005) *Choosing Better Oral Health: An oral health plan for England* (London: Department of Health), available at: http://www.dh.gov.uk/assetRoot/04/12/32/53/04123253.pdf.

[9] National Statistics (2004) *Executive Summary of preliminary findings: 2003 Children's Dental Health Survey*, available at: http://www.statistics.gov.uk/downloads/theme_health/Executive_Summary-CDH.pdf.

[10] National Statistics (2005) *Children's Dental Health in the United Kingdom, 2003 Summary Report*, available at: http://www.statistics.gov.uk/CHILDREN/dentalhealth/downloads/cdh_Summary.pdf.

[11] Pitts NB, Boyles J, Nugent ZJ, Thomas N and Pine CM (2007) The dental caries experience of 5-year-old children in Great Britain (2005/6). Surveys co-ordinated by the British Association for the Study of Community Dentistry *Community Dent Health* **24**: 59–63; Pitts NB, Boyles J, Nugent ZJ, Thomas N and Pine CM (2006) The dental caries experience of 11-year-old children in Great Britain. Surveys coordinated by the British Association for the Study of Community Dentistry in 2004 / 2005 *Community Dent Health* **23**: 44–57; Pitts NB, Boyles J, Nugent ZJ, Thomas N and Pine CM (2004) The dental caries experience of 14-year-old children in England and Wales. Surveys co-ordinated by the British Association for the Study of Community Dentistry in 2002/2003 *Community Dent Health* **21**: 45–57.

Water fluoridation

Background to fluoride and water fluoridation

7.4 The chemical element fluorine is found combined with other elements to form fluoride compounds in soil, rock, air and water.[12] Although all water contains dissolved fluoride, the concentrations at which it is present naturally in water vary considerably, from less than 0.5 parts per million (ppm) to, rarely, as high as 25 ppm.[13] Fluoride can also be present in various food and drink products that people may consume, in particular tea.[14]

7.5 Fluoride is a mineral. It is unclear whether, in biological terms, it should be considered an essential mineral,[15] but it does appear to be of benefit in the prevention of tooth decay, or dental caries (see Box 7.2). This benefit was first suggested in the 1930s and 1940s when researchers in the USA compared areas with different levels of natural fluoride in the water.[16] In 1945 the first water fluoridation scheme was implemented in the USA, and this was followed by further schemes in the USA, the UK and elsewhere. The water fluoride level used in these schemes, and still widely used today, was 1 ppm. This was suggested to be a suitable level at which the prevalence of dental caries was reduced and adverse effects were rare.[17]

Box 7.2: How does fluoride work?

Current research suggests that fluoride affects demineralisation and remineralisation of the tooth, and has anti-bacterial effects. These properties alter the process by which dental caries may occur.[18] It is estimated that most, if not all, anti-caries effects of fluoride occur through the presence of fluoride in the mouth, and that maintaining adequate levels of fluoride in the mouth is essential for preventing and controlling decay.[19] It is unclear whether there is a systemic effect from fluoride that is ingested.[20]

Benefits and harms of water fluoridation

7.6 The purpose of water fluoridation, where it is implemented, is to reduce dental caries. However, the extent of any reduction has been difficult to quantify on the current evidence. Some of the early studies on water fluoridation suggested that the measure was highly beneficial. For example, research into the scheme begun in 1945 concluded that water

---

[12] European Food Safety Authority (2005) Opinion of the Scientific Panel on Dietetic Products, Nutrition and Allergies on a request from the Commission related to the tolerable upper intake level of fluoride *European Food Safety Authority Journal* **192**: 1–65, available at:
http://www.efsa.europa.eu/etc/medialib/efsa/science/nda/nda_opinions/851.Par.0001.File.dat/nda_op_ej192_fluoride_corrigendum1.pdf.

[13] Expert Group on Vitamins and Minerals (2001) *Review of Fluoride*, available at:
http://archive.food.gov.uk/committees/evm/papers/evm0103.pdf. Consuming water with very high fluoride levels can be harmful (see paragraphs 7.7, 7.31–7.33 and Box 7.3), and consequently in some places the fluoride level in the drinking water supply is reduced. In the UK, the maximum level of fluoride permitted is 1.5 ppm under the Water Supply (Water Quality) Regulations 2000 and Water Supply (Water Quality) (Scotland) Regulations 1990. In the USA the guideline maximum contaminant level goal is 4 ppm, although there are some calls for this to be reduced. Committee on Fluoride in Drinking Water, National Research Council of the National Academies (2006) *Fluoride in Drinking Water* (Washington, DC: National Academies Press).

[14] European Food Safety Authority (2005) Opinion of the Scientific Panel on Dietetic Products, Nutrition and Allergies on a request from the Commission related to the tolerable upper intake level of fluoride *European Food Safety Authority Journal* **192**: 1–65, available at:
http://www.efsa.europa.eu/etc/medialib/efsa/science/nda/nda_opinions/851.Par.0001.File.dat/nda_op_ej192_fluoride_corrigendum1.pdf.

[15] Essential minerals are those that are required for human health, either for growth or to sustain life, and as such if insufficient amounts are consumed adverse health effects occur. It is unclear whether fluoride should be categorised as an essential mineral. Expert Group on Vitamins and Minerals (2003) *Safe Upper Levels for Vitamins and Minerals* (London: Food Standards Agency), available at: http://www.food.gov.uk/multimedia/pdfs/vitmin2003.pdf.

[16] Lennon MA (2006) One in a million: the first community trial of water fluoridation *Bull World Health Org* **84**: 759–60.

[17] *Ibid*.

[18] Clarkson J (Ed) (2000) International collaborative research on fluoride *J Dent Res* **79**: 893–904.

[19] *Ibid*.; Aoba T and Fejerskov O (2002) Dental fluorosis: chemistry and biology *Crit Rev Oral Biol Med* **13**: 155–70.

[20] Clarkson J (Ed) (2000) International collaborative research on fluoride *J Dent Res* **79**: 893–904

fluoridation was "remarkably effective" in reducing the prevalence of dental caries among children.[21] However, in many of the studies on fluoridation, particularly the early ones, the methodologies used have not been of high quality. A major review of the evidence on water fluoridation was published in 2000 by the Centre for Reviews and Dissemination at the University of York (hereafter referred to as the York review).[22] It concluded that the best available evidence suggested that fluoridation of drinking water reduced the prevalence of caries, but found that the reduction was difficult to quantify from the evidence available.

7.7 Drinking fluoridated water can have adverse effects, the risks of which increase with higher levels of consumption. Dental fluorosis, a defect of the tooth enamel that causes visible markings on the teeth, is the most well known and frequently studied negative effect of fluoridation (see also Box 7.3).[23] It can vary from mild speckling to more substantial staining and pitting of the teeth, and may have a psychological effect on the children concerned. Estimates of the prevalence of fluorosis among people receiving fluoridated water vary. The York review and a report by the Medical Research Council suggested prevalences of 12.5% and 3–4%, respectively, for fluorosis serious enough to cause aesthetic concern at a fluoridation level of 1 ppm (see also paragraph 7.32).[24] Besides fluorosis, some have suggested other harms may be associated with water fluoridation, including bone fractures and cancer, although the evidence for such effects is generally weak; we discuss these further later (see paragraph 7.31).

7.8 We have not, in this chapter, sought to re-assess the evidence on fluoridation. In our discussions we have drawn on expert assessments by others, and in particular the York review, because this represents the most recent major review in this area.[25] We do, however, note a comment made by authors of the York review that: "Given the level of interest surrounding the issue of public water fluoridation, it is surprising to find that little high quality research has been undertaken".[26] This is particularly surprising as fluoridation has been implemented as an intervention in some areas of the country, and has been considered as a policy option in others, over several decades. Later in the chapter we return to consider further the reported benefits and harms of fluoridation in relation to the ethical principles and the stewardship model established in Chapter 2 (paragraphs 2.41–2.44, 7.29–7.33).

---

[21] Lennon MA (2006) One in a million: the first community trial of water fluoridation *Bull World Health Org* **84**: 759–60.

[22] McDonagh M, Whiting P, Bradley M *et al.* (2000) *A Systematic Review of Public Water Fluoridation* (York: NHS Centre for Reviews and Dissemination).

[23] Committee on Fluoride in Drinking Water, National Research Council of the National Academies (2006) *Fluoride in Drinking Water* (Washington, DC: National Academies Press).

[24] McDonagh M, Whiting P, Bradley M *et al.* (2000) *A Systematic Review of Public Water Fluoridation* (York: NHS Centre for Reviews and Dissemination); Medical Research Council (2002) *Water Fluoridation and Health* (London: MRC).

[25] For more information on the methods used in the York review and for discussion of the rigorous approach taken, see: McDonagh M, Whiting P, Bradley M *et al.* (2000) *A Systematic Review of Public Water Fluoridation* (York: NHS Centre for Reviews and Dissemination); Medical Research Council (2002) *Water Fluoridation and Health* (London: MRC); Wilson PM and Sheldon TA (2006) Muddy waters: evidence-based policy making, uncertainty and the 'York review' on water fluoridation *Evidence and Policy* **2**: 321–31.

[26] McDonagh M, Whiting P, Bradley M *et al.* (2000) *A Systematic Review of Public Water Fluoridation* (York: NHS Centre for Reviews and Dissemination).

> **Box 7.3: Fluorosis**
>
> Dental fluorosis is a defect of the tooth enamel, typically characterised by visible effects on the teeth. The condition develops during tooth formation (from birth up to the age of about eight years) and is permanent. Several different types, with different ranges of severity, can be distinguished. Although mild fluorosis is often considered to be of fairly minor concern, for example involving mild whitish speckling on the teeth, more severe fluorosis, which is much less common, can cause serious aesthetic concern and there is some evidence of this leading to adverse psychological and social effects in those affected.[27] Severe fluorosis may require medical attention such as restorative treatments or fillings for pits. If enamel fluorosis affects the structure of the teeth, for example if pitting is present, the ability of the enamel to protect the internal structures of the tooth from decay and infection may be reduced.[28]
>
> Some respondents to our consultation commented on skeletal fluorosis, a condition characterised by skeletal abnormalities and joint pain, which is caused by long-term exposure to large amounts of fluoride. WHO suggests that skeletal fluorosis is observed when water fluoride levels are above 3 ppm, and the most severe form occurs when the level is over 10 ppm.[29] In the USA, where 2% of the population receives a water supply with a natural fluoride level at or above 4 ppm, a recent study found that the most severe form of skeletal fluorosis "appears to be a rare condition", although it could not be determined whether a less severe form of skeletal fluorosis was associated with a fluoride level of 4 ppm.[30] In the UK the highest water fluoride level permitted is 1.5 ppm,[31] and the Committee on Toxicity has advised that "there is no evidence of clinical skeletal fluorosis arising from exposures in the UK."[32]

Extent of water fluoridation in the UK and worldwide

7.9 Water fluoridation schemes are in place in around 30 countries, and it is estimated that more than 350 million people receive a fluoridated water supply worldwide (see Appendix 5).[33] However, in some countries, fluoridation schemes have been suspended and/or alternative dental health measures, such as the fluoridation of salt, have been adopted (see Appendix 5 and Box 7.4). In most areas where water is fluoridated, 1 ppm is still the target concentration, although in Ireland this has been reduced to 0.7 ppm.[34]

7.10 Data from 2004 indicate that around six million people in the UK (10% of the population) receive a water supply that is either fluoridated to 1 ppm or is naturally fluoridated.[35] A small area of Scotland has a naturally fluoridated water supply, but all other areas receiving artificially or naturally fluoridated water are, at the time of writing, in England. The largest number of people receiving artificially fluoridated water is in the West Midlands and the North East of England.[36] In some areas, other fluoridation measures are in operation, such as schoolchildren receiving a daily portion of fluoridated milk.[37] Several organisations, including the British Dental Association and the British Fluoridation Society, have argued that water

---

[27] Committee on Fluoride in Drinking Water, National Research Council of the National Academies (2006) *Fluoride in Drinking Water* (Washington, DC: National Academies Press).

[28] *Ibid.*

[29] World Health Organization (2004) *Fluoride in Drinking Water*, available at: http://www.who.int/water_sanitation_health/dwq/chemicals/fluoride.pdf.

[30] Committee on Fluoride in Drinking Water, National Research Council of the National Academies (2006) *Fluoride in Drinking Water* (Washington, DC: National Academies Press).

[31] Committee on the Toxicity of Chemicals in Food, Consumer Products and the Environment (2003) *COT Statement on Fluorine in the 1997 Total Diet Study*, available at: http://www.food.gov.uk/multimedia/pdfs/fluoride.pdf.

[32] *Ibid.* The Committee on Toxicity concluded in 2003 that: "based on the current information available and the dietary intakes estimated from the 1997 TDS [Total Diet Study], no adverse effects other than mild to moderate dental fluorosis would be expected to be associated with fluoride intake from food, either in adults or in children, at the intake levels in the UK."

[33] Jones S and Lennon K (2004) *One in a Million: The facts about water fluoridation*, 2nd Edition (London: The British Fluoridation Society, The UK Public Health Association, The British Dental Association and The Faculty of Public Health).

[34] This move followed a report by the Forum on Fluoridation, a group established by the Minister for Health and Children, and was due to concerns over exposure to multiple sources of fluoride, increased rates of fluorosis and decreased rates of dental decay. Forum on Fluoridation (2002) *Forum on Fluoridation* (Dublin: The Stationery Office); Whelton H, Crowley E, O'Mullane D, Cronin M and Kelleher V (2003) *Children's Oral Health in Ireland 2002: Preliminary results. A north–south survey coordinated by the Oral Health Services Research Centre, University College Cork* (Dublin: Department of Health and Children Dublin), available at: http://www.dohc.ie/publications/pdf/coral.pdf?direct=1.

[35] Jones S and Lennon K (2004) *One in a Million: The facts about water fluoridation*, 2nd Edition (London: The British Fluoridation Society, The UK Public Health Association, The British Dental Association and The Faculty of Public Health).

[36] *Ibid.* For a map of the areas receiving fluoridated water, see http://www.dwi.gov.uk/consumer/concerns/fluoridemaps.pdf.

[37] This is, for example, in operation in parts of Yorkshire° and the Humber: see Department of Health (2007) *2006 Annual Report of the Chief Medical Officer: On the State of Public Health*, available at: http://www.dh.gov.uk/en/Publicationsandstatistics/Publications/AnnualReports/DH_076817.

fluoridation should be extended to other areas where dental disease levels are high, to cover around 25–35% of the population.[38]

7.11 Where fluoridation schemes are in operation in the UK, fluoridation is performed at water treatment works, using hexafluorosilicic acid or its sodium salt, disodium hexafluorosilicate, as the source of fluoride. These chemicals are produced from co-products of the manufacture of phosphate fertilisers and are specifically manufactured to required standards.[39] The chemical is injected into the water at a suitable rate to achieve the concentration of 1 ppm, and a system of continuous monitoring (linked to an alarm and automated shut-down programme) protects against the fluoride concentration becoming too high.[40] The Drinking Water Inspectorate, whose responsibility is to monitor and check the quality of water in England and Wales, has published a code of practice on water fluoridation.[41]

7.12 The current legislative framework for fluoridation is the Water Industry Act 1991 and the Water Act 2003. The law requires water providers to fluoridate supplies where this is requested by strategic health authorities.[42] These, in turn, must follow certain procedures, which include carrying out a consultation, before making such requests. The health authority has to bear the cost of the measure and of indemnifying the water supplier against any liabilities incurred.

Alternative fluoride-based measures

7.13 Other means of providing fluoride include adding it to salt or milk for consumption, fluoride supplements and topical applications such as toothpastes. We consider these alternatives further in Box 7.4, while Appendix 5 gives an overview of the international situation, outlining interventions adopted by different countries.

Box 7.4: Other means of using fluoride for dental health purposes

Alternative ways of providing fluoride include ingested interventions such as salt, milk and supplements, and topically applied interventions, including fluoride toothpastes.

Fluoridation of salt for human consumption

Typically, fluoride levels of 250–350 ppm are used. The proportion of salt that is fluoridated varies between 35% and over 90% in different countries. Fluoridated salt may be available just for use in the home, or may be used by the food industry also. Fluoridated salt is estimated to be available to almost 200 million people worldwide.[43]

A review article, which considered evidence from early and more recent studies from around the world, suggested that salt fluoridation "was as effective as water fluoridation" but noted that: "The full potential of salt fluoridation … is reached when most of the salt for human consumption is fluoridated".[44] In Switzerland, where 87% of salt is fluoridated, data suggest that this measure decreases the prevalence of caries by around 30%.[45]

One advantage of fluoridated salt is that the potential for consumer choice is, to some extent, retained where non-fluoridated salt can still be obtained. However, research has shown that a consequence of such consumer choice is that those from higher socio-economic groups are more likely to choose fluoridated salt, and hence this measure does not necessarily reach the whole population, and may miss those who are most likely to develop dental caries.[46] In terms

---

[38] Jones S and Lennon K (2004) *One in a Million: The facts about water fluoridation*, 2nd Edition (London: The British Fluoridation Society, The UK Public Health Association, The British Dental Association and The Faculty of Public Health).

[39] British Fluoridation Society, *Technical Aspects of Fluoridation*, available at: http://www.bfsweb.org/facts/tech_aspects/chem.htm.

[40] Drinking Water Inspectorate (2005) *Code of Practice on Technical Aspects of Fluoridation of Water Supplies 2005*, available at: http://www.dwi.gov.uk/regs/infolett/2005/0505fluoridationCOP.pdf.

[41] *Ibid*.

[42] Before the amendment in 2003, water providers were not obliged to provide fluoridation when requested to do so. In several cases they had refused to accede to such requests and the courts upheld their right to do so. *R v Northumbrian Water Ltd ex p. Newcastle and North Tyneside Health Authority* [1999] Env LR 715.

[43] National Fluoride Information Centre *Salt Fluoridation – The facts*, available at: http://www.fluorideinformation.com/topic.aspx?main=6&sub=601.

[44] Marthaler TM and Petersen PE (2005) Salt fluoridation – an alternative in automatic prevention of dental caries *Int Dent J* **55**: 351–8.

[45] Marthaler TM (2005) Increasing the public health effectiveness of fluoridated salt *Schweiz Monatsschr Zahnmed* **115**: 785–92.

[46] *Ibid*.

of cost, it has been suggested that the start-up costs for salt fluoridation are similar to those for water fluoridation, and the running costs are 10–100 times lower.[47]

WHO favours fluoridation of water over salt, in part because this measure generally ensures that all consumers receive the fluoridated product.[48] However, it recognises that fluoridation of salt may be more appropriate in some circumstances, for example, in places where people tend to drink bottled water rather than tap water, or where fluoridation of water is unsuitable for political reasons or for technical reasons such as in some rural areas. Various medical authorities in the UK have opposed the fluoridation of salt, in part because of the possibility of this leading to people consuming more salt, which can have adverse effects on health.[49] However, in countries that have been using fluoridated salt for some time, such changes in salt consumption have not been seen.[50]

Fluoridation of milk

Examples of schemes for fluoridation of milk include: providing a daily portion of fluoridated milk or yoghurt to children, usually through schools, and distributing powdered fluoridated milk for young children through health clinics.

A systematic review of fluoridated milk as a means of preventing caries concluded that: "There are insufficient studies with good quality evidence examining the effects of fluoridated milk in preventing dental caries. However, the included studies suggested that fluoridated milk was beneficial to school children, especially to their permanent dentition."[51]

Fluoride supplements

Generally the use of fluoride supplements is not encouraged except for children at a high risk of developing caries, although in a few countries fluoride tablets are recommended, with the dosage dependant on the fluoride level of the drinking water.[52]

Topical application of fluoride

Examples of topically applied fluorides include fluoridated toothpastes and mouth rinses, and professionally applied fluoride gels and varnishes.

A systematic review of topically applied fluoride products found that: "children aged 5 to 16 years who applied fluoride in the form of toothpastes, mouth rinses, gels or varnishes had fewer decayed, missing and filled teeth regardless of whether their drinking water was fluoridated," and concluded that "benefits of topical fluorides have been firmly established on a sizeable body of evidence".[53]

Fluoride toothpaste

A systematic review that compared fluoride toothpastes, mouth rinses and gels found that they all "reduce tooth decay in children and adolescents to a similar extent". However, it indicated that toothpastes were more likely to be regularly used, suggesting that this made them more advantageous.[54]

Fluoride toothpastes are the most widely used of the topical applications, and their use is endorsed by various medical and dental organisations around the world including WHO and the British Dental Association.[55] They are endorsed regardless of whether fluorides are also ingested in water, salt or milk.

---

[47] Gillespie GM and Marthaler TM (2005) Cost aspects of salt fluoridation *Schweiz Monatsschr Zahnmed* **115**: 778–84.

[48] Marthaler TM and Petersen PE (2005) Salt fluoridation – an alternative in automatic prevention of dental caries *Int Dent J* **55**: 351–8; Petersen PE & Lennon MA (2004) Effective use of fluorides for the prevention of dental caries in the 21st century: the WHO approach *Community Dent Oral Epidemiol* **32**: 319–21.

[49] National Fluoridation Information Centre, *Salt Fluoridation – Safety and Effectiveness*, available at: http://www.fluorideinformation.com/topic.aspx?main=6&sub=602.

[50] National Fluoridation Information Centre, *Salt Fluoridation – Safety and Effectiveness*, available at: http://www.fluorideinformation.com/topic.aspx?main=6&sub=602. For example, in Germany, Bergmann KE and Bergmann RL (1995) Salt fluoridation and general health *Adv Dent Res* **9**: 138–43.

[51] Yeung CA, Hitchings JL, Macfarlane TV, Threlfall AG, Tickle M and Glenny AM (2005) Fluoridated milk for preventing dental caries *Cochrane Database of Systematic Reviews* Issue 3. Art. No.: CD003876. DOI: 10.1002/14651858.CD003876.pub2.

[52] European Food Safety Authority (2005) Opinion of the Scientific Panel on Dietetic Products, Nutrition and Allergies on a request from the Commission related to the tolerable upper intake level of fluoride *European Food Safety Authority Journal* **192**: 1–65, available at: http://www.efsa.europa.eu/etc/medialib/efsa/science/nda/nda_opinions/851.Par.0001.File.dat/nda_op_ej192_fluoride_corrigendu m1.pdf; Árnadottír IB, Ketley CE, van Loveren C *et al.* (2004) A European perspective on fluoride use in seven countries *Community Dent Oral Epidemiol* **32** (Suppl. 1): 69–73; Committee on Fluoride in Drinking Water, National Research Council of the National Academies (2006) *Fluoride in Drinking Water: A Scientific Review of EPA's Standards* (Washington, DC: The National Academies Press).

[53] Marinho VCC, Higgins JPT, Logan S and Sheiham A (2003) Topical fluoride (toothpastes, mouthrinses, gels or varnishes) for preventing dental caries in children and adolescents *Cochrane Database of Systematic Reviews 2003*, Issue 4. Art. No.: CD002782. DOI: 10.1002/14651858.CD002782.

[54] *Ibid.*

[55] Petersen PE and Lennon MA (2004) Effective use of fluorides for the prevention of dental caries in the 21st century: the WHO approach *Community Dent Oral Epidemiol* **32**: 319–21; British Dental Association (2003) *Seven Point Plan for Healthy Teeth Launched*, available at: http://www.bda.org/advice/news.cfm?ContentID=938.

Ethical considerations in fluoridation of water

7.14 The fluoridation of water supplies illustrates how tensions can arise between competing principles and values within the stewardship model developed in Chapter 2 (paragraphs 2.41–2.44). Here we set out three main principles that might justify fluoridation (reducing risks of ill health, protecting the vulnerable and reducing inequalities), and three further principles that might be referred to in opposing it (not coercing people to live healthy lives, respecting important personal values and the requirement of consent). These principles touch on many of the issues on water fluoridation raised by respondents to our consultation (see Box 7.5). We then present the Working Party's analysis of the merits and weights of the different arguments.

Box 7.5: Quotations from respondents to the consultation

"There are two principal issues – firstly, the balance between the population good and the risk of individual harm and secondly, the matter of individual choice. Fluoridation of water is particularly contentious … because the ubiquity of the water supply severely curtails individual choice and there is the possibility, albeit small, of individual harm." *MRC Human Nutrition Research*

"It is reasonable to restrict the freedom of individuals [in order] to protect the health of children, but only when the health threat is serious. I don't think fluoridation qualifies." *Anon*

"Those from the more vulnerable sections of the community are likely to experience more tooth decay and thus potentially receive the greatest benefit from water fluoridation. […] Being provided with water containing 1 ppm fluoride does not infringe any human right … although some people may have an individual preference with regard to the concentration of fluoride in their water. Where parliament has determined that a measure should be permitted and consultation demonstrates public acceptance then a restriction of personal choice is acceptable for the sake of the common good." *British Fluoridation Society*

"As water is one of the most vital elements of life, surely our water supply should only be treated with chemicals that are necessary to make it safe to drink." *Anon*

Principles that may be used in favour of water fluoridation

Reduction of risks of ill health

7.15 One of the arguments that could be made in favour of fluoridation is that the liberal state has a duty to provide interventions that reduce ill health, as outlined in paragraphs 2.8–2.9 and 2.41–2.44. However, for this principle to carry weight, several empirical questions need to be considered, including the extent of the benefits to health and of any risks or harms. We noted above (paragraphs 7.6–7.7) that evidence in relation to these questions is not straightforward to interpret, and we consider this further in our discussion below (paragraphs 7.29–7.33).

7.16 In Chapter 2 we discussed the principle of reducing of ill health in particular through ensuring environmental conditions that sustain good health (paragraph 2.38). This could potentially be called upon in the fluoridation of mains water. We noted in Chapter 1 the considerable contribution made to public health through housing and sanitation programmes in the 19th and early 20th Centuries, and noted in Chapter 5 the importance of infrastructural policies such as cycle lanes or pedestrian zones as components of strategies to reduce obesity. Along similar lines, it could be argued that the fluoridation of water might be a way of improving environmental conditions in such a way as to promote people's health. Just as water may be treated in several ways to improve safety, such as by adding chlorine to kill bacteria and by filtering out harmful substances (see Box 7.8), the claim could be made that it would be legitimate to alter the quality of drinking water by adding fluoride, if it were shown to promote improved health for the population.

Special care for the health of children

7.17 Children represent an especially vulnerable group in many public health contexts (see paragraphs 2.16, 2.44). This is true in the area of dental health, because they are susceptible to dental caries, are less able to make informed choices about their dental health, and are dependent on parents and carers to assist with or promote preventative measures such as tooth brushing.

7.18 The discussions on vaccinations, obesity, and smoking and alcohol (Chapters 4, 5 and 6) has demonstrated that despite the vulnerability of children, for ethical and policy reasons, it is usually not appropriate for the state to seek to promote the health of children in such as way that would infringe on the liberties of their parents (see paragraphs 4.30–4.32, 5.39, 6.14–6.15). However, water fluoridation may be a special case in which children could be reached directly without major infringements on their parents' liberties.

Reducing health inequalities

7.19 As we have seen in paragraph 7.3 and Figure 7.1, there are considerable inequalities in dental health in the UK, which, for example, vary according to socio-economic group and geographical area. In Chapter 2 we noted that reducing health inequalities should be considered central to the goals of public health, and prioritarian programmes that address inequalities can, in principle, be ethically justified (see paragraphs 2.27–2.32). This justification could be used for fluoridation of water given that it may potentially improve dental health across the population including in lower socio-economic groups.[56]

Principles that may be used against water fluoridation

Not intervening without the consent of those affected

7.20 We noted in Chapter 2 the importance of consent in medical interventions, especially where there is the possibility of a risk to the health of the person involved (paragraphs 2.22–2.25). For water fluoridation it could be argued that this measure is only acceptable if all those receiving fluoridated water agree individually to whatever level of risk there may be, both for themselves, and for those in their care, especially children. Here, drinking fluoridated water might be perceived in the same way as taking a medicine, and represent 'forced medication' of the population if consent is not obtained from everyone (see Box 7.6). However, because of the nature of the intervention it is not possible to provide each individual affected with a choice. This is both because its implementation across whole areas means that it would not be possible to accommodate the differing choices of every individual in that area, and because people from outside the area who visit or move there after its introduction would be affected by the measure. Considerations about consent could hence be used to argue that the measure should not be introduced either where some individuals, however few, were opposed to it, or where individuals who had not agreed to it might be affected by it, such as those from outside the area. However, this would presuppose clear evidence about risks of harms and in the absence of such evidence give too much weight to the importance of choice and consent, allowing them automatically to override any collective good that might be achieved through the measure. Further to our general observations on individual consent and procedural justice arrangements in Chapter 2, we consider in our discussion below how the requirement for consent might be addressed (see paragraphs 7.38–7.41).

---

[56] All Party Parliamentary Group on Primary Care and Public Health (2003) *Inquiry into Water Fluoridation*, available at: http://www.bfsweb.org/APPCPH%20report.pdf.

> ### Box 7.6: Fluoridated water – food or medicinal product
>
> Several respondents to our consultation raised concerns over whether fluoridated water was a fortified food or a medicinal product, and where this fitted within the regulatory system in the UK. The legal situation is that while in principle drinking water is considered a food, the addition of fluoride is not considered a food supplementation process. This is because, from a legal viewpoint, water provided by the local water supply is only considered a food once "it emerges from the taps that are normally used for human consumption",[57] and because water is not considered a food at the point at which fluoride is added, the process is not considered supplementation of food.[58]
>
> The UK Medicines and Healthcare Products Regulatory Agency (MHRA), which licenses medicinal products in the UK, has indicated that fluoridation of water is not within its remit: "As drinking water is quite clearly a normal part of the diet the MHRA does not regard it to be a medicinal product."[59] Fluoridation of water at the water treatment stage also does not fall within the remit of the Food Standards Agency as a fortified food, because it is not legally considered to be such a food, as outlined above.[60] However, this is not to say that the content of drinking water is unregulated, because it is covered by legislation on water quality, which includes levels of fluoride and processes for implementation of fluoridation. Drinking water safety and quality, including the water fluoride level, is checked by the UK Drinking Water Regulators.[61] Policy on water fluoridation is determined by the Department of Health in England, the Welsh Assembly Government in Wales and by the Scottish Executive in Scotland.[62]

Minimise interventions that affect important areas of personal life

7.21 Another argument that might be made against fluoridation is that, although individual consent may not be required, the intervention could be seen to restrict the choices of individuals in some significant way (see paragraphs 2.19, 2.44), because individuals are able to exercise little choice over the water they consume. Fluoridation might thus be seen to interfere with important values of personal life, but the precise nature of these values may not always be clear. For some, the value may relate to being able to have a choice about what to ingest.[63] For others, the value may be about a certain conception of health, or water may be considered to be 'special'. For example, some respondents to the consultation suggested that water could be regarded as intrinsically pure and natural, or as a public good that should be provided in as 'neutral' a form as possible (see Box 7.7).

> ### Box 7.7: Is water special?
>
> Several respondents to our consultation suggested that water fluoridation measures were, or could appear to be, different to those of food fortification because water was in some way 'special' or different from other foods.
>
> "I believe that people have an emotional attachment to the purity of water [...] However, with food, people are often more than happy to tolerate quite extensive manipulation." *Mr Robert Warwick*
>
> "Water is unique among nutrients. It makes up nearly three quarters of the human body and brain. It is essential to life and there is no substitute for water." *Elizabeth A McDonagh*
>
> "Water is not for supplementing. Water ... is primarily an essential for life on this planet. [...] Without water we die very quickly." *Richard Carruthers*

---

[57] Regulation (EC) No. 178/2002 of the European Parliament and of the Council laying down the general principles and requirements of food law, establishing the European Food Safety Authority and laying down procedures in matters of food safety, available at: http://europa.eu.int/eur-lex/pri/en/oj/dat/2002/l_031/l_03120020201en00010024.pdf; Council Directive 98/83/EC on the quality of water intended for human consumption, available at: http://europa.eu.int/eur-lex/pri/en/oj/dat/1998/l_330/l_33019981205en00320054.pdf.

[58] Several respondents to our consultation raised concerns about the currently used source of fluoride for water fluoridation, fluorosilicates, not being included in the list of permitted vitamins and minerals for food supplementation that is found in EU legislation. Some suggested that this meant that fluoridation by this means was illegal; however, as described in the text above the process is not legally considered to be supplementation of food. Regulation (EC) No 1925/2006 of the European Parliament and of the Council of 20 December 2006 on the addition of vitamins and minerals and of certain other substances to foods (see Annex II), available at: http://eur-lex.europa.eu/LexUriServ/site/en/oj/2006/l_404/l_40420061230en00260038.pdf.

[59] Personal communication, MHRA.

[60] Personal communication, FSA. Furthermore, the FSA's Expert Group on Vitamins and Minerals concluded that drinking water and dental products containing fluoride were "neither foods or food supplements"; Expert Group on Vitamins and Minerals (2003) *Safe Upper Levels for Vitamins and Minerals* (London: Food Standards Agency), available at: http://www.food.gov.uk/multimedia/pdfs/vitmin2003.pdf.

[61] This includes the Drinking Water Inspectorate for England and Wales, the Drinking Water Quality Regulator for Scotland and the Drinking Water Inspectorate for Northern Ireland. For further information see: Drinking Water Inspectorate, *Fluoridation of Drinking Water*, available at: http://www.dwi.gov.uk/consumer/concerns/fluoride.shtm.

[62] Department of Health, *Oral Health*, available at: http://www.dh.gov.uk/en/Aboutus/Chiefprofessionalofficers/Chiefdentalofficer/DH_4138822; Welsh Assembly Government, *Information Briefing on Fluoridation*, available at: http://new.wales.gov.uk/topics/health/professionals/dental/oral-health/programmes/fluoridation/?lang=en; Scottish Executive (2002) *Towards Better Oral Health in Children*, available at: http://www.scotland.gov.uk/consultations/health/ccoh.pdf.

[63] However, few people would probably follow up this argument by maintaining that naturally occurring fluoride should be removed from water supplies in areas where this occurs at low levels.

Not coercing ordinary adults to lead healthy lives

7.22 In presenting the stewardship model we noted that it can be acceptable to require members of society to sacrifice some freedom in order to secure benefits for those who cannot make effective choices about their health, but that it should not normally be considered acceptable to restrict freedoms in such a way as to force individuals into leading healthy lives (paragraphs 2.44–2.45). The acceptability of a public health intervention should therefore depend on the amount of freedom to be sacrificed and how this relates to the extent of the benefits across society (see paragraphs 3.18, 3.37–3.38). In the case of fluoridation the question is whether the intervention is overly coercive, given the potential benefits to certain groups within society.

Discussion of arguments

7.23 Having outlined the different arguments for and against fluoridation, we now consider these further, and engage them with each other, where relevant.

Personal values

7.24 The arguments about not coercing ordinary adults to lead healthy lives and minimising interventions that affect important areas of personal life both, in this context, relate to the degree to which it is acceptable to modify water for the purposes of health benefits for the population. We find the argument that water is 'special', and that it should never be altered (paragraph 7.21), to be problematic. The composition of tap water varies from one place to another and is already altered in various respects during the water treatment processes, for example by the removal of potentially harmful chemicals and adding chlorine to kill bacteria (see Box 7.8).[64] It seems unlikely that those who argue that 'water is special' would maintain that it should never be treated, but instead be provided in its untreated form.

Box 7.8: Treatment of water

Some of the water treatment processes that are most commonly used include the following.[65]

Clarification for the removal of silt, algae, colour, manganese and aluminium, and some pathogens from raw water. A coagulant is added to the water, usually an iron or aluminium salt, which combines with these other materials to form larger particles that can then be removed.

Filtration removes any particles remaining in raw water after clarification and is used on ground water to remove iron and manganese. There are different types of filter; the most common is a gravity filter, which uses a bed of sand to filter the water.

Disinfection to kill bacteria. In the UK the most common method of disinfection is the use of chlorine, but can include the use of ozone and ultraviolet light. In all cases, however, chlorine remains in the water after it leaves the treatment works to keep the water free of bacteria as it is distributed through the water supply.

Ion exchange to remove nitrate from ground water, and in some cases for softening of water. Ion exchange is similar to the process used in water softeners in the home, in which water is passed through special particles.

Activated carbon and ozone to remove organic substances, for example from pesticides. The substances are broken down by the ozone and then adsorbed on the surface of the carbon.

7.25 **The principles of avoiding coercive interventions and minimising interventions in personal life could be used to argue against the addition of any substance to the water supply. However, we do not accept that the addition of potentially beneficial substances to the water supply should always be prohibited. Rather, we seek to identify the situations in which this may be appropriate.**

---

[64] Drinking Water Inspectorate, *Tap water*, available at: http://www.dwi.gov.uk/pubs/tap/index.htm.
[65] *Ibid.*

7.26 We note that a distinction could be made between adding chlorine to avoid harms that could be caused by the water itself, and adding fluoride to promote benefits that are unrelated to the water. The Working Party members were divided over whether the distinction between these different intentions was ethically relevant or not. However, we agree that **the acceptability of any public health policy involving the water supply should be considered in relation to: (i) the balance of risks and benefits; (ii) the potential for alternatives that rank lower on the intervention ladder to achieve the same intended goals; and (iii) the role of consent where there are potential harms**. In the case of fluoridation of water, there are considered to be potential benefits in reducing ill health and inequalities, although currently these are difficult to quantify (see paragraph 7.31). There are also potential harms (see paragraphs 7.32–7.33), and there is therefore a need to consider in what sense consent is relevant, as well as the possibility of alternative approaches (Box 7.4).

Reducing inequalities

7.27 We noted above that considerable inequalities in dental health remain (see paragraph 7.3 and Figure 7.1),[66] and therefore the potential for water fluoridation to reduce inequalities could, in principle, be an important argument in favour of the intervention. It could be argued conceptually at least that those expected to have lower levels of dental health had a greater potential to benefit, and that inequalities in outcome might therefore be reduced. However, the evidence on this point is not clear-cut. The York review of 2000 found that "The research evidence is of insufficient quality to allow confident statements about … whether there is an impact on social inequalities".[67] It concluded that "[although] the available evidence… appears to suggest a benefit in reducing the differences in the severity of tooth decay, … the quality of evidence is low and based on a small number of studies".[68] For now, we note that based on the best available evidence it is not straightforward to conclude that water fluoridation reduces dental health inequalities as measured by outcomes.

7.28 On inequalities in access, because water fluoridation is an intervention that is provided directly to everyone owing to the mechanism by which it is distributed, it is an intervention that, in principle, provides equal access for all. However, this principle needs to be weighed against other considerations, in particular the potential for harms, and the likelihood and extent of benefits.

Reducing ill health by ensuring environmental conditions that sustain health, and caring for the health of children

7.29 Another strong argument, in principle, in favour of water fluoridation would be that of reducing ill health, particularly given that children could be some of those to benefit. Figure 7.2 and our discussion in paragraph 7.3 above show that there have been improvements in oral health in recent decades in the UK. An analysis of data from 14 European countries (see Figure 7.2) shows that oral health has improved across all these countries over the past 30 years, and the average levels of decayed, missing or filled teeth are now similar irrespective of whether water (or salt) fluoridation is in operation.[69] It would seem, therefore, that the potential for benefit from fluoridation of water may have decreased, although this may vary in different areas given the regional variations in dental health (paragraph 7.3).

---

[66] Note also that just 10% of the UK population have received artificially or naturally fluoridated water; Jones S and Lennon K (2004) *One in a Million: The facts about water fluoridation*, 2nd Edition (London: The British Fluoridation Society, The UK Public Health Association, The British Dental Association and The Faculty of Public Health).

[67] McDonagh M, Whiting P, Bradley M *et al.* (2000) *A Systematic Review of Public Water Fluoridation* (York: NHS Centre for Reviews and Dissemination).

[68] *Ibid.*

[69] Cheng KK, Chalmers I and Sheldon TA (2007) Adding fluoride to water supplies *Br Med J* **335**: 699–702.

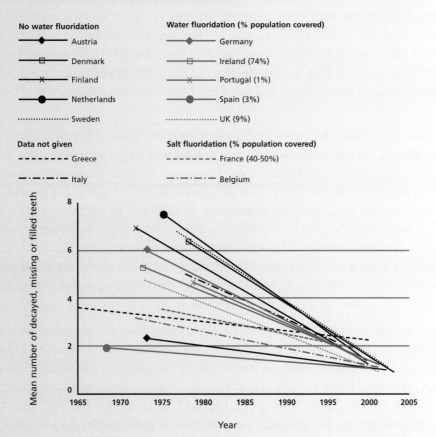

Figure 7.2: Mean number of decayed, missing or filled teeth in 12 year olds in European Union countries (1965–2003)*

*Source: Cheng KK, Chalmers I and Sheldon TA (2007) Adding fluoride to water supplies *Br Med J* **335**: 699–702. Figure reproduced with permission from the BMJ Publishing Group.

7.30 The York review concluded that: "The best available evidence suggests that fluoridation of drinking water does reduce caries prevalence".[70] However, the degree to which it was found to be reduced was "not clear from the data", with results of individual studies ranging from a substantial reduction in caries prevalence to a slight increase in prevalence. Of the 30 studies assessed, twelve had not detected a statistically significant difference between the populations receiving fluoridated and non-fluoridated water. An average of the studies included in the York review suggested that water fluoridation may lead to an additional 14.6% of the child population having no caries.

7.31 In relation to whether any harms result from the fluoridation of water, the York review investigated fluorosis, bone fractures and other bone problems, cancer and other possible adverse effects. The York review study group concluded (from analyses of almost 30 studies most of which were assessed as being of low quality) that on the basis of the best available evidence no clear association could be established between either bone problems or cancers and fluoridation.[71] However, both a review of the evidence and a large study published shortly after the York review suggested that fluoridated drinking water did not adversely

---

[70] McDonagh M, Whiting P, Bradley M *et al.* (2000) *A Systematic Review of Public Water Fluoridation* (York: NHS Centre for Reviews and Dissemination).

[71] *Ibid.*

affect bones.[72] The York group also found a small number of studies on other health risks, including Alzheimer's disease, malformations and mental retardation, but concluded that: "interpreting the results of the other possible negative effects is very difficult because of the small number of studies that met inclusion criteria on each specific outcome, the study designs used and the lower study quality".[73] For several reasons, it may be difficult to determine whether particular harms are caused by fluoridation,[74] for example because of the presence of other confounding factors, because of the difficulties in estimating people's total fluoride exposure and where there is a long lag time between exposure and occurrence of harm.

7.32 The York review included 88 studies that investigated the association between fluorosis and water fluoridation, of which almost all were considered to be of low quality. A significant dose-response relationship was found to exist between fluoride levels and the prevalence of fluorosis. It was estimated that with a water fluoride level of 1 ppm[75] the overall prevalence of fluorosis would be 48%, and the prevalence of fluorosis of aesthetic concern would be 12.5%.[76] However, a later report by the Medical Research Council suggested a lower estimate of fluorosis of aesthetic concern of 3–4%.[77] In the York review it was also estimated that for roughly every six people receiving water fluoridated to 1.0–1.2 ppm, one extra person would have some form of dental fluorosis compared with those receiving water with a fluoride level of 0.4 ppm, and a quarter of these individuals would have fluorosis of aesthetic concern.

7.33 In summary, on the benefits and risks to health of fluoridation, we conclude that there is evidence to show that fluoridation programmes are associated with benefits, although these are difficult to quantify, particularly in the context of the current historically low population caries levels. Similarly, there is evidence of harm, although there is debate over the extent and significance of the harm. This gives rise to the potential for two alternative, and opposing, applications of the precautionary approach (paragraphs 3.15–3.19). On the one hand, it could be suggested that because fluoridation offers the possibility of some benefits to health, it should be implemented. Conversely, given that fluoridation raises the possibility of some risks to health, perhaps its implementation should be prohibited as a precaution. However, in our discussion of the precautionary approach and proportionality (see paragraphs 3.15–3.19), we also highlighted the need to compare the policy in question with alternative approaches, and we consider these next.

Alternatives to water fluoridation

7.34 Box 7.4 provided details on several other means of administering fluoride, including through toothpastes and mouth rinses, and supplementation of salt. These alternatives all rank lower than water fluoridation on the intervention ladder that we introduced in Chapter 3 (paragraphs 3.37–3.38). Implementing measures that may be perceived as coercive can have a major effect on the acceptability of public health measures more generally, contributing unhelpfully to concerns about the 'nanny state', and this may influence policy decisions. For water fluoridation to be acceptable it must be shown that there is justification for this level

---

[72] Phipps KR, Orwell ES, Mason JD and Cauley JA (2000) Community water fluoridation, bone mineral density, and fractures: prospective study of effects in older women *Br Med J* **321**: 860–4; Demos LL, Kazda H, Cicuttini FM, Sinclair MI and Fairley CK (2002) Water fluoridation, osteoporosis, fractures—recent developments *Aust Dent J* **46**(2): 80–7.

[73] McDonagh M, Whiting P, Bradley M *et al.* (2000) *A Systematic Review of Public Water Fluoridation* (York: NHS Centre for Reviews and Dissemination).

[74] Cheng KK, Chalmers I and Sheldon TA (2007) Adding fluoride to water supplies *Br Med J* **335**: 699–702.

[75] This is the level generally proposed in artificial fluoridation schemes.

[76] McDonagh M, Whiting P, Bradley M *et al.* (2000) *A Systematic Review of Public Water Fluoridation* (York: NHS Centre for Reviews and Dissemination).

[77] Medical Research Council (2002) *Water Fluoridation and Health* (London: MRC).

of intervention. Factors to consider include the costs, benefits, harms and effectiveness of the different options in comparison to any reduction in liberty. Water fluoridation is considered to be relatively cost-effective,[78] but how does it otherwise compare with the alternatives?

7.35 The lowest-ranking fluoride interventions are those of fluoride-containing dental products, such a toothpastes, mouth rinses and tablets. Many of these products have been widely used in the UK and other industrialised countries since the early 1970s, and it might be questioned whether such measures negate any need for other fluoridation interventions. The York review sought to establish whether health benefits of water fluoridation were still reported after this time, in order to determine whether water fluoridation had a beneficial effect over and above these interventions. The conclusion, based on the findings of ten studies of "moderate quality", was that: "a beneficial effect of water fluoridation was still evident in spite of the assumed exposure to non-water fluoride in the populations studied."[79] We note also that water fluoridation has the advantage over toothpaste and mouth rinse of ensuring complete uptake of the measure, and of not requiring individuals to change their behaviour, which can be difficult to achieve (see paragraph 2.33).

7.36 The strongest case for an alternative intervention ranking lower than water fluoride can perhaps be made for salt fluoridation (see Box 7.4). This has been suggested to be "as effective" as water fluoridation if a large enough proportion of the salt is fluoridated,[80] and is typically similar to or lower than water fluoridation in setting-up and running costs.[81] One particular advantage is that it allows consumer choice to be retained, to some extent, if non-fluoridated salt can still be obtained by consumers who wish to do so. However, some groups may then choose against fluoridated salt, and hence this measure can miss groups that are likely to develop dental caries.[82] The concern may also be raised that salt fluoridation could cause individuals to increase their salt intake, which can be unhealthy, although in other countries that have been using fluoridated salt for some time, changes in overall salt consumption have not been reported.[83]

7.37 We note that a range of alternative interventions that rank lower on the 'intervention ladder' exist, and that the relative costs and benefits both to population health and individual liberty should be assessed when considering water fluoridation. We previously discussed the variation in dental health across different areas of the UK, and note here that the alternatives should be considered in terms of the context in which they may be applied, because, for example, greater health need of a particular subgroup of the population may play an important role in justifying a higher-ranking intervention.

Consent

7.38 The nature of water fluoridation measures is such that whole areas either receive fluoridated water or do not, and it is therefore not possible to provide each individual with a choice. Some might argue that the impossibility of individual consent must, in principle, rule out a

---

[78] An analysis on the cost-effectiveness of water fluoridation notes that the financial benefits, such as reduced treatment costs, can be greater than the financial costs, although the costs vary for example according to the size of the population and the level of caries present and case-by-case assessment is needed. York Health Economics Consortium (1998) *Water Fluoridation – An Economic Perspective* (York: York Health Economics Consortium).

[79] McDonagh M, Whiting P, Bradley M *et al.* (2000) *A Systematic Review of Public Water Fluoridation* (York: NHS Centre for Reviews and Dissemination).

[80] Marthaler TM and Petersen PE (2005) Salt fluoridation – an alternative in automatic prevention of dental caries *Int Dent J* **55**: 351–8.

[81] Gillespie GM and Marthaler TM (2005) Cost aspects of salt fluoridation *Schweiz Monatsschr Zahnmed* **115**: 778–84.

[82] Marthaler TM (2005) Increasing the public health effectiveness of fluoridated salt *Schweiz Monatsschr Zahnmed* **115**: 785–92.

[83] National Fluoridation Information Centre, *Salt Fluoridation – Safety and Effectiveness*, available at: http://www.fluorideinformation.com/topic.aspx?main=6&sub=602. For example, in Germany: Bergmann KE and Bergmann RL (1995) Salt fluoridation and general health *Adv Dent Res* **9**: 138–43.

proposed intervention (paragraph 7.20). As we have observed in Chapter 2 and subsequent case study chapters (see paragraphs 2.22–2.25, 4.38–4.40 and Box 4.4), requirements for individual consent can sometimes be over-emphasised in the context of public health. This is especially problematic where there is a very low risk of harm to a person and where refusal to give consent would prevent others from accessing important benefits.

7.39 This is not to say that reducing choices requires no justification. As we have said (paragraph 2.25), procedural justice arrangements can form an appropriate means of reconciling different preferences within a population, even if the final policy does not meet with everyone's approval. However, consideration needs to be given to the situations in which it would be acceptable to replace individual consent with such an approach, and whether fluoridation of water qualifies. We consider these questions in relation to two hypothetical situations for fluoridation.

7.40 First, if there were robust evidence that fluoridation of water was associated with a substantial likelihood of significant harm to individuals, individual consent would certainly be required. Alternatively, if there are no harms, but clear benefits, it might be argued that fluoride should be added by default without individual consent, in the same way as chlorine. Neither of these situations represents the current situation, in which there is some evidence of possible harms, and some evidence of benefits, though both are difficult to quantify. Thus, both action (adding fluoride) and inaction (not adding it) might disadvantage some groups of people, either through limiting personal choice or through preventing individuals from receiving any possible health benefits of the measure. Overall, the prevalence of caries has reduced considerably over recent decades, but inequalities between regions persist, and therefore the extent to which these costs materialise varies in different regions. **The most appropriate way of deciding whether fluoride should be added to water supplies is to rely on democratic decision-making procedures. These should be implemented at the local and regional, rather than national level,[84] because the need for, and perception of, water fluoridation varies in different areas. Account should be taken of relevant evidence, and of alternative ways of achieving the intended benefit in the area concerned. Whatever policy is adopted, dental health and any adverse effects of fluoridation should be monitored.**

7.41 We commented in Chapter 2 that procedural justice approaches are characterised by: transparency of decision-making processes; a focus on rationales that those affected recognise as being helpful in meeting health needs fairly; and involvement of individuals and stakeholder groups in decision-making processes, with opportunities to challenge such interventions (paragraph 2.25). These will typically involve: publishing plans for fluoridation programmes in ways and formats that are suitable for the public; a period of consultation; and a response to the issues raised during the consultation. The outcome should be a justification of a policy proposal which engages the scientific and health-related evidence on the benefits of water fluoridation for the respective regions in relation to alternative approaches, the consultation responses and relevant ethical considerations. Two important elements that feature in the process are the evidence base for an intervention (and its alternatives) and the availability of information for policy makers and individuals, particularly where they are to be asked to vote or contribute to policy decisions through these approaches.

Evidence and information

Evidence

7.42 We noted in Chapter 3 the importance of taking an evidence-based approach to public health policy (paragraphs 3.3–3.12). We also commented above on the lack of high quality

---

[84] Within the constraints of the water supply network.

research on fluoridation, which is particularly noteworthy given the interest in this intervention and the length of time over which it has been considered and implemented as a policy option (paragraphs 7.8, 7.29–7.33). Nevertheless, we recognise that, as in the case of obesity (Chapter 6), and in many other areas of public health more generally, inconclusive evidence by itself is not necessarily a sufficient reason to halt an otherwise promising strategy. Such strategies may be pursued as long as there is mandate for the intervention and appropriate monitoring is conducted. Therefore, **the UK health departments should monitor the effects of water fluoridation, including the incidence and severity of fluorosis and other possible harms**.[85] We note also that other research priorities have previously been suggested in the York review, and by the MRC, WHO and National Research Council of the National Academies in the USA.[86] These have included investigating total fluoride exposure, and how this relates to harm, and the impact of using lower levels of fluoride in water. **Water fluoridation policy should be objectively reviewed by the UK health departments on a regular basis in light of the findings of ongoing monitoring and further research studies. Furthermore, the conclusions and their basis should routinely be published.**

Information

7.43 In Chapter 3 we highlighted the importance of considering the robustness of scientific evidence, of not over-interpreting it, and of accurately portraying the current evidence. The need for accurate reporting of the evidence is especially important for debates such as the one about fluoride where the public would otherwise have great difficulty in establishing the benefits and the risks of the intervention.

7.44 There have been particular problems with the communication of the results of the York review (see paragraphs 7.27, 7.30–7.32).[87] These have been used by both proponents and opponents of fluoridation to support their case, by focusing on different aspects or interpretations of the findings. Soon after the report's publication (in 2000), its authors began to draw attention to their view that the report had been "widely misinterpreted."[88] The York review team sought to correct the record and expressed their concern over statements by groups including the British Fluoridation Society, British Dental Association, and the National Alliance for Equity in Dental Health which "mislead the public about the review's findings".[89] The reported problems included overstating the potential benefits of fluoridation, understating the potential harms, and the inaccurate claim that the review concluded water fluoridation to be "safe".[90]

7.45 One example is that of *One in a Million: The facts about water fluoridation*, which was funded by the British Fluoridation Society (BFS), and published in a second edition in 2004 by

---

[85] Consideration should, however, be given to possible difficulties in detecting harms, as noted above (see paragraph 7.31).

[86] McDonagh M, Whiting P, Bradley M *et al.* (2000) *A Systematic Review of Public Water Fluoridation* (York: NHS Centre for Reviews and Dissemination); Medical Research Council (2002) *Water Fluoridation and Health* (London: MRC); WHO (2002) *Environmental Health Criteria 227* Fluoride (Geneva: WHO); Committee on Fluoride in Drinking Water, National Research Council of the National Academies (2006) *Fluoride in Drinking Water* (Washington, DC: National Academies Press).

[87] McDonagh M, Whiting P, Bradley M *et al.* (2000) *A Systematic Review of Public Water Fluoridation* (York: NHS Centre for Reviews and Dissemination).

[88] *Hansard* text of letter from Professor Trevor Sheldon, Chair of the Advisory Group for the systematic review on the effects of water fluoridation at the University of York; *Hansard* (29 January 2001) column 146, available at: http://www.publications.parliament.uk/pa/cm200001/cmhansrd/vo010129/debtext/10129-40.htm.

[89] *Ibid*.

[90] For example, on safety, Professor Trevor Sheldon comments: "The review did not show fluoridation to be safe. The quality of the research was too poor to establish with confidence whether or not there are potentially important adverse effects in addition to the high levels of fluorosis." Further examples of discrepancies between the findings of the review and other groups' reporting of the findings have been noted, and can be found at: *Hansard* (29 January 2001), column 148–149, available at: http://www.publications.parliament.uk/pa/cm200001/cmhansrd/vo010129/debtext/10129-40.htm. See also: NHS Centre for Reviews and Dissemination (2003) *What the York Review on the fluoridation of drinking water really found*, available at: http://www.york.ac.uk/inst/crd/fluoridnew.htm.

the BFS, the UK Public Health Association, the British Dental Association and the Faculty of Public Health.[91] On the benefits and harms of fluoridation, the executive summary states that: "Many studies have confirmed that water fluoridation reduces tooth decay, and has no harmful side effects." The main discussion on the York review describes its conclusions without sufficiently drawing out of the degree of cautiousness that was central to the report's findings.[92] As such, the publication gives a potentially misleading account of the state of the evidence on fluoridation. This is disappointing given that the members of the York review team had previously raised their concerns about misinterpretation of the report, and that this specific issue had been raised in the House of Lords in 2001, where Lord Hunt, on behalf of the Government, said: "We accept that the York review identified a need for more good-quality evidence and have asked the British Fluoridation Society to ensure that this is reflected in future briefings."[93] It is of particular concern that at the time of the publication of this report the BFS was receiving Government funding,[94] and we consider that as such its publications bore a special responsibility for accurately informing debate.

7.46 At the same time, in the view of the Working Party, some of the information materials of groups opposed to fluoridation could be considered to overstate the risks of the intervention, and this too is problematic. For example the National Pure Water Association website reports that fluoride "causes" brain damage and lowered IQ in children, and abnormalities to sperm and eggs,[95] where other groups have been considerably more cautious. The York review noted in relation to IQ that there was not "enough good quality evidence ... to reach conclusions";[96] and the National Research Council of the National Academies in the USA noted in relation to reproductive and developmental effects that although existing studies showed that "high concentrations" of fluoride "might" have negative effects, "design limitations make those studies insufficient for risk evaluation."[97]

7.47 **Neither the public nor policy makers are helped by information that makes it difficult for the non-expert to obtain a good understanding of current evidence.[98] All the groups involved in the fluoridation debate should ensure that the information they produce presents a balanced account of risks and benefits, and indicates accurately the strengths and weaknesses of the evidence base.** As in the case of inaccurate reporting on the alleged link

---

[91] Jones S and Lennon K (2004) *One in a Million: The facts about water fluoridation*, 2nd Edition (London: The British Fluoridation Society, The UK Public Health Association, The British Dental Association and The Faculty of Public Health).

[92] *Ibid.*, p.4; Wilson PM and Sheldon TA (2006) Muddy waters: evidence-based policy making, uncertainty and the 'York review' on water fluoridation *Evidence and Policy* 2: 321–31.

[93] *Hansard* (12 Feb 2001), column WA16, available at: www.publications.parliament.uk/pa/ld200001/ldhansrd/vo010212/text/10212w04.htm.

[94] The BFS has received grants from the Department of Health for England, the Scottish Executive Health Department, the National Assembly for Wales and the Northern Ireland Health Department, given "to support the BFS in promoting the benefits of the fluoridation of water in reducing tooth decay". Between 1998 and 2005 these grants totalled between £90,000 and £104,500 per financial year. We note, however, the Department of Health for England, which was the largest contributor, has ceased to give these grants; the last, of £90,000, was in 2005–6. Department of Health (8 Feb 2007) *Grants, resources or donations to dental bodies*, available at: www.dh.gov.uk/en/Publicationsandstatistics/Freedomofinformationpublicationschemefeedback/FOIreleases/DH_4111162; *Hansard* (8 March 2007), column 2205W, available at: www.publications.parliament.uk/pa/cm200607/cmhansrd/cm070308/text/70308w0020.htm; *Hansard* (18 April 2006), column 216W, available at: http://www.publications.parliament.uk/pa/cm200506/cmhansrd/cm060418/text/60418w57.htm.

[95] National Pure Water Association, *Adverse effects of fluoride*, available at: http://www.npwa.freeserve.co.uk/adverse_effects.html.

[96] McDonagh M, Whiting P, Bradley M *et al.* (2000) *A Systematic Review of Public Water Fluoridation* (York: NHS Centre for Reviews and Dissemination).

[97] Committee on Fluoride in Drinking Water, National Research Council of the National Academies (2006) *Fluoride in Drinking Water* (Washington, DC: National Academies Press).

[98] Cheng KK, Chalmers I and Sheldon TA (2007) Adding fluoride to water supplies *Br Med J* **335**: 699–702.

between MMR and autism (paragraphs 4.33–4.34 and Box 4.3), **we consider that researchers, journalists and others who report research have a duty to communicate findings in a responsible manner. Those who report research should take account of the Guidelines on Science and Health Communication published by the Social Issues Research Centre, the Royal Society and the Royal Institution of Great Britain.[99] In particular we emphasise that the source and the status of scientific evidence alluded to should be identified (including, for example, whether it is preliminary or based on a conference presentation, and whether it has been peer reviewed).**

Summary

7.48 Water fluoridation has the potential to contribute to three central goals of the stewardship model: first, the principle of reducing health inequalities between different regional and socio-economic groups; secondly, the possibility of reducing ill health through environmental measures; and thirdly, concern for the health of children, who constitute a vulnerable group. Although the best available evidence suggests that fluoridation is beneficial, the evidence on the extent of benefits and harms is weak overall, particularly in the context of the current historically low levels of caries in the population; these are therefore difficult to fully evaluate and quantify.

7.49 The principles of consent, minimising interventions that affect important areas of personal life, and not coercing adults to lead healthy lives could in principle be used to argue against water fluoridation. We reject the view that, on the basis of arguments about interference in personal life and coercing ordinary adults, the fluoridation of water should be prohibited outright. Instead the acceptability of any policy involving the water supply should be considered in relation to the balance of risks and benefits, the potential of alternatives, and, where there are harms, to the role of consent.

7.50 Regarding consent, it is clear that an approach requiring individual consent is not feasible in practice. However, both the decision to introduce fluoridation programmes and a decision not to do so would require justification. Both action and inaction are policy options with the potential to have advantages and disadvantages to some groups of people. Therefore, a mechanism is needed for considering the views of the public in providing a mandate for either option. We suggest the adoption of local decision-making procedures that take into account the context in each area in which a decision is to be taken. In particular the health needs, the degree of benefit anticipated in a given community, the local perceptions of the measure, and possible alternatives need to be considered. The latter is particularly important as there are potential alternatives that rank lower on the intervention ladder, although the evidence on these is also limited.

7.51 Evidence, and information materials conveying that evidence, are important in any policy decisions, but particularly so when scientific knowledge is complex and a procedural justice approach involving the public is to be taken. We noted that the evidence base for fluoridation is not strong, and that as such ongoing monitoring and further research, particularly on risks, are recommended. Policy makers and the public need to have access to clear and accurate information, and uncertainties and the strength or weakness of the evidence should be explicitly recognised.

---

[99] Social Issues Research Centre, the Royal Society and the Royal Institution of Great Britain (2001) *Guidelines on Science and Health Communication*, available at: http://www.sirc.org/publik/revised_guidelines.pdf.

Chapter 8
General and
overarching conclusions

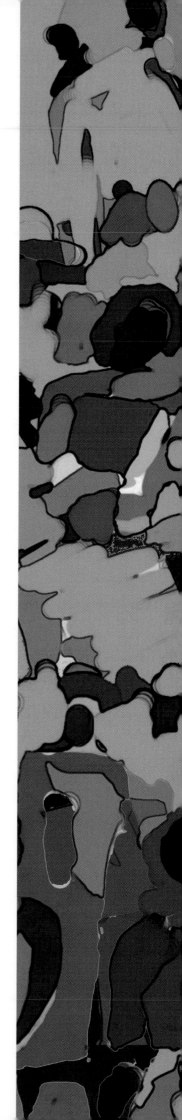

General and overarching conclusions

Introduction

8.1 In Chapters 2 and 3, we presented general ethics and policy considerations before examining, in Chapters 4–7, a range of more specific issues arising in relation to infectious disease, obesity, tobacco and alcohol, and fluoridation of water. We have drawn specific conclusions and made recommendations in each of the case study chapters. In this final chapter we review recurrent themes and identify several overarching and cross-cutting issues.

8.2 We first consider whether, having examined the case studies, there are lessons that can be learned for the stewardship model established in Chapter 2. Is there a hierarchy of ethical principles that should guide policy makers? Are there some principles that are more significant than others? Secondly, we take up some of the thoughts initially presented in Chapter 3. We review in what ways our findings can inform discussions about the relationship between public health interventions and general health and safety regulations; the use and communication of evidence; consistency in different areas of public health policy; and issues arising from targeting and monitoring.

Ethics: observations

Hierarchy of principles

8.3 It might seem desirable, at the conclusion of a report on the ethics of public health, to be able to set out a 'hierarchy' of ethical principles, or to state which principle should be the guiding one, 'trumping' all others. However, **in our view, the case studies have shown that a fixed set of ethical norms is unlikely to be an appropriate tool for solving the central ethical problems of public health.** Some principles are more relevant than others in different types of situation, but most can be invoked to differing degrees. In our view, **the role of the principles that we set out in Chapter 2 is that they, first, provide obligations that should ideally not be infringed. Secondly, where an infringement is seen as necessary, sound justification is required. In this sense, the Report establishes a framework rather than a set of rules for dealing with particular issues.**

8.4 Although it is attractive to argue that, wherever possible, specific principles should never be eroded, we recognise that that there are situations in which some infringement might be justified. We have, for example, considered cases where autonomy should be balanced against other values, such as protecting vulnerable people (paragraphs 4.28–4.29) or prevention of harm (paragraphs 6.10–6.15, 6.23–6.25). These values are not commensurable with each other, which illustrates further that it is unhelpful to think of a strict hierarchy. Thus, there may be circumstances where there are good reasons that one, or several, of the principles included in the stewardship model might not be fully respected. Autonomy therefore, although important, is not always paramount (see also paragraphs 2.22–2.25). The law, which is strongly rooted in personal autonomy, already recognises that the competing value of public health may sometimes override personal privacy. For example, in Article 8 of the European Convention on Human Rights, the right to respect for private and family life is limited by the interests of public health and the rights and freedoms of others; and, provided certain considerations are satisfied, the Data Protection Act (1998) recognises 'health purposes' as a justification for the use of sensitive personal data without the need for consent.

8.5 Nonetheless, it is possible to identify several principles that are of special importance, either because infringing them can have significant consequences, or because they are of particular relevance to public health interventions. We highlight the classical harm principle, care of the vulnerable, and autonomy and consent.

Harm principle

8.6 In Chapter 2, we introduced the classical harm principle, according to which, state intervention could be appropriate where the actions of one person negatively affect the well-being or interests of one or more others (paragraphs 2.13–2.14). The case studies illustrated that there are degrees of harm: severe harm was most prominently demonstrated in the case of alcohol, where injury might be caused directly to 'innocent' third parties. Here, the classical harm principle has had a crucial role in justifying policies that protect third parties, even though these entail restrictions of choice or freedoms (see paragraphs 6.6, 6.11–6.15). The classical harm principle was also the basis for legislation on notifiable diseases, and on powers to isolate and quarantine people known or suspected to be carrying a serious infectious disease and those they have been in contact with (paragraphs 4.41–4.43 4.58–4.62). In the case of obesity and smoking we noted that there may be cases where an intervention in the home may be justified where the behaviour of adults puts the health of children at significant risk (paragraphs 5.39, 6.14–6.15).

Caring for the vulnerable

8.7 A principle that featured to different extents in almost all the case studies was that of caring for the vulnerable. Vulnerability might first mean lacking capacity to make informed judgements for oneself, being socially or economically disadvantaged, or secondly be the result of other factors that contribute to a lack of autonomy.

8.8 In all our case studies we have seen clear correlations between socio-economic status and health, and we noted that, although there are exceptions, poorer health is generally associated with lower income and social status (see also paragraphs 3.23–3.28). Drawing on the discussion about the value of the community, respect for vulnerable people and the stewardship model, we argued that aiming to reduce inequalities through prioritarian strategies should be a primary goal of health policy (paragraphs 2.27–2.32). The more detailed discussion in the case studies illustrated some of the potential problems with such strategies, such as the potential risk of stigmatisation that may arise from targeting (see paragraphs 4.45, 5.12, 5.30–5.31, 5.34, 5.38, 5.42, 6.16, 8.28–8.29). In the case of obesity we saw that sometimes two desirable goals may pull in opposite directions; for example where information is used disproportionately by people of higher socio-economic status, the result may be that inequalities are increased, rather than decreased (see paragraphs 5.12, 5.25, 5.31, 5.34). A similar kind of tension may arise from prioritarian approaches that seek to increase access for disabled people. For example, some initiatives, such as escalators and lifts, may have the unintended consequence of reducing physical activity levels among other people, thus contributing to obesity. Clearly, the possibility that one intervention may have several different consequences often cannot be avoided. **It is important, therefore, to assess the implications of particular public health measures at the planning stage, and to monitor initiatives in terms of their effectiveness, in particular in reducing health inequalities.**

8.9 Vulnerable people include not only children, the elderly or the socially disadvantaged, but also those without sufficient healthcare-related knowledge to act as fully autonomous citizens. We noted the obligation of healthcare professionals (paragraph 4.19), campaigning groups (paragraphs 7.43–7.47) and the media (paragraphs 4.33–4.35) to be aware of this imbalance, and not to exploit the vulnerable position in which people with insufficient or inadequate knowledge may find themselves. Information that neither over- nor understates risks and benefits is of crucial importance for a climate of trust, which, in turn, plays a central role in information and education campaigns, rightly favoured by many as the least intrusive of public health strategies (see also paragraphs 8.19–8.23).

Autonomy and consent

8.10 In Chapter 2 we highlighted the importance of individual consent, which is often regarded as paramount. We noted that the concept had different meanings in the contexts of clinical and population-level bioethics (paragraphs 2.22–2.25). Chapter 4 illustrated that it would be wrong to require explicit individual consent for all public health interventions. If consent requirements were interpreted stringently, a considerable amount of important healthcare data might not be accessible, and effective control of highly infectious diseases could be jeopardised (paragraphs 4.38–4.43). We have therefore argued that requirements for consent need to be scrutinised carefully to ensure that the risks are proportionate to the benefits of a given intervention. In Chapter 7 we gave a more detailed illustration of the limitations of the concept of consent in the context of water fluoridation. We noted that local decision-making (procedural justice) arrangements can provide a valid alternative mandate for fluoridation programmes (paragraphs 2.25, 7.38–7.41).[1]

8.11 These examples show that in some situations both consent and autonomy may have to be accorded less importance in public health ethics than they would in, for example, clinical medicine. Existing bioethics frameworks are often, therefore, not well suited to address the problems that arise in public health. Much of the literature on ethics in clinical medicine and research tends to focus on the protection of the *individual*, whereas in the examples considered in this Report, conflicts arise when the behaviour of some individuals has an impact on others. Thus, bioethical discussions should take ethical issues arising at the level of the *population* equally seriously.

8.12 The individual-centred approach that has often dominated bioethical and political discussions has meant that considerations of the 'greater good' are often swept aside as somehow unethical, because they are viewed as incompatible with respect for individuals and their autonomy. However, in Chapter 2 and in the case studies we have shown that there are other theoretical frameworks and principles by which people can accept some personal restrictions or inconveniences in the interest of the wider population. These may be based on respect for the vulnerable, the value of community or other facets of the stewardship model (paragraphs 2.34, 2.41–2.44). This has been accepted historically where policy has focused on ensuring healthy and safe work and living environments, but it may be more difficult in the context of personal behaviour and health, as the examples in this Report have shown.

Collective efforts of society versus individual action

8.13 A focus on the population raises the question of whether health should be protected and promoted through the personal efforts of the individuals that make up society, or whether the emphasis should be on strengthening infrastructural factors and, more generally, on the organised efforts of society. In our earlier discussions we noted that the concepts of 'lifestyle' and genuinely free choice are problematic, because social, commercial or other external factors can limit or influence people's choices and behaviours (paragraphs 1.4, 3.20–3.21). In this context the food, drinks and tobacco industries play a major role, as may schools (see paragraphs 5.35–5.36, 6.18–6.27). Moreover, an undue focus on individual responsibility can result in 'victim blaming' (paragraphs 5.42, 6.16): attributing responsibility to those who are already disadvantaged by social and structural arrangements. There is also a question of efficacy: while emphasising individual action may be one way of improving population health, in our view the benefits of the organised efforts of society may often be greater than the aggregate sum of the efforts of individuals.

---

[1] See also: Cassell J and Young A (2002) Why we should not seek individual informed consent for participation in health services research *J Med Ethics* **28**: 313–7.

8.14 We have emphasised in this Report the ethical duty of the state to create conditions that help to maintain and improve the health of those under its jurisdiction (paragraphs 2.41–2.44). At the same time, although the organised efforts of society can provide opportunities for leading a healthy life, no measures are likely to succeed without a contribution from the individual. Environments may be more or less conducive to healthy behaviour, but ultimately people need to take up the opportunities provided. It would be wrong, therefore, to place responsibility for health either solely on the state or solely on individuals.

Conflicts involving third parties

8.15 We have commented in Chapters 5 and 6 on initiatives that industries pursue under the heading of 'corporate social responsibility' (paragraphs 2.47–2.50, 5.15–5.25, 6.18–6.27). However, there is often a fundamental conflict of interest, most clearly illustrated by the tobacco industry. There is an element of the absurd in seeking to devise marketing strategies to sell a product that is known to be very harmful, while at the same time seeking to play an effective role in reducing harms (see paragraph 6.23). Industries will usually consider changes in product ranges or marketing strategies only if they are expected to be advantageous for the business. At the same time, if market advantage can be obtained by innovation (for example, by selling low-fat or low-salt products for which there is demand) or diversification (where, for example, a soft drink company buys another firm producing 'healthy' fruit juices), then industry may purport to be taking voluntary measures to promote population health, although such initiatives may be perceived merely as part of sophisticated marketing strategies (see also paragraph 5.17).[2]

8.16 **Irrespective of the different motivations that companies may have for pursuing corporate social responsibility strategies, the corporate sector has obligations that go beyond simply complying with relevant laws and regulations. The alcohol, tobacco and food industries have a significant role to play in minimising harms, and by analogy the same goes for other producers, marketers and vendors of products that may have negative health effects.** Although most liberal states strive to ensure a free market, many also intervene to protect important goods, such as the environment, and the health of workers and consumers, for example by banning certain types of ingredients in foods. We commented earlier that such measures are part of the stewardship function of the state, and that regulation should not merely be seen as an enemy of the market, as it can often act as a driver of innovation. Nonetheless, if corporate social responsibility were taken more seriously, some of these interventions might not be necessary at all.

Specific policy issues

Paternalism, public health policy, and health and safety policy

8.17 People are often sensitive about state intervention in health policy where it relates to personal behaviour. The media are quick to criticise any measure that might be seen as telling people how to live their lives as unacceptable forms of paternalism (see paragraphs 2.35–2.40) or 'nannying'. However, although measures that infringe on liberties do indeed require careful consideration, it is also fallacious to think that there can be a completely 'nannying-free' world. *Any* regulation, including no regulation, implies the making of value judgements,[3] and it is important to identify those that are most compatible with the obligations of the stewardship-guided state. This is true both for explicit public health

---

[2] See Jordan A and Lunt A (Editors) (2006) *Whose Responsibility? The role of business in delivering social and environmental change* (London: Smith Institute).

[3] Sunstein CR and Thaler RH (2003) Libertarian paternalism *American Economic Review* **93**: 175–9.

programmes, and for apparently neutral ones, such as the design of towns or buildings. Throughout our discussions we were struck by an imbalance in acceptability between explicit public health measures, as opposed to general health and safety policies, many of which rank highly on what we have called the intervention ladder (paragraphs 3.37–3.38 and Box 3.3). The introduction of mandatory seat-belt wearing is instructive in this respect: there are clear health benefits associated with the policy, and the 'costs' are primarily that wearing a seat-belt might be considered a nuisance. However, this example does illustrate that although many people are initially reluctant to change their behaviour, this resistance can turn into acceptance and even approval if the intervention is perceived to be beneficial, even if some degree of personal autonomy is reduced (see Box 8.1).

Box 8.1: Compulsory use of seat-belts in cars and wearing of cycle helmets

Compulsory use of seat-belts in cars, initially only in front seats, later also for child passengers and subsequently for all, was introduced by law during the 1980s and 1990s in the UK. This followed campaigns by various groups, including the Royal Society for Prevention of Accidents (RoSPA), who believed that such a change would reduce the number of deaths and injuries caused by road accidents. In 1979 William Rodgers, the then Secretary of State for Transport, stated that: "On the best available evidence of accidents in this country … compulsion could save up to 1,000 lives and 10,000 injuries a year".[4]

It was estimated at that time that each year in Britain 2,500 car occupants died and 155,000 more were injured in road accidents.[5] Government figures suggest that between 1983 and 2003 the compulsory wearing of front seat-belts alone has prevented 50,000 deaths, 590,000 serious casualties and 1,590,000 minor casualties.[6]

At the same time, standards for what counts as an acceptable trade-off between comfort and safety vary internationally. For example, although most countries require wearing seat-belts in cars, in the USA there is no federal mandatory seat-belt legislation applicable in all states.

Similarly, although cycle helmets must be worn by law in Australia, New Zealand, Spain, the Czech Republic (for those aged under 16), Canada (for those aged under 18) and 20 States in the USA, few other countries, including most of the EU Member States, have such a requirement. The evidence suggests that wearing helmets significantly reduces overall risk of brain injury and the incidence of facial injuries.[7]

8.18 The case studies considered in this Report show that acceptance of restrictive strategies, policies or legislation can be difficult to achieve. This can, for example, be because some behaviours, such as those relating to food and drink consumption are considered to be more private. Perception of risk may also play a role: the risks to health caused by examples such as water fluoridation are less straightforward and more long-term than those encountered on the roads; and for vaccinations we noted that not everyone may be persuaded of their need to be vaccinated if there are high levels of population immunity, as people may perceive the risks associated with the vaccination to be higher than those of the disease that the vaccine protects against (see paragraph 4.15, also Box 3.1).

Use and communication of evidence

8.19 We have commented on a range of different issues related to the use and interpretation of evidence, including the role of the media, and highlighted problems caused by the selective use of evidence.

---

[4] *Hansard* (22 March 1979) column 1720.

[5] John Adams (1982) *The Efficacy of Seat Belt Legislation* The Society of Automotive Engineers, available at: http://www.geog.ucl.ac.uk/~jadams/PDFs/SAE%20seatbelts.pdf.

[6] Think Road Safety! UK Department for Transport (2003) *20 Facts for the 20th Anniversary of Front Seat Belt Wearing*, available at: http://www.thinkroadsafety.gov.uk/usergroups/factsheets/12.htm. We note, however, that there is some debate over whether the comparisons made are relevant, and it has been argued that making the wearing of seat-belts compulsory has increased the numbers of cyclists and pedestrians involved in accidents. See: Bjerklie D (2006) The hidden danger of seat-belts *Time* 30 November, available at: http://www.time.com/time/nation/article/0,8599,1564465,00.html.

[7] British Medical Association (2004) *Legislation for the Compulsory Wearing of Cycle Helmets*, available at: http://www.bma.org.uk/ap.nsf/Content/cyclehelmetslegis.

8.20 We concluded in Chapter 7 that, on the available evidence, fluoridation of water appears to have some benefits, although it is difficult to quantify these accurately. The same assessment appears to be true for possible harms. We argued that, provided that these uncertainties are openly acknowledged and appropriate monitoring measures are in place, democratic decision-making procedures at a local or regional level can provide the necessary mandate to implement the measure. However, there are problematic examples where findings are quoted selectively, or the strength of the evidence is overstated to support a particular case (paragraphs 7.43–7.47).

8.21 The selective use of evidence is especially problematic where it is difficult for the public to evaluate the claim being made, for example because the underlying science is complex. Moreover, not only might evidence be incomplete, ambiguous or conflicting, but different forms of evidence are valued differently by different individuals and groups. In the fluoridation debate, for example, one contentious issue is how much value should be attached to evidence from research trials of differing quality. The Cochrane Collaboration has made its value hierarchy explicit, but not all stakeholders in the debate about fluoridation would accept this hierarchy. Some may attach a higher value and credibility to personal testimony from an individual who claims to have been harmed by fluoridated water, while others may value the opinion of a designated 'expert', whether or not this is supported by empirical evidence.[8]

8.22 Although it is important to acknowledge this variation, the Working Party rejects the notion of evidence being essentially relativistic. Instead, **we emphasise the importance of presenting available evidence in a way that is as fair and accurate as possible** (paragraphs 3.13–3.14, 7.47). Any information advanced by stakeholders should always be scrutinised with sound scepticism, and the public should always ask the question 'who is speaking?' in order to be aware of possible bias or distortion. At the same time, it is clearly unreasonable to expect people to carry out comprehensive research to ascertain that the data and conclusions being presented are indeed reliable. The Chief Scientific Advisor's Guidelines on providing and responding to scientific advice to underpin policy lay out clearly the obligations of those involved.[9]

8.23 Finally regarding evidence and information, we considered the media. We commented in Chapter 3 on the adversarial nature of much media reporting (see paragraphs 3.7–3.9). The preference for portraying a polarised for-and-against picture may be intended to present a balanced approach. However, in practice particular views may be over-represented, where the two opinions do not have equal support among relevant scientific, medical or other communities (see paragraph 3.44). Also, there may be uneven scrutiny of the evidence base on which the claims of both sides rest. The example of media coverage over the safety of the MMR vaccination provided an illustration of this (see Box 4.3). A more responsible approach by the media would assist in reducing undue worry and misleading interpretations of the evidence. The cases of both infectious disease and water fluoridation illustrated the importance of providing adequate information, and we highlighted the need to take account of the *Guidelines on Science and Health Communication* published by the Social Issues Research Centre, the Royal Society and the Royal Institution of Great Britain[10] (see paragraphs 4.34–4.35, 7.43–7.47).

---

[8] See Elliott H and Popay J (2000) How are policy makers using evidence? Models of research utilisation and local NHS policy making *J Epidemiol Community Health* **54**: 461–8; Majone G (1989) *Evidence, Argument and Persuasion in the Policy Process* (New Haven, CT: Yale University Press).

[9] May R (2000) *Guidelines 2000: Scientific Advice and Policy Making*, available at http://www.berr.gov.uk/science/page15432.html. The principal points made in these guidelines have also been included in other reports, including: House of Commons Science and Technology Committee (2006) *Scientific Advice, Risk and Evidence Based Policy Making*, available at: http://www.publications.parliament.uk/pa/cm200506/cmselect/cmsctech/900/900-i.pdf.

[10] Social Issues Research Centre, the Royal Society and the Royal Institution of Great Britain (2001) *Guidelines on Science and Health Communication*, available at: http://www.sirc.org/publik/revised_guidelines.pdf.

Consistency and conditions of enforceability

8.24 Ethical arguments should be applied consistently in different areas of public health policy. We pointed out that although alcohol and tobacco are not directly comparable in terms of the nature of the harms involved, it is striking that there are several significant inconsistencies in policies on them, with more stringent measures being applied recently to tobacco (paragraphs 6.12–6.13, 6.29–6.33). The consumption of alcohol has long been embedded in social practices, and powerful industries seek to maximise their profits from the production, marketing and sale of alcohol products. These factors may *explain* the difference in approaches towards tobacco and alcohol, but they do not necessarily *justify* it exhaustively. We noted the significant degree of harm caused by excessive consumption of alcohol and that evidence has shown that measures such as tax and price changes, and advertising strategies can be effective in reducing these harms (see paragraph 6.29). We suggested that it would be justifiable, in ethical terms, to be more stringent in harm prevention strategies for alcohol. At the same time, such measures need to respect proportionality, and the 'social costs' of any measure need to be considered carefully. For example, it would be difficult to implement a ban on the consumption of alcohol in public premises.

International dimensions of public health

8.25 The issue of consistency in policies on alcohol and tobacco is also relevant at an international level. We argued that companies involved in producing, selling and advertising harmful products such as alcohol or tobacco in different countries should take seriously their commitment to corporate social responsibility (paragraphs 2.47–2.50) by implementing a voluntary code of practice that universalises best practice in terms of consumer protection. One example would be to adhere worldwide to standards that have been shown to be most effective concerning advertising standards (paragraphs 6.26–6.27). It was confirmed to us in one of our fact-finding meetings (see Appendix 1) by an industry representative that the industry does not follow this practice.

8.26 Chapter 4 gave another example of the international dimension of public health, illustrating that public health problems can transcend national borders, affecting states at different stages of development and with differing political systems and regulations. We commented on the case of infectious disease pandemics and the significant ethical problems that can arise from inequalities in the capacity for disease surveillance, vaccine development and access to vaccines. Applying the stewardship model at the global level, we identified obligations of WHO and the pharmaceutical industry to contribute to effective public health surveillance and reducing health inequalities at the global level, guided by the stewardship model (paragraphs 4.51–4.55, 4.66).

Targeting

8.27 We outlined in Chapter 3 the advantages of different types of targeting and concluded that, generally, a population-wide approach should be pursued, as this is least likely to lead to stigmatisation and discrimination (paragraphs 3.22, 3.29–3.34). However, we also observed that although universal measures may not *aim* to target particular groups, they often have the *consequence* that some groups benefit more than others, and hence these groups might be targeted indirectly.

8.28 When targeting is used it may take the form of mandatory measures, for instance quarantine, or information campaigns directed at particular at-risk groups. Any targeting programme carries with it potential benefits but also particular risks, such as stigmatisation and 'driving a disease underground' (see paragraph 4.45).

Monitoring

8.29 Finally, regardless of whether or not a programme is targeted, its efficacy and effectiveness should be monitored over a suitable timeframe. Monitoring may be complicated by factors such as people moving in an out of areas in which certain public health programmes are trialled, and many interventions, such as changing the food available in schools, relate to deeply engrained social habits which are difficult to change in the short term. These examples illustrate that care and patience are required in compiling and evaluating data on the efficacy and effectiveness of public health programmes (see paragraphs 4.37, 4.43, 4.50, 5.25, 5.30, 5.36, 6.29, 7.40, 7.42).

Appendices

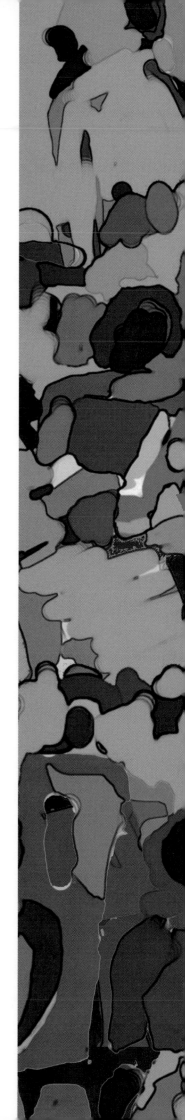

Appendix 1: Method of working

In July 2004, the Council held a workshop that addressed ethical issues relating to public health. Subsequently, in January 2006, the Working Party on the ethics of public health was established. Nine meetings of the Working Party were held over a period of 18 months.

As part of its work, the Working Party held five fact-finding meetings, each of which took the form of discussions with experts and stakeholders. Further details of these meetings are provided below.

From May to September 2006, the Working Party held a consultation, to which 112 individuals and organizations responded. A list of respondents and a summary of their responses is at Appendix 2.

During the progress of the Working Party, the Council worked with Ecsite-UK, the UK Network of Science Centres and Museums, to develop workshops for young people on the issues surrounding vaccinations. The Working Party provided advice on the content of the workshop materials. A total of 503 people aged 14–19 took part in debates about vaccinations in schools and four science centres around the country between April and September 2006. A summary of the discussions was provided to the Working Party in October 2006.

An earlier version of the Report was peer reviewed by ten individuals with expertise in the areas covered. These were Professor Dan Brock, Professor Alex Capron, Niall Dickson, Professor Ian Gilmore, Professor Larry Gostin, Professor Gerard Hastings and Professor Alan Jackson, Professor Philip James, Stephen John and Professor Theresa Marteau.

The Working Party is extremely grateful to all those who took the time and contributed to its work, provided valuable insights and helped to clarify the complexities of scientific, regulatory, social and ethical issues raised by public health.

Fact-finding meetings[2]

26 May 2006, London

Meeting with individuals and organisations with an interest in **obesity** held as part of the third meeting of the Working Party

Dr Bryony Butland
Head, Foresight Obesity Project, Office of Science and Technology,

Ms Gaynor Bussell
State Registered Nutritionist, Food and Drink Federation

Professor Chris Riddoch
Head of London Sports Institute, Middlesex University

Dr Susan Jebb
Head of Nutrition and Health Research, MRC Human Nutrition Research

[1] The consultation paper is available for download at: http://www.nuffieldbioethics.org/go/ourwork/publichealth/page_811.html.
[2] Institutional affiliations at the time of the meeting are listed.

18 July 2006, London

Meeting with individuals and organisations with an interest in **fluoridation of water and fortification of food** held as part of the fourth meeting of the Working Party

Dr John Beal
Vice Chairman, British Fluoridation Society, and Consultant in Dental Public Health, South Leeds Primary Care Trust

Douglas Cross
Advisor, National Pure Water Association

The Earl Baldwin of Bewdley
Member of the Advisory Board of the York Review, and Joint Chairman, All Party Parliamentary Group Against Water Fluoridation

Professor Judy Buttriss
Science Director, British Nutrition Foundation

26 October 2006, London

Meeting with individuals and organisations with an interest in **alcohol use**

Professor Chris Cook
Professorial Research Fellow, Durham University, and Fellow, Institute of Alcohol Studies

Mr Rob Hayward OBE
Chief Executive, British Beer and Pub Association

Dr Jane Marshall
Consultant Psychiatrist, South London and Maudsley NHS Trust

Meeting with individuals and organisations with an interest in **tobacco use**

Dr Amanda Sandford
Research Manager, Action on Smoking and Health (ASH)

Dr Chris Procter
Head of Science and Regulation, British American Tobacco (member, Tobacco Manufacturers' Association)

Meeting with individuals and organisations with an interest in **infectious disease**

Mrs Karpasea-Jones
Director, Vaccination Awareness Network UK

Dr Barry Evans
Health Protection Agency Centre for Infections

Professor Brian Duerden
Inspector of Microbiology, Department of Health

Dr Elaine Gadd
Senior Medical Officer, Department of Health

Professor Andrew Hall
Professor of Epidemiology, London School of Health and Tropical Medicine

Appendix 2: Wider consultation for the Report

To gain the views of interested professionals, organisations and members of the public, the Council held a consultation shortly after the Working Party was established. This was based on a Consultation Paper that contained background information and a set of nine questions for respondents to answer.[1] The Council sent copies of the Paper to individuals and organisations with an interest in this area, and publicised the consultation through email discussion lists, its website and a widely circulated press release. In total 1,100 copies of the Paper were sent to healthcare and professional organisations, religious and interest groups, academics, medical experts and interested individuals; it was also available online.

In total 112 responses were received, 57% of which were from individuals and 43% from organisations. The Working Party would like to thank everyone who contributed to the consultation. The figure below shows the proportions of respondents by category:

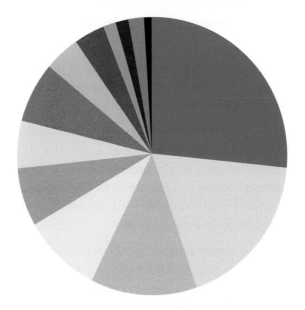

■ Interest group or member of such a group
Academic institution or individual
Other/not specified individuals
Individual with other professional interest
■ Professional body or society
Health professional
■ Government and NHS bodies and departments
Health-related organisations
■ Other/not specified organisations
■ LRECs and LREC members
■ Funding bodies
■ School
■ Companies or organisations with a commercial interest

All responses received were sent to the members of the Working Party and discussed in meetings. A summary of the responses, prepared by the Council's secretariat and approved by the Working Party, is set out below, followed by a list of respondents. Many respondents agreed to make their full submissions publicly available and their comments can be found at the Council's website.[2]

---

[1] The consultation paper is available to download at: http://www.nuffieldbioethics.org/go/ourwork/publichealth/page_811.html.
[2] See: http://www.nuffieldbioethics.org/go/ourwork/publichealth/introduction.

Summary of consultation responses

The following summary outlines some of the key points raised by the individuals and organisations that responded to our consultation. We received 112 responses in total, and are unable to relay all the points made; however, we have tried to broadly reflect the opinions expressed and to highlight salient points. Because the consultation was open to anyone to respond, rather than being conducted as a survey or poll, the responses cannot be considered to be representative of the population, and should not be interpreted as such.

We begin by considering the responses relevant to the case studies in the Report, and then discuss some of the general ethical and policy issues raised.

Fluoridation of water and fortification of foods

Some respondents commented broadly on the acceptability of fortification of food or drink, for example:

> "We feel that, in general, subject to a sensible procedure for risk assessment, there is nothing objectionable in the supplementation of food and water. If we can expect substantial benefits and there is no (or a very low) risk of harm from the supplementation of food and water, then such supplementation ought to go ahead." *Public Health Genetics Unit, Cambridge*

A significant number of the respondents commented solely or particularly on water fluoridation, and some expressed strong views on this topic. Some favoured the widespread implementation of such schemes, whereas others opposed them, for example:

> "The evidence that water fluoridation improves oral health and narrows health inequalities is such that we feel it should be widely introduced across the UK. [...] We consider it a duty of the government as fluoridation is a safe process which confers benefits on human beings … and is an example of beneficence. [...] Failure to fluoridate will result in suffering for many individuals and if viewed this way fluoridation is an example of non-maleficence." *British Association for the Study of Community Dentistry*

> "Given the state of all-round uncertainty in the evidence…; given the recommendations for substantial research to plug the gaps in knowledge…; we believe this is a strong reason not to impose on unwilling patients… an unproven medical intervention." *All-Party Parliamentary Group Against Fluoridation*

Other reasons given against fluoridation included claims of harms caused or uncertainties over harms caused, that it involved providing a 'medication' without individual consent, and suggestions that fluoride was toxic, corrosive and/or dangerous to transport to water treatment sites. Fluoridation of water raised particular issues over individual choice and freedoms:

> "In the case of fluoridation of water the consumer is left with no alternative easily and freely available [...] There are other ways of protecting children's teeth than the fluoridation of water. Acceptance of supplements to water would be determined by necessity – the *only* choice – and of major importance to all health aspects and to the vast majority of the population." *National Council of Women of Great Britain*

> "You're not restricting choice at all. If a parent wants their child not to have fluoridated water, by all means let them buy bottled water." *Dr Paul Wicks*

It also raised issues about the decision-making process for population-wide measures such as this. Comments included:

> "[For] fluoridation where there is possibly … mistrust on the issue, a public consultation would be justified. A referendum may not be justified as public health could be considered

a 'public good' that is greater than the sum total of 'individual goods' (therefore decisions should not be dependent on individual votes which could be influenced by individual concerns)." *PR Myles*

"We believe that decisions openly made by Parliament are sufficient democratic instruments for such measures." *Anon*

"No local authority, Parliamentary or other collective decision-making process is in any way appropriate in this instance [...] I have not vested in my MP, my local councillor or my neighbour the authority to decide what is good for me or my child." *Anne Butcher*

"It is correct to think that choices about public goods have to be made collectively, although [I'm] dubious whether any one method is best." *Professor Onora O'Neill*

Vaccinations, quarantine and isolation

On infectious diseases too, respondents expressed strong opinions over the acceptability of public health interventions. Regarding childhood vaccination, three main views were put forward. Some felt that this was "an entirely inappropriate and erroneous procedure" and that there was "no justification for the vaccination of anybody" (Ms Magda Taylor). Meanwhile, others felt that vaccinations for children were appropriate where parents decided to accept them, but that "children should not be vaccinated against the wishes of the parent" (Karen Stack). Some, however, felt that in certain, mostly exceptional, circumstances vaccinations could be made compulsory and children could be vaccinated against the wishes of their parents, depending on factors such as the severity of the disease and whether effective treatments were available.

On quarantine and isolation, some respondents expressed the view that "substantial risks of harm to others might be sufficient justification for infringement of civil liberties" (Dr V Larcher); this respondent noted other circumstances in which restrictions on behaviour are imposed in order to reduce harms, such as seatbelt and crash helmet legislation. Another commented that:

> "If an individual has a contagious infection and does not comply with treatment maybe then it would be appropriate to enforce quarantine. While it is an individual's choice to accept or not accept treatment, their choice has to have limits when it impinges on another person's right to health." *Fiona Reynolds*

Others, however, found such measures to be unacceptable. For example Richard Carruthers commented that quarantine "may be regarded as an infringement of civil liberties [and] also indicates a lack of persuasion by the health authority." Several respondents made comments about ensuring that people were well-informed about vaccines and infectious disease control, and that education and voluntary policies on these issues were preferable to compulsory vaccination and quarantine.

Smoking

Several respondents commented on bans on smoking in public places. Some felt that these were incompatible with individuals' human rights, for example the right to respect for private and family life, while others supported such measures, for example on the basis that smoking exposes others to harmful substances. Regarding smoking in the home or private places, more of the respondents felt that this should be left up to the individual, although some suggested that consideration needed to be given to children exposed to smoke in the home.

Regarding the role of the state in imposing restrictions on smoking, some expressed views along the lines that:

> "it is the role of the state to protect [individuals'] freedoms, not to remove them or to make such decisions on an individual's behalf." *Imperial Tobacco Group Plc*

Others suggested "it is only right to protect the public ... from the harmful behaviour of those who smoke" (Anon). Another view was that:

> "The state has a duty to educate people about the dangers of smoking; to help people who wish to stop smoking; and ... to deter children from starting to smoke. [...] However, the basic right for adults to smoke (in a private place or where the smoke is not going to affect other people) still remains." *Action on Smoking and Health*

Many of the respondents agreed that the state should act strongly to prevent children from smoking. Some of the responses received from school pupils commented on smoking; many of the children thought it was appropriate for the state to intervene to prevent smoking, but a few suggested that it "is the smoker's choice", and others suggested problems with people obtaining cigarettes illegally and that such measures would cost the government in taxes.

Alcohol

In public health terms alcohol was perceived to be different from tobacco in a several ways. First, respondents suggested that the relationship between alcohol and health is more complicated, for example in that there are:

> "There are some health benefits from moderate consumption ... and a great deal of perceived social benefit [...] the causal connection between heavy drinking and injury to others is complex and difficult to fully quantify." *Public Health Group, Institute of Health and Society, University of Newcastle upon Tyne*

Secondly, respondents suggested that alcohol is "far more integrated into society's culture and rituals than smoking" (MRC Human Nutrition Research). Other factors that particularly applied to alcohol included its importance in some religions and cultures, and that alcohol consumption, unlike smoking, is common in higher socio-economic groups, and these groups include the policy makers themselves, and other politically influential sectors of the population. Respondents commented on the difficulty of constructing public health policy in this area:

> "the goal has been to persuade the public not to desist from the activity but, rather, to practice it 'sensibly', a much more complicated task, especially as there is some uncertainty and confusion about what counts as sensible drinking. The result is that the public message on alcohol has not been as clear or as credible as it might have been." *Institute of Alcohol Studies*

Many respondents outlined public health measures relating to alcohol that they thought to be acceptable, for example relating to marketing, labelling, taxation and pricing of alcoholic drinks, and education. However, it was noted that severe restrictions on alcohol, and indeed tobacco, may have counterproductive consequences, as exemplified by 'prohibition' in America.

Obesity

In relation to obesity policy, MRC Human Nutrition Research made the following comments in their response:

> "Policy decisions must be based on evidence, but here, as elsewhere, the evidence is never complete or perfect. [...] Policy makers must develop a proportionate response that strikes a balance between the strength of evidence available and the likelihood of success, against the appropriate and acceptable degree of infringement of personal choice or commercial freedom."

A health visitor commented:

> "Individuals are responsible for their dietary choices but we cannot as a society fail to give education and opportunity to learn about food, ... minimise facilities for exercise, provide

poor food in institutions particularly schools, [and] allow advertising for fat laden and high sugar foods to be directed at children. [...] There is a need to empower people to take responsibility for health choices and equally for organisations and government to acknowledge they also have a responsibility to provide a suitable environment." *Mrs A King*

A hospital consultant commented:

"A libertarian approach suggests that competent adults have a right to make informed choices about lifestyle provided that they do not pose harms to others. The issue is therefore whether the consequences of the mortality and morbidity associated with obesity do harm others and what pressures might be exerted to overcome them." *Dr V Larcher*

Many respondents suggested measures that could be implemented to tackle obesity by schools, industry and government and other stakeholders, including initiatives for reducing energy intake in the diet and increasing exercise and activity levels, and including structural changes and initiatives promoting or enabling behaviour change. Some suggested that a comprehensive and coherent strategy was needed across these sectors, and others advocated the idea of a 'balanced' or healthy lifestyle overall. Some also commented on ways in which policies in other areas can contribute to obesity, for example, transport policy and the design of the built environment, which can affect how much people walk or take exercise, and policy on sport and food education in schools. The British Medical Association commented that:

"whilst ... as an absolute minimum, information both about the kinds of choices that lead to obesity and the health impact of obesity must be made available, the extent to which more intrusive or coercive measures are justified is unclear."

Corporate agents

The topics of obesity, alcohol and smoking all raised issues around the roles and responsibilities of corporate agents in public health. Respondents expressed a variety of opinions on this. For example:

"The food industry are ultimately there to make money and with the high demand for junk foods and drinks I cannot imagine that they would discontinue many of their lines to reduce obesity." *Ms Magda Taylor*

"Producers have a responsibility to their shareholders, to market their products and promote the image of the product and the company, and they do so with great success. Retailers have responsibility to their shareholders to compete successfully on price and availability, and they do so with great success. Both of these main influences act against the health interest, unless Government intervention compels them to present a less contentious and more balanced view of the consequences of drinking to excess." *Royal College of Physicians of Edinburgh*

"The government needs to regulate schools, the food industry, and school-foods providers ... They've all been given a chance at self-regulation, and they've all failed." *Dr Paul Wicks*

"The plethora of different food labelling systems in the UK is confusing to consumers, and ... is a clear example of those with money and power (food industry) winning over those with the least power to influence things (individual and low income consumers), which is unethical. Legislation to make one standard labelling system compulsory for all food manufacturers selling food in the UK would serve to remove this inequality, and create a level playing field for the greater good of society." *Heart of Mersey*

"The food industry, in its broadest sense,... sets the food environment in which individuals select their diets and has a crucial role both in determining food availability and cost, as well as driving consumer preferences through diverse marketing activities." *MRC Human Nutrition Research*

Role of government or state

Respondents also expressed a variety of opinions on the role of the government in public health. These included the following:

> "If [the] State ... attempts to tackle the problem it is criticised as generating a nanny state. If it does nothing, it is criticised for not helping the population." *Fiona Reynolds*

> "The government does not always know best and should intrude into people's lives as little as possible." *AR&CR Smith*

> "Society and government have responsibilities to deal with issues (such as smoking) that cause ill-health even if there is a considerable element of free choice as regards whether people choose to smoke. While this has been characterized as the 'nanny state', it would be an abrogation of our responsibilities to ignore it. ... A caring society cannot be one which simply 'allows' free choice despite knowing the consequences." *Health Protection Agency*

> "When removing any ... freedom, a burden of the highest order is placed on the law maker to examine such risks from a factual point of view and to satisfy itself that the risk is; a) real; b) of a quality which has led to similar restrictions for other risks; c) incapable of being managed in another way which does not restrict personal authority... This must be a minimum expectation for any state which attaches value to the sovereignty of the individual." *Imperial Tobacco Group Plc*

Choice

The tension between personal freedom and curtailing choice in order to provide public health benefits arose in several of the case studies included in the consultation, and various viewpoints were expressed on this. Some consultation respondents felt it was important that public health measures did not infringe on freedoms, or did so as little as possible, whereas others suggested that infringements on freedom could be justified in some circumstances. One respondent said "there are no circumstances in which it is acceptable to restrict the choice of individuals to protect the health of children" (Vaccination Awareness Network (VAN) UK), whereas another said "restricting individual choice could be justified by a view that achieving the greatest good for greatest number morally justifies an action" (Anon), and another said "Freedom of choice is overridden by the responsibility not to cause harm to others" (National Institute for Health and Clinical Excellence (NICE) quoting its Citizens Council). Other points raised included:

> "Autonomy cannot be totally unrestrained or unrestricted in any society if that society is to survive. Our individual autonomies interrelate and must therefore be limited by the autonomies of others. The autonomy of one individual cannot 'claim' precedence over that of another. If this is not to be so, and everyone can simply do what they like, then society becomes impossible." *Dr IM Jessiman*

> "Compulsion should be used only as a last resort and with full backing of the vast majority of a community. [...] It is a far more favourable outcome if people can be persuaded to change behaviour voluntarily, to take up or persist with desired behaviour." *National Social Marketing Centre for Excellence*

Problems with the concept of choice

Several respondents suggested that the addictive nature of alcohol and tobacco, and the role of genetics in obesity meant that decisions made in these areas should not necessarily be considered true free choices. Other respondents commented on further problems about choice:

> "While ... decisions about food consumption, exercise uptake and the use of cigarettes and alcohol are to a large extent personal, it is clear ... that factors to a greater or lesser extent outside an individual's control – such as socio-economic status, gender and geographical

location – influence the likelihood that individuals will make lifestyle choices that harm their health." *British Medical Association*

"Behaviour in health contexts is often conceptualised in policy and contemporary psychology as reflecting individual choice. [...] The majority of smokers want to quit. The majority of those who are overweight want not to be so. Yet for most people these so-called choices are not realised." *Professor Theresa Marteau*

"Individual decisions are not made in a vacuum and are very much affected by the environments in which people live and work. In the case of obesity, although it might be easy to place responsibility with the individual, it is important to recognise that the individual is part of a community where physical activity is generally declining and convenience foods tend to have a high calorific and salt content." *Academy of Medical Sciences*

Personal responsibility for personal choices?

We asked for views on whether individuals with health problems that in some way related to lifestyle or personal choice should be less eligible for treatment on the NHS or should pay more for it, and received a variety of responses. Here again respondents raised problems with the notion of choice and people's freedoms to make individual choices. Others felt that such an approach was impractical or unfair, was not consistent with the ethos of the NHS, would be subject to a 'slippery slope', or overlooked the multiplicity of factors contributing to ill health. It was also noted that smokers already pay extra in taxes on tobacco, some of which go into healthcare. However, some respondents supported such an approach, and others suggested that the manufacturers and other companies making money from cigarettes and other unhealthy products should provide the extra resources needed to deal with the health effects they contribute to. Others felt that it was appropriate to require individuals to, for example, stop smoking or lose weight, in order to receive treatment, and/or suggested that those who were obese or smoked or drank could be refused treatments only where it gave rise to issues of clinical or cost effectiveness.

Factors affecting public health

One of the questions we asked was whether the following five factors were the main influences affecting public health: environment, social and economic factors, lifestyle, genetic background, and preventative and curative health services. Some respondents agreed with these, whereas some suggested other influences such as education, as well as historical, political, cultural and psychological factors. Several commented on the inclusion of 'lifestyle': some thought that this needed to be defined, or that 'behaviour' was a better term, whereas others felt that lifestyle was adequately covered by the other factors. Although some respondents suggested that certain factors were more important than others, there was little consensus over which these were, and some felt that this would vary, for example, "for different health problems and different geographical areas" (University of Glasgow, Section of Public Health and Health Policy). Another view was that it was unhelpful to try to assess which factors were more important, but that they should be considered to be inter-dependent.

Ethical principles

In the consultation paper we discussed the concepts of autonomy, solidarity, fair reciprocity, the harm principle, consent and trust, and asked which might be considered more important, and whether these could be ordered into a hierarchy. Although some respondents thought one or several of the principles to be more important, there was no consensus over which these should be. Some respondents considered that these were all important, some suggested other principles, including beneficence, justice, honesty and responsibility, and a few suggested that the 'four principles of biomedical ethics' should be used instead.

A few of the respondents suggested how the principles might be ordered, but more were of the opinion that this could not be done, and instead preferred to consider that they were all equally important, that they should be weighed up against one another, or that they should form a matrix rather than a hierarchy.

Responses to the Consultation

The Working Party wishes to thank the following individuals and organisations for their responses. Where the respondents have given permission, the Council has published their responses on its website.[3]

List of respondents

Organisations

Anonymous (2)

Academy of Medical Sciences

Action on Smoking and Health (ASH)

All-Party Parliamentary Group against Fluoridation

Bedford Allergy Support Group (BASG)

British Association for the Study of Community Dentistry

British Fluoridation Society

British Medical Association

British Psychological Society

Centers for Disease Control and Prevention, Public Health Ethics Committee

Commission for Racial Equality

Ethox Centre, Division of Public Health and Primary Care, University of Oxford

European Commission, Directorate-General Environment

Expert Advisory Group on AIDS (EAGA)

Food Standards Agency

Dr Peter Mansfield, Good HealthKeeping (responding both personally and on behalf of the organisation)

Health Protection Agency

Heart of Mersey

Imperial Tobacco Group Plc

Institute of Alcohol Studies

Institute of Biology

Institute of Public Health in Ireland

JABS (Justice, Awareness and Basic Support)

Ministry of Defence

---

[3] See http://www.nuffieldbioethics.org/go/ourwork/publichealth/introduction

Emma L Morgan, Emerald Holistics (responding both personally and on behalf of the organisation)

Medical Research Council (MRC)

MRC Human Nutrition Research

MRC Population Health Sciences Research Network

National AIDS Trust

National Council of Women of Great Britain

National Institute for Health and Clinical Excellence (NICE)

National Register of Children with Dental Fluorosis

National Social Marketing Centre for Excellence

Newstead Wood School for Girls (multiple responses from students)

NHS Health Scotland

NHS Lanarkshire

Public Health Genetics Unit, Cambridge

Public Health Group, Institute of Health and Society, University of Newcastle upon Tyne

Royal College of Paediatrics and Child Health

Royal College of Physicians of Edinburgh

Safe Water Campaign for Avon, Gloucestershire and Wiltshire

SENSE (UK Deafblind Charity)

South Birmingham Primary Care Trust

Terrence Higgins Trust

University of Glasgow Section of Public Health and Health Policy

VAN UK (Vaccination Awareness Network)

Wellcome Trust

Individuals

Anonymous (9)	Les Dundon	Dr V Larcher
Elizabeth Booth	Rachel Flowers	Dr Stefano Lazzari
Mrs Kate Boulton	Evelyn Gloyn	Dr Peter Lucas
Mr M Bowman	Dr David S Gordon	Elizabeth A McDonagh
Mrs Janet Brears	Mrs Linda Halliday	Dr McFarlane
Anne Butcher	Dr Patrick Hill	Professor Theresa Marteau
C Buckley & S Nolan	Mrs Esther Hollands	Professor B Mepham
Richard Carruthers	Dr I M Jessiman	Clifford G Miller
Dr David Chappel	Mrs A King	Professor David Morton
Dr Richard Cookson	Rudolf Kirst	PR Myles

Professor Onora O'Neill

IE Packington

J Parfitt

Mr Michael Parkes

Dr S Parlour

John Powles

Mr C V Praveen

Mrs Penny S Pullen

Mike Rayner

Bridget Reader

Fiona Reynolds

Mrs Marijke Roberts

Ms Sarah Rowett

Bernard J Seward

Professor Darren Shickle

AR & CR Smith

Sukhvinder Sohpal

Karen Stack

Dr Allison Streetly

Ms Magda Taylor

Professor Dame Margaret Turner-Warwick

Professor Paul Wainwright

Mr Robert Warwick

Dr Paul Wicks

Mrs Anne Wilks

Mr & Mrs R Woodward

Appendix 3: Vaccination policy – the international context

Childhood vaccination policies vary considerably in different countries, for example which vaccines are included, and the means of promoting or ensuring vaccine uptake. Here we set out some of the policies that operate in various countries around the world.[1] We also give the coverage rates for three vaccines: the third dose of polio (P), the third dose of Hib (H) and the third dose of the combined diphtheria, tetanus and pertussis (DTP).[2]

Voluntary vaccination policies

Country	Policy and comments
UK	All vaccination schemes are voluntary;[3] some are incentivised (see below). Eleven diseases are routinely vaccinated against. The British Medical Association and an Expert Group for the Scottish Executive have indicated that they do not support compulsory vaccination in the UK.[4] (P, 91; H, 91; DTP, 91.)
Canada	Vaccinations are not mandatory, but some states require proof of vaccination status for a child to enrol for school, such that the child must either have been vaccinated or have documentation to indicate that their parents have actively refused vaccination. Throughout Canada unvaccinated children can be excluded from school during outbreaks of vaccine-preventable disease. (P, 89; H, 83; DTP, 94.)
Sweden	All vaccination schemes are voluntary. Nine diseases are routinely vaccinated against during childhood, and children at high risk of infection are offered vaccines against two further diseases (tuberculosis and hepatitis B). Some of the highest levels of coverage across all vaccines in Europe are seen. (P, 99; H, 98; DTP, 99.)

[1] British Medical Association Board of Science and Education (2003) *Childhood Immunisations: A guide for healthcare professionals* (London: BMA Publications); Moran NE, Shickle D, Munthe C *et al.* (2006) Are compulsory immunisations and incentives to immunise effective ways to achieve herd immunity in Europe? in *Ethics and Infectious Disease*, Selgelid MJ, Battin MP and Smith CB (Editors) (Malden MA: Blackwell Publishing), pp.215–31; Wellborn AA (2005) *Mandatory Vaccinations: Precedent and current laws*, available at: www.fas.org/sgp/crs/RS21414.pdf Achat H, McIntyre P and Burgess M (1999) Health care incentives in immunisation *Aust N Z J Public Health* **23**: 285–8; Swedish Institute for Infectious Disease Control (2006) *The Swedish Vaccination Programme*, available at: http://www.smittskyddsinstitutet.se/in-english/activities/the-swedish-vaccination-program/ National Advisory Committee on Immunization (Canada) (2006) *Canadian Immunization Guide*, 7th Edition, available at: http://www.phac-aspc.gc.ca/publicat/cig-gci/index.html; Antona D, Bussière E, Guignon N, Badeyan G and Lévy-Bruhl D (2003) Vaccine coverage of pre-school age children in France in 2000 *Euro Surveill* **8**: 139–44; available at: www.eurosurveillance.org/em/v08n06/0806-224.asp.

[2] Coverage rates are given as the percentage of the target population vaccinated; data use are WHO-UNICEF estimates for 2005, see World Health Organization (2006) *WHO Vaccine-Preventable Diseases: monitoring system – 2006 global summary*, available at: http://www.who.int/vaccines-documents/GlobalSummary/GlobalSummary.pdf.

[3] Although we note that some nurseries and schools require children to have received certain vaccinations before admission. British Medical Association Board of Science and Education (2003) *Childhood Immunisations: A guide for healthcare professionals* (London: BMA Publications).

[4] British Medical Association Board of Science and Education (2003) *Childhood Immunisations: A guide for healthcare professionals* (London: BMA Publications); Scottish Executive MMR Expert Group (2002) *MMR: Report of the MMR Expert Group*, available at: http://www.scotland.gov.uk/Resource/Doc/46905/0014171.pdf.

Mandatory vaccination policies

Country	Policy and comments
Belgium	Vaccination against polio is mandatory by the age of 18 months. Parents who do not comply can receive a prison sentence or a fine. Other vaccines are voluntary. (P, 97; H, 95; DTP, 97.)
Italy	Childhood vaccination against diphtheria, tetanus, polio and hepatitis B are mandatory. Parents who do not comply can receive fines, which differ depending on which vaccine has not been received. Until 1999, certain vaccinations were required for school attendance; this changed when a Presidential Decree ruled that every child was entitled to an education regardless of immunisation status. (P, 97; H, 95; DTP, 96.)
Poland	Some vaccinations are mandatory during childhood, including measles. Those who do not receive the vaccines may be fined. However, in practice it is suggested that fines are only applied if vaccine coverage decreases and threatens herd immunity. (P, 99; H, 22[5]; DTP, 99.)
USA	All states have laws requiring children to be vaccinated before starting private or public school, although many provide exemptions for medical reasons, and sometimes also for reasons of religion or philosophy. (P, 92; H, 94; DTP, 96.)

Vaccination policies involving incentives for parents

Country	Policy
Australia	Certain benefits are only paid if the child is up-to-date with their vaccinations. (P, 92; H, 94; DTP, 92.)
Austria	Mothers used to be given €1,100 if they attended ten scheduled health visits, during which immunisations were offered. This amount was subsequently reduced, leading to a reduction in immunisation coverage, and the scheme has now ended, having been replaced by other policies. In one part of Austria, €370 is given to mothers who complete the childhood vaccination programme. (P, 86; H, 86; DTP, 86.)
USA	In some areas 'lottery-style' incentives have been tried, whereby parents who get their children vaccinated can be entered into a draw to win a prize. Research from a scheme in which a US$50 food voucher could be won showed that those given this incentive where significantly more likely to be immunised than those in a control group.[6] (P, 92; H, 94; DTP, 96.)

---

[5] In Poland the Hib vaccine is only given to children living in orphanages or who have two or more siblings.

[6] Achat H, McIntyre P and Burgess M (1999) Health care incentives in immunisation *Aust N Z J Public Health* **23**: 285–8.

Vaccinations involving incentives to healthcare providers

Country	Policy
UK	GPs are eligible for two bonus payments when over 70% and over 90% of children registered at their practice are immunised against several diseases. The percentage of GPs reaching 90% coverage increased from 55% to 70% in a year when this policy was introduced, although this may also have been influenced by other factors.[7] (P, 91; H, 91; DTP, 91.)
Australia	GPs receive a payment for notifying the authorities that a child has been vaccinated and a bonus relating to the percentage of children under six who are fully immunised. (P, 92; H, 94; DTP, 92.)
Ireland	For each child immunised GPs receive a payment while a deduction is made for each child that does not receive the MMR vaccine by the age of two, and an additional bonus is paid if an uptake rate of 95% or more is achieved, excluding children whose parents have actively refused. (P, 90; H, 90; DTP, 90.)

---

[7] Moran NE, Shickle D, Munthe C *et al*. (2006) Are compulsory immunisations and incentives to immunise effective ways to achieve herd immunity in Europe? in *Ethics and Infectious Disease*, Selgelid MJ, Battin MP and Smith CB (Editors) (Malden MA: Blackwell Publishing), pp.215–31.

APPENDIX 3 VACCINATION POLICY – THE INTERNATIONAL CONTEXT

Appendix 4: Obesity policy – the international context

World Health Organization (WHO)

Member States of the European section of WHO adopted a *Charter on Counteracting Obesity* in 2006, aimed at providing political guidance to strengthen action in Europe.[1] It is intended that a *European Action Plan* covering nutrition and physical activity will provide more specific action and monitoring mechanisms. The Charter includes principles for guiding action on reducing the level of obesity across Europe, including:

- "Action against obesity should be linked to overall strategies to address noncommunicable diseases and health promotion activities, as well as to the broader context of sustainable development. Improved diet and physical activity will have a substantial and often rapid impact on public health, beyond the benefits related to reducing overweight and obesity.

- "A balance must be struck between the responsibility of individuals and that of government and society. Holding individuals alone accountable for their obesity should not be acceptable.

- "Special attention needs to be focused on vulnerable groups such as children and adolescents, whose inexperience or credulity should not be exploited by commercial activities."

WHO has also adopted a *Global Strategy on Diet, Physical Activity and Health*, endorsed by Member States at the World Health Assembly 2004.[2] The goal of this prevention-based strategy is to improve public health through healthy eating and physical activity. The Assembly "urged" Member States to implement and evaluate the actions recommended in the strategy and to promote healthy behaviours amongst other measures.

European Union

The European Union, driven by concerns about the adverse effects of obesity on the health of citizens and its contribution to the number of premature deaths, has adopted several strategies to try to reduce its prevalence.[3] These include:

- Nutrition Policy: The European Commission has a 'Nutrition Policy' stating its commitment to the promotion of healthy diets and physical activity as a part of healthy lifestyles. It would like to see the development of multi-stakeholder approaches and action at local, regional, national and European levels. Its long-term objective is to work towards the establishment of a coherent and comprehensive *Community Strategy on Diet, Physical Activity and Health*.

- Public Health Action Programme (2003–2008): The Programme aims to address health determinants through supporting health promotion and disease prevention measures.

- Diet, Physical Activity and Health – EU Platform for Action: Launched in 2005, the European Commission's Platform is aimed at stimulating initiatives at national, regional or local level.

---

[1] WHO European Ministerial Conference on Counteracting Obesity (2006) *European Charter on Counteracting Obesity*, available at: http://www.euro.who.int/Document/E89567.pdf.

[2] World Health Organization *Global Strategy: Overall goal and guiding principles*, available at: http://www.who.int/dietphysicalactivity/goals/en/.

[3] European Commission *Nutrition and Physical Activity*, available at: http://ec.europa.eu/health/ph_determinants/life_style/nutrition/nutrition_en.htm.

Members, which include industry associations, have agreed a set of 96 pledges to tackle obesity across the EU, including information campaigns to promote healthy behaviours, reducing amounts of sugar and salt in food, improving nutritional information on packages and not marketing directly to children.

■ In May 2007, the European Commission published the *White Paper on A Strategy for Europe on Nutrition, Overweight and Obesity-related Health Issues*[4], following a consultation period. The purpose of the White Paper is to "set out an integrated EU approach to contribute to reducing ill health due to poor nutrition, overweight and obesity." The Paper notes that actions need to be taken at a local or national level, although it includes information on the following EU-wide measures:

– the Commission is reviewing the options for nutrition labelling;

– a best practice model for self-regulation of food advertising for children has been introduced;

– the Commission will promote the supply of surplus fruit and vegetables to children;

– proposal of a study in 2008 to explore the potential for the reformulation of foods to reduce the levels of fats, salt and sugar; and

– consideration of the promotion of physical activity in daily life during the development of transport policy.

APPENDIX 4 OBESITY POLICY – THE INTERNATIONAL CONTEXT

---

[4] Available at: http://ec.europa.eu/health/ph_determinants/life_style/nutrition/documents/nutrition_wp_en.pdf.

Appendix 5: Fluoride for dental health – the international context

In Box 7.4 we outlined the alternatives means of providing fluoride for dental health purposes. Here we give an overview of the international situation, outlining the interventions adopted by different countries.

Fluoridation measure	Examples of countries in which measure is employed	Used in the UK?	Policies	Other comments
Water fluoridation	USA, Ireland, Australia, Spain, Brazil, Singapore, and Malaysia;[1] over 30 countries in total	Yes, some areas	Typical target fluoridation level of 1 ppm, but lower in Ireland[2]	Estimated that over 350 million people receive a fluoridated water supply worldwide;[3] In some areas water fluoridation schemes have been discontinued[4]
Salt fluoridation	Austria, France, Germany, Jamaica, Ecuador and Mexico;[5] around 15 countries in total	No	In Mexico all salt is fluoridated; in France 35% of all salt is fluoridated;[6] in Germany 75% of salt for use in the home is fluoridated	Estimated that the total amount of fluoridated salt ingested per person per day is around 3 grams in France and 2 grams in Germany;[7] Estimated to be available to almost 200 million people worldwide[8]

[1] Jones S and Lennon K (2004) *One in a Million: The facts about water fluoridation*, 2nd Edition (London: The British Fluoridation Society, The UK Public Health Association, The British Dental Association and The Faculty of Public Health).

[2] In Ireland the target level was recently reduced from 1 ppm, following a report by the Forum on Fluoridation, a group established by the Minister for Health and Children, which stated "In the light of both international and Irish research which shows that there is an increasing occurrence of dental fluorosis, the Forum recommends the lowering of the fluoride level in drinking water to a range of 0.6 to 0.8 ppm, with a target of 0.7 ppm." *Forum on Fluoridation* (2002) Forum on Fluoridation (Dublin: Stationery Office).

[3] Jones S and Lennon K (2004) *One in a Million: The facts about water fluoridation*, 2nd Edition (London: The British Fluoridation Society, The UK Public Health Association, The British Dental Association and The Faculty of Public Health).

[4] Instances where water fluoridation schemes have been abandoned include the following; please note that this list is not exhaustive. Basle in Switzerland discontinued water fluoridation in around 2003 and switched to a salt fluoridation scheme, as was already in place in the rest of Switzerland. A scheme in Finland ceased when the equipment used needed to be repaired, and was not restarted. Meanwhile in the Netherlands, fluoridation of water was withdrawn by the Government. In Sweden, legislation was brought in permitting water fluoridation in 1962, but was withdrawn in 1971 before any schemes had been implemented; in 1977 a Fluoride Commission opposed legislation on the basis that dental caries had declined by other means and further preventative measures could be obtained voluntarily and by 1985 it was declared that there was no intention of raising the issue again. Jones S and Lennon K (2004) *One in a Million: The facts about water fluoridation*, 2nd Edition (London: The British Fluoridation Society, The UK Public Health Association, The British Dental Association and The Faculty of Public Health); Martin B (1991) *Scientific Knowledge in Controversy: the social dynamics of the fluoridation debate* (New York: State University of New York Press).

[5] Jones S and Lennon K (2004) *One in a Million: The facts about water fluoridation*, 2nd Edition (London: The British Fluoridation Society, The UK Public Health Association, The British Dental Association and The Faculty of Public Health).

[6] European Food Safety Authority (2005) Opinion of the Scientific Panel on Dietetic Products, Nutrition and Allergies on a request from the Commission related to the tolerable upper intake level of fluoride *European Food Safety Authority Journal* **192**: 1–65, available at: http://www.efsa.europa.eu/etc/medialib/efsa/science/nda/nda_opinions/851.Par.0001.File.dat/ nda_op_ej192_fluoride_corrigendum1.pdf.

[7] *Ibid.*

[8] National Fluoride Information Centre *Salt Fluoridation – The facts*, available at: http://www.fluorideinformation.com/topic.aspx?main=6&sub=601.

Fluoridation measure	Examples of countries in which measure is employed	Used in the UK?	Policies	Other comments
Milk fluoridation	Russia, Bulgaria, China, Chile, and Thailand[9]	Yes, some areas[10]	Fluoridated milk, yoghurt or powdered milk provided to children (see Box 7.4)	Over 650,000 children estimated to receive fluoridated milk
Fluoride supplements	Few countries have population-wide policies, including Portugal and the USA	Not generally encouraged, except for children at a high risk of developing caries	In Portugal and the USA, fluoride tablets are recommended for children, with dosage dependant on fluoride level of drinking water and age of the child[11]	
Topical application	Fluoride toothpastes used in many countries. Fluoride-rinsing schemes exist in some schools in Ireland, Iceland and Portugal;[12] In various European countries dentists will provide fluoride varnish or gel treatments for children at a high risk of developing caries[13]	Fluoride toothpastes widely recommended; Fluoride varnish or gel treatments may be provided for children at a high risk of developing caries	Recommended toothpaste doses and fluoride levels vary in different countries[14]	In Europe, toothpastes with various fluoride levels are available, although none are allowed to exceed 1,500 ppm and specific guidance is given for young children to prevent excessive levels of ingestion

[9] The Borrow Foundation, *International Programme*, available at: http://www.borrowfoundation.org/html/programme.asp.

[10] The UK programme currently involves over 42,000 children aged 3–11 years from 16 local authority districts. It involves the daily consumption of a carton of milk with 0.5mg of added fluoride. The Borrow Foundation, *International Programme*, available at: http://www.borrowfoundation.org/html/programme.asp.

[11] European Food Safety Authority (2005) Opinion of the Scientific Panel on Dietetic Products, Nutrition and Allergies on a request from the Commission related to the tolerable upper intake level of fluoride *European Food Safety Authority Journal* **192**: 1–65, available at: http://www.efsa.europa.eu/etc/medialib/efsa/science/nda/nda_opinions/851.Par.0001.File.dat/nda_op_ej192_fluoride_corrigendum1.pdf; Árnadóttir IB, Ketley CE, van Loveren C et al. (2004) A European perspective on fluoride use in seven countries *Community Dent Oral Epidemiol* **32** (Suppl. 1): 69–73; Committee on Fluoride in Drinking Water, National Research Council of the National Academies (2006) *Fluoride in Drinking Water: A Scientific Review of EPA's Standards* (Washington, DC: National Academies Press).

[12] Árnadóttir IB, Ketley CE, van Loveren C et al. (2004) A European perspective on fluoride use in seven countries *Community Dent Oral Epidemiol* **32** (Suppl. 1): 69–73.

[13] *Ibid.*

[14] *Ibid.*

Appendix 6: Alcohol and tobacco policy – the international context

International efforts to reduce the harm caused by alcohol

European Union

In 2006, the European Commission published *An EU strategy to support Member States in reducing alcohol related harm*. This Communication identified several priority areas and described how the Commission intended to contribute to measures to address what it described as a "major public health concern". Such measures included financing public health and research projects, exchanging good practice on issues such as curbing under-age drinking, exploring cooperation on information campaigns and tackling drink-driving. The Commission proposed that Member States and stakeholders should use this Communication as a basis for their own interventions as it does not itself intend to implement the strategy through specific new legislative proposals.[1]

International efforts to reduce the harm caused by smoking

World Health Organization

The WHO Framework Convention on Tobacco Control (WHO FCTC) is a global treaty that came into force in February 2005. Among its many measures, the treaty requires countries that adopt it to: impose restrictions on tobacco advertising, sponsorship and promotion; set rules for packaging and labelling of tobacco products; establish clean indoor air controls; and strengthen legislation to address tobacco smuggling. At the time of writing there are 168 signatories to the WHO FCTC, including the UK.[2]

European Union

In 2001, an EU Directive on the manufacture, presentation and sale of tobacco products set maximum tar, nicotine and carbon monoxide yields for all cigarettes circulated, marketed or manufactured in the EU. It also stipulated that health warnings of a certain size should appear on packets of tobacco products. Other measures were enacted including a requirement on manufacturers and importers to make available lists of ingredients of tobacco products, and terms that suggested that a particular tobacco product was less harmful than others (such as 'light' or 'mild') were banned on the packaging. The Directive was introduced on the basis of health protection.[3] A further EU Directive was passed in 2003 which banned tobacco advertising in the print media, on radio and the internet from August 2005.[4]

---

[1] Commission of the European Communities (2006) Communication from the Commission to the Council, the European Parliament, the European Economic and Social Committee and the Committee of the Regions *An EU Strategy to Support Member States in Reducing Alcohol Related Harm*, available at: http://eur-lex.europa.eu/LexUriServ/site/en/com/2006/com2006_0625en01.pdf.

[2] See World Health Organization *Smoking*, available at: http://www.who.int/topics/smoking/en/.

[3] Directive 2001/37/EC on the approximation of the laws, regulations and administrative provisions of the Member States concerning the manufacture, presentation and sale of tobacco products, available at: http://eur-lex.europa.eu/LexUriServ/site/en/oj/2001/l_194/l_19420010718en00260034.pdf.

[4] European Commission (2005) *Questions and Answers on Tobacco Advertising*, available at: http://europa.eu.int/rapid/pressReleasesAction.do?reference=MEMO/05/274&format=HTML&aged=1&language=EN&guiLanguage=en.

Appendix 7: Reports by other organisations

Academy of Medical Sciences (2004) *Calling Time: The nation's drinking as a major health problem* (London: Academy of Medical Sciences).

Academy of Medical Sciences (2005) *Response to House of Commons Health Committee Inquiry into the Government's Public Health White Paper* (London: Academy of Medical Sciences).

Acheson D (1998) *Independent Inquiry into Inequalities in Health Report* (London: The Stationery Office).

Babor T, Caetano R, Casswell S *et al.* (2003) *Alcohol: No ordinary commodity – Research and public policy* (Oxford: Oxford University Press).

Baggott R (2000) *Public Health: Policy and politics* (Basingstoke: Palgrave Macmillan)

British Medical Association (2002) *Asylum Seekers: Meeting their healthcare needs* (London: BMA Publications).

Cabinet Office (2004) *Alcohol Harm Reduction Strategy for England* (London: Strategy Unit).

Cabinet Office (2004) *Personal Responsibility and Changing Behaviour: the state of knowledge and its implications for public policy* (London: Strategy Unit).

de Neeling JND (2003) *Cost-Utility Analysis* (The Hague: Health Council of the Netherlands).

Department for International Development (2007) *Working Together for Better Health* (London: Department for International Development).

Department of Health (1998) *Smoking Kills. A White Paper on tobacco* (London: The Stationery Office).

Department of Health (2004) *Choosing Health: Making healthy choices easier* (London: The Stationery Office).

Department of Health (2005) *Alcohol Needs Assessment Research Project (ANARP): The 2004 national alcohol needs assessment for England* (London: Department of Health).

Department of Health (2005) *Tackling Health Inequalities: Status Report on the Programme for Action* (London: Department of Health).

Department of Health (2006) *Immunisation against Infectious Disease: The Green Book* (London: The Stationery Office).

Department of Health (2007) *Health is Global* (London: Department of Health).

Department of Health, Home Office, Department for Education and Skills and Department for Culture, Media and Sport (2007) *Safe. Sensible. Social. The next steps in the National Alcohol Strategy* (London: Department of Health).

Food Ethics Council (2005) *Getting Personal: Shifting responsibilities for dietary health* (Brighton: Food Ethics Council).

Foresight (2006) *Infectious Diseases: Preparing for the future* (London: Office of Science and Innovation).

Foresight (2007) *Tackling Obesities: Future choices project*, available at: http://www.foresight.gov.uk/Obesity/Obesity.htm.

Foresight Obesity Project (2005) *Report from the Scoping Workshops* (Edinburgh: Waverley Management Consultants).

Forum on Fluoridation (2002) *Forum on Fluoridation* (Dublin: The Stationery Office).

Gostin L (2006) Public health strategies for pandemic influenza *J Am Med Assoc* **295** (14): 1700–4.

House of Commons Health Select Committee (2004) *Obesity* (London: The Stationery Office).

House of Commons Health Select Committee (2005) *Smoking in Public Places* (London: The Stationery Office).

House of Lords Science and Technology Committee (2003) *Fighting Infection* (London: The Stationery Office).

International Obesity Taskforce (2002) *Obesity in Europe: the case for action*, available at: http://www.iotf.org/popout.asp?linkto=http://www.iotf.org/media/euobesity.pdf.

Jones S and Lennon K (2004) *One in a Million: The facts about water fluoridation*, 2nd edition (London: The British Fluoridation Society, The UK Public Health Association, The British Dental Association and The Faculty of Public Health).

Lader D and Goddard E (2005) *Smoking-related Behaviour and Attitudes, 2004* (London: Office for National Statistics).

McDonagh M, Whiting P, Bradley M *et al.* (2000) *A Systematic Review of Public Water Fluoridation* (York: NHS Centre for Reviews and Dissemination).

Medical Research Council (2002) *Water Fluoridation and Health* (London: Medical Research Council).

National Audit Office (2001) *Tackling Obesity in England* (London: The Stationery Office).

National Institute for Health and Clinical Excellence (2005) *Social Value Judgements: Principles for the development of NICE guidance* (UK: National Institute for Health and Clinical Excellence).

Committee on Fluoride in Drinking Water, National Research Council of the National Academies (2006) *Fluoride in Drinking Water* (Washington, DC: National Academies Press).

NHS Immunisation Information (2004) *MMR The facts* (London: Department of Health Publications).

Parliamentary Office of Science and Technology (2004) *Vaccines and Public Health* (London: Parliamentary Office of Science and Technology).

Plant M and Plant M (2006) *Binge Britain: Alcohol and the national response* (Oxford: Oxford University Press).

Royal College of Physicians (2005) *Going Smoke-free: The medical case for clean air in the home, at work and in public places* (London: Royal College of Physicians).

Scientific Advisory Committee on Nutrition (2006) *Folate and Disease Prevention* (London: The Stationery Office).

Scientific Advisory Committee on Nutrition (2003) *Salt and Health* (Norwich: The Stationery Office).

Scottish Executive (2002) *Plan for Action on Alcohol Problems* (Edinburgh: Scottish Executive).

The Hastings Center (2006) *Flu Pandemic and the Fair Allocation of Scarce Life-Saving Resources: How can we make the hardest of choices?* (New York: Hastings Center).

Wanless Report (2002) *Securing our Future Health: Taking a long-term view* (London: HM Treasury).

Wanless Report (2004) *Securing Good Health for the Whole Population* (London: The Stationery Office).

World Health Organization (2003) *Social Determinants of Health: The solid facts*, 2nd edition, Wilkinson R & Marmot M (Editors) (Copenhagen: WHO).

World Health Organization (2003) *WHO Framework Convention on Tobacco Control* (Geneva: WHO).

World Health Organization (2004) *Global Status Report on Alcohol 2004* (Geneva: WHO)

World Health Organization (2005) *The European Health Report 2005: Public health action for healthier children and populations* (Copenhagen: WHO).

York Health Economics Consortium (1998) *Water Fluoridation – An Economic Perspective* (York: York Health Economics Consortium, University of York).

Zaninotto P, Wardle H, Stamatakis E, Mindell J and Head J (2006) *Forecasting Obesity to 2010*, available at: http://www.dh.gov.uk/en/Publicationsandstatistics/Publications/PublicationsStatistics/DH_4138630.

APPENDIX 7 REPORTS BY OTHER ORGANISATIONS

175

Glossary

Accountability: To be responsible and required to account for one's conduct.

Acquired immune deficiency syndrome (AIDS): A deficiency of cellular immunity induced by infection with the **human immunodeficiency virus** (HIV).

Aggregate: A collection of, or the total of, disparate elements.

Altruism: Benefiting or helping others, even at major costs to oneself.

Alzheimer's disease: A brain disease involving the loss, usually progressive, of cognitive and intellectual functions, without impairment of perception or consciousness.

Anonymise: Here: to remove from biological material or data any immediately identifying information that would enable the holder of the material or data to identify the person from whom the data or material has come.

Antibiotic: A substance that inhibits the growth of bacteria.

Antimicrobial: Tending to destroy pathogens, to prevent their multiplication or growth or to prevent their pathogenic action.

Asthma: An inflammatory disease of the lungs characterised by reversible (in most cases) obstruction of the airways.

Autism: A mental disorder characterised by severely abnormal development of social interaction and verbal and non-verbal communication skills.

Autonomy: Self-governance or self-determination.

Avian influenza: An influenza virus infection that is found naturally in birds which can, rarely, be transmitted to humans. The most serious sub-type of the disease for human health at present is H5N1.

Best interests: Here: principle that requires that in all matters affecting a child, his or her best interests should be an important consideration. Although there are different interpretations of scope and status, the principle is central to medical practice, child protection and disputes about child custody.

'Binge' drinking: Drinking a large amount of alcohol over a short period of time, typically leading to drunkenness. According to a Government definition: drinking more than eight units of alcohol for men and six units or more for women in a day.[1]

Bioethics: The study of ethical issues raised in the context of human, animal and plant life, typically concerning medical and biological research.

Blood-alcohol level: The amount of alcohol present in a person's blood stream, recorded in milligrams of alcohol per 100 millilitres of blood.

Body mass index (BMI): The body mass index measurement is an approximate guide to **overweight** and **obesity**. It is a measurement of weight relative to height, see paragraph 5.2.

Cancer: General term frequently used to indicate any of various types of malignant tumour or growth, most of which invade surrounding tissues.

Carbohydrates: A large group of energy-producing organic compounds.

---

[1] Department of Health, Home Office, Department for Education and Skills and Department for Culture, Media and Sport (2007) *Safe. Sensible. Social. The next steps in the National Alcohol Strategy* (London: Department of Health Publications).

Chlamydia: A bacterial sexually transmitted infection.

Chlorine: A chemical element commonly added during water treatment to kill bacteria in the water.

Chronic: Referring to a health-related state lasting for a long period of time.

Cirrhosis: Disease of the liver that can develop as a result of long-term drinking of excessive amounts of alcohol.

Civil liberty: Freedom of action and speech subject to the law.

Civil society: Voluntary and social organisations and institutions that contribute to providing services needed by society.

Classical harm principle: Ethical principle which states that coercive, liberty-infringing state interference can be acceptable where the purpose is to prevent harm to others (see paragraph 2.14).

Coercion: The act of persuading or forcing.

Collectivists: Those who view groups (of varying sizes) as the fundamental units of society, rather than the individual (see: paragraph 2.3ff).

Consent: Here: voluntary agreement of an individual to medical treatment or measures that infringe **civil liberties**. The purpose is to ensure absence of coercion, force or duress (see paragraphs 2.22ff).

Coronary heart disease: A disorder of the blood vessels of the heart.

Crohn's disease: A chronic, episodic, inflammatory condition of the gastrointestinal tract.

Curative: Tending or able to heal an injury.

Democracy/Democratic: Literally: rule of the people. Here: a form of government or decision-making seeking to ensure equality through fair, open and transparent participatory processes (see paragraph 2.25).

Dental caries: Tooth decay; a disease that progressively destroys the structure of the teeth and is caused by bacteria in the mouth.

Dental fluorosis: A defect of the tooth enamel that causes visible markings on the teeth, and can lead to problems with tooth enamel. It can vary from mild speckling to more substantial staining and pitting.

Dentition: The natural teeth, considered collectively.

Diphtheria: A bacterial infectious disease that produces degeneration in nerves, heart muscle and other tissues.

Disability-adjusted life year (DALY): A measure of the burden of disease in a population, based on adjustment of life expectancy to take into account long-term disability.

Efficacy: The degree to which an intervention can have a desired effect, in principle (or in ideal circumstances).

Effectiveness: The degree to which an intervention has a definite or desired effect in a specific context.

Egalitarianism/egalitarian: A doctrine advocating the principle of equal rights and opportunities for all.

Emphysema: A condition in which the air sacs of the lungs enlarge, causing breathlessness.

Empirical: Based on observation or experiment rather than theory.

Enamel: The hard substance covering the exposed portion of the tooth.

Epidemic: The widespread occurrence of significantly more cases of a disease in a community or population than expected over a period of time.

Epidemiology: The study of the distribution and determinants of health-related states or events in specified populations, and the application of this study to the control of health problems.

Equitable: Here: distribution of goods or access to services in a fair or just way.

Externalities: Costs resulting from a transaction between two parties that primarily affect a third party not involved in or benefiting from the transaction.

Fiscal: Of public revenue.

Fluoride/Fluoridation: Fluoride is a mineral that is found naturally in some food and drink products, including tea, and in varying concentrations in water. Synthetic forms are sometimes added to the water supply, toothpastes and dental products with the intention of providing benefits in protecting against **dental caries**.

Fluorosis: See **Dental fluorosis** and **Skeletal fluorosis**.

Folate: A B vitamin that is essential to health. Insufficient levels during early pregnancy of folate or its synthetic substitute, **folic acid**, can lead to neural tube defects in the newborn.

Folic acid: See **folate**.

Fortification: Here: the addition of nutrients to foods and drinks.

Gradient: A rate of inclination or decline.

Harm principle: See **Classical harm principle**.

Health inequalities: Inequalities in health between different population subgroups, for example according to socio-economic status or ethnic background. Inequalities are typically measured in terms of mortality, life expectancy or health status.

Heterodox: Of an opinion that is held in contrast to generally accepted views or beliefs.

Homogeneous: Of the same kind.

Human immunodeficiency virus (HIV): A retrovirus which causes **AIDS**.

Incentivised: Involving incentives for people who comply with the recommended policy in order to encourage uptake.

Incubation period (of a disease): The period between exposure to an infection and the appearance of the first symptoms.

Infectious period: The time period during which an individual can transmit an infection.

Influenza: An acute infectious respiratory disease caused by influenza viruses.

Infrastructural: To possess the basic structural foundations of a society or enterprise.

Interdisciplinary: Of or between more than one branch of learning.

Intrinsic: Inherent, essential.

Isolation: Separation of individuals infected with a communicable disease from those who are not for the period they are likely to be infectious in order to prevent further spread. Compare **Quarantine**.

Liberalism: A political theory which favours individual liberty and equality, see egalitarianism.

Libertarians: Defenders of what they term 'natural' rights of man: life, liberty and property. Advocates of a minimal state that protects natural rights but, in particular, does not seek to redistribute wealth.

Mandate: Political authorisation for certain policies or measures given in a **democratic** system by a group of people to their representatives.

Mandatory: Compulsory. See also **quasi-mandatory**.

Measles: An acute infectious viral disease marked by fever and red spots on the skin.

Meningitis: Inflammation of the brain or spinal cord.

MMR (measles, mumps and rubella): A combined vaccination administered in childhood against measles, mumps and rubella.

Morbidity: A diseased state.

Mortality: A fatal outcome. Mortality rates refer to the rate of death in a given population.

Mumps: An acute infectious and contagious disease.

Nicotine: A substance in **tobacco** that is responsible for many of its effects, including its addictiveness.

Normative: Concerning moral or legal obligations of people.

Obese: Defined by WHO as having a **BMI** of ≥30.

Obesogenic: An environment or substance that is conducive to weight gain.

Overweight: Defined by WHO as having a **BMI** of ≥25.

Pandemic: A worldwide epidemic – an influenza pandemic occurs when a new strain of influenza virus emerges that causes human illness and is able to spread rapidly within and between countries because people have little or no immunity to it. Compare **Epidemic**.

Paradigm: A representative example or pattern, especially one underlying a theory or viewpoint.

Passive smoking: The involuntary inhaling of smoke (sometimes called environmental tobacco smoke) from others' cigarettes, cigars or pipes.

Paternalism: "Interference of a state or an individual with another person, against their will, and justified by a claim that the person interfered with will be better off or protected from harm"[2] (see paragraph 2.35ff).

Pathogen: An agent that causes disease.

Per capita: Literally: 'per head'; for each person.

Pharmacological: Relating to the branch of medicine that deals with the uses, effects and modes of the action of drugs.

Polio (poliomyelitis): An infectious viral disease that affects the central nervous system and which can cause temporary or permanent paralysis.

Precautionary approach: Dynamic set of interacting criteria considered in making policy decisions under uncertainty (see paragraphs 3.15–3.16).

Prevalence: Total number of cases (for example, of a disease) in a population at a given time.

Preventative: That which stops or hinders an occurrence.

Prioritarian: Approach focusing on reducing inequalities in health by raising the levels of the most

---

[2] Dworkin R (2002) Paternalism, in Stanford Encyclopedia of Philosophy, available at: http://plato.stanford.edu/entries/paternalism/.

disadvantaged (see paragraph 2.31).

Procedural justice: Approach that focuses on fair, open and transparent procedures to ensure negotiation of substantive disagreement about, for example, practices or policies (see paragraph 2.25).

Prognostic: A prediction or forecast.

Proportionality: Here: criterion for judging whether a particular policy is an appropriate response in relation to a public health problem (see paragraph 3.18).

Psychosocial: Of or involving the influence of social factors or human interactive behaviour.

Public service agreement (PSA): Measurable targets that are agreed for each government department for a Spending Review period.

Quarantine: Separation of those who are thought to have been exposed to a communicable infection but are well, from others who have not been exposed in order to prevent further spread. Compare **Isolation**.

Quasi-mandatory: 'Almost mandatory'; in the context of vaccinations, strategies in which individuals are required to be vaccinated unless they qualify for an exemption and where there are penalties for those who do not comply.

Rubella: An acute but mild disease caused by rubella virus; a high incidence of birth defects in children results from maternal infection during the first trimester of pregnancy.

Sanitation: The maintenance or improvement of conditions that affect health, especially with regard to dirt and infection.

Satiety: The condition of having had enough to eat, or of not being hungry.

Sedative: A drug that tends to calm or soothe.

Severe acute respiratory syndrome (SARS): A serious infectious disease that was first reported in China in November 2002, caused by a virus.

Skeletal fluorosis: A condition characterised by skeletal abnormalities and joint pain that is caused by long-term exposure to large amounts of fluoride.

Small pox: An acute eruptive contagious disease caused by a virus.

Snus: A form of tobacco that comes either loose or in tiny sachets which are placed under the upper lip.

Social contract: An implicit or explicit agreement among members of a society to cooperate for certain benefits, e.g. by sacrificing some individual freedom for state protection (see paragraphs 2.5–2.7).

Socio-economic group: A commonly used classification of socio-economic group in the UK is as follows: I, professional occupations; II, managerial and technical occupations; III, skilled occupations; IV, partly skilled occupations; V, unskilled occupations.

Social marketing: "The systematic application of marketing techniques and approaches to achieve specific behavioural goals, to improve health and reduce health inequalities."[3]

Statistically significant: Indication that an event occurred with a likelihood that is above pure chance probability.

Stewardship: "A function of a government responsible for the welfare of the population, and concerned with the trust and legitimacy with which its activities are viewed by the citizenry. [...] Stewardship is the overarching function that determines the success or failure of all other

---

[3] French J and Blair Stevens C (2005) *Social Marketing Pocket guide*, 1st Edition (London: National Social Marketing Centre for Excellence).

functions of the health system. It places the responsibility back on government and calls for the strengthening of ministries of health"[4] (see paragraphs 2.41–2.44).

Stigmatisation: Literally, 'to brand'; to describe or mark a person or people as unworthy or disgraceful, usually because of certain characteristics or features they possess.

Subgroups: A subset of a group.

Supplementation: See **Fortification**.

Surveillance (of disease): The ongoing scrutiny of the occurrence and spread of disease in order to inform and direct public health action.

Syphilis: An acute and chronic infectious bacterial disease transmitted by direct contact, usually through sexual intercourse.

Tobacco: A plant of American origin, with narcotic leaves used for smoking, chewing or snuff.

Tooth decay: See **Dental caries**.

Topically applied fluoride product: A fluoride product which is applied externally to the teeth (rather than being ingested), for example toothpaste.

Totalitarianism: A system of government that tolerates only one political leader or party to which all other institutions are subordinated, and which usually demands the complete subservience of the individual.

Toxicologist: A scientist who studies poisonous properties of entities.

Transmission: The spread of an infectious agent from a source or reservoir (including another person) to a person.

Tuberculosis: A disease caused by infection with the tubercle bacillus which can affect almost any tissue or organ of the body, most commonly affecting the lungs.

Typhoid: A bacterial infectious disease characterised by a high fever, septicaemia and intestinal ulceration.

Unit of alcohol: A unit of alcohol is 10 millilitres of pure alcohol. Guidance on drinking typically uses this measure to distinguish between different levels of drinking, and to suggest sensible drinking levels.[5]

Urbanisation: To destroy the rural quality of a district.

Utilitarianism: A theory that focuses on promoting those rules or actions that produce the most overall happiness or pleasure.

Vaccination: Vaccinations involve treating a healthy person with a substance that is derived from (or similar to) a particular infectious disease agent. The purpose is to induce a response by the body that leads to enhanced immunity, and consequent protection, when exposed to the disease in the future.

Variant Creutzfeldt-Jakob disease (vCJD): A form of transmissible spongiform encephalopathy in humans caused by an infectious agent.

Virus: An infectious agent that is only able to multiply within the living cells of a host.

Whooping cough: An infectious bacterial disease, especially in children, with a series of short violent coughs followed by a whoop.

---

[4] World Health Organization (2000) *World Health Report 2000* (Geneva, Switzerland: WHO).
[5] Department of Health (2007) *Alcohol and Health*, available at: http://www.dh.gov.uk/en/PolicyAndGuidance/HealthAndSocialCareTopics/AlcoholMisuse/AlcoholMisuseGeneralInformation/DH_4 062199.

List of abbreviations

AIDS	Acquired immune deficiency syndrome
ANARP	Alcohol Needs Assessment Research Project (ANARP)
ASA	Advertising Standards Authority
ASH	Action on Smoking and Health
BFS	British Fluoridation Society
BMA	British Medical Association
BMI	Body mass index
CAP	Committee of Advertising Practice
CDC	Centers for Disease Prevention and Control (USA)
DALY	Disability-adjusted life year
ECDC	European Centre for Disease Prevention and Control
ETS	Environmental tobacco smoke
EU	European Union
FSA	Food Standards Agency
GDA	Guideline daily amounts (of nutrients)
GP	General practitioner
HFSS	High in fat, salt and sugar
HiB	*Haemophilus influenzae* type b
HIV	Human immunodeficiency virus
IQ	Intelligence quotient
ISD	Information Services Division
MHRA	Medicines and Healthcare products Regulatory Authority
MMR	Measles, mumps and rubella
MRC	Medical Research Council
NATA	National Anonymous Tonsil Archive
Ofcom	Office of Communications
NGO	Non-governmental organisation
NHS	National Health Service
NICE	National Institute for Health and Clinical Excellence
PSA	Public service agreement
SACN	Scientific Advisory Committee on Nutrition
SARS	Severe acute respiratory syndrome
STI	Sexually transmitted infection
TB	Tuberculosis

TDS	Total diet study
VAN UK	Vaccination Awareness Network UK
VAT	Value added tax
vCJD	variant Creutzfeldt-Jakob disease
WHA	World Health Assembly
WHO	World Health Organization
WMA	World Medical Association

Index